Nutrition in Women's Health

DEBRA A. KRUMMEL, MS, PhD, RD
Assistant Professor
Community Medicine
West Virginia University
School of Medicine
Morgantown, West Virginia

PENNY M. KRIS-ETHERTON, MS, PhD, RD
Professor of Nutrition
Nutrition Department
The Pennsylvania State University
University Park, Pennsylvania

AN ASPEN PUBLICATION®
Aspen Publishers, Inc.
Gaithersburg, Maryland
1996

Library of Congress Cataloging-in-Publication Data

Nutrition in women's health/
[edited by] Debra A. Krummel,
Penny M. Kris-Etherton.
p. cm.
Includes bibliographical references and index.
ISBN 0-8342-0682-X
1. Women—Nutrition. 2. Nutritionally induced diseases.
3. Pregnancy—Nutritional aspects.   I. Krummel, Debra A.
II. Kris-Etherton, P.M.
[DNLM: 1. Women's Health.   2. Nutrition.   WA 309 N976 1995]
QP143.N894   1995
613.2'082—dc20
DNLM/DLC
for Library of Congress
95-24231
CIP

Editorial Resources: Amy Myers-Payne

Library of Congress Catalog Card Number: 95-24231
ISBN: 0-8342-0682-X

Printed in the United States of America

1   2   3   4   5

This book is dedicated to improving the health and well-being of women through optimal nutritional practices.

Table of Contents

          Lactation** 212
          Cheryl Lovelady

          Dietary Intake 212
          Energy Balance 213
          Nutritional Issues....................................222
          Promotion of Lactation To Improve Maternal Health........228
          Summary 228

Chapter 8— Vegetarianism for Women 232
          Johanna T. Dwyer

          Who Are Vegetarian Women? 232
          Special Challenges that Vegetarian Eating Styles Present to
             Women 234
          Food Guidance for Vegetarian Women 236
          Planning Ahead: Life Cycle-Related Concerns............238
          Disease Prevention 248
          Conclusions..256

Chapter 9— Nutrition for the Female Athlete 263
          Louise Burke

          Goals of the Training Diet...........................263
          Nutrient Intakes of Female Athletes 264
          Issues of Body Fat...................................265
          Nutrient Needs.......................................270
          Competition Diet.....................................279
          Summary 288
          Appendix 9-A 294

Chapter 10—Nutritional Needs of Elderly Women 299
          Ronni Chernoff

          Energy Needs 300
          Macronutrients 302
          Fluid Requirements...................................305
          Vitamins 306
          Minerals...310
          Trace Minerals.......................................311
          Future Research Needs 313

Contributors

Irene Alton, MS, RD
Director of Nutrition Services
Health Start, Inc.
St. Paul, Minnesota

Louise Burke, PhD, RD
Sports Dietitian
Australian Institute of Sport
Canberra, Australia

Elizabeth R. Burrows, MS, RD
Nutrition Intervention and Training Supervisor
Women's Health Initiative Clinical Coordinating Center
Fred Hutchinson Cancer Research Center
Seattle, Washington

Catherine M. Champagne, PhD, RD, LDN
Assistant Professor, Research
Nutrient Data Systems Scientist
Pennington Biomedical Research Center
Louisiana State University Agricultural and Mechanical College
Baton Rouge, Louisiana

Ronni Chernoff, PhD, RD
Associate Director
Geriatric Research Education and Clinical Center
John L. McClellan Memorial Veterans Hospital
Professor, Nutrition and Dietetics
College of Health Related Professions
University of Arkansas for Medical Sciences
Little Rock, Arkansas

Ann M. Coulston, MS, RD
Senior Research Dietitian
Stanford University Medical Center
General Clinical Research Center
Stanford, California

Johanna T. Dwyer, DSc, RD
Director
Frances Stern Nutrition Center
New England Medical Center
Professor of Medicine
Tufts University School of Medicine
Professor of Nutrition
Tufts University School of Nutrition
Boston, Massachusetts

Jo L. Freudenheim, PhD, RD
Associate Professor
Department of Social and Preventive Medicine
State University of New York at Buffalo
School of Medicine and Biomedical Sciences
Buffalo, New York

Pamela S. Haines, DrPH, RD
Associate Professor
Department of Nutrition
University of North Carolina at Chapel Hill
School of Public Health
Chapel Hill, North Carolina

Robert P. Heaney, MD, FACP, FAIN
John A. Creighton University Professor
Creighton University
Omaha, Nebraska

Holly Henry, MS, RD
Research Nutritionist
Women's Health Initiative Clinical Coordinating Center
Fred Hutchinson Cancer Research Center
Seattle, Washington

Rachel K. Johnson, PhD, MPH, RD
Assistant Professor
Department of Nutritional Sciences
The University of Vermont
Burlington, Vermont

Betty G. Kirkley, PhD
Associate Clinical Professor
Department of Psychiatry
University of North Carolina at Chapel Hill
Chapel Hill, North Carolina

Penny M. Kris-Etherton, PhD, RD
Professor of Nutrition
Nutrition Department
The Pennsylvania State University
University Park, Pennsylvania

Debra A. Krummel, PhD, RD
Assistant Professor
Community Medicine
West Virginia University
School of Medicine
Morgantown, West Virginia

Judith H. LaRosa, PhD, RN, FAAN
Clinical Professor of Public Health
Department of Applied Health Sciences
Tulane University
School of Public Health and Tropical Medicine
New Orleans, Louisiana

Barbara Levin, MD, ABFP
Health Officer
Monroe County Health Department
Medical Director
Monroe County Maternity Center
Madisonville, Tennessee

Cheryl Lovelady, PhD, MPH, RD
Assistant Professor
Department of Food, Nutrition, and Food Service Management
The University of North Carolina at Greensboro
Greensboro, North Carolina

Jennifer R. McDuffie, MPH, RD
Nutritionist
Eating Disorders Clinic
Department of Psychiatry
University of North Carolina at Chapel Hill
Chapel Hill, North Carolina

Ruth E. Patterson, PhD, RD
Associate in Cancer Prevention
Cancer Prevention Research Program
Fred Hutchinson Cancer Research Center
Affiliate Instructor
Department of Epidemiology
University of Washington
Seattle, Washington

Nancy Potischman, PhD
Senior Staff Fellow
Nutritional Epidemiology Section
Environmental Epidemiology Branch
Division of Cancer Etiology
National Cancer Institute
Bethesda, Maryland

Joan W. Rupp, MS, RD
Assistant Clinical Professor
Department of Family and Preventive Medicine
University of California–San Diego
La Jolla, California

Stanley R. Shane, MD
Professor and Chair
Department of Medicine
University of Nevada School of Medicine
Reno, Nevada

Lori J. Silverstein, PhD, RD
Assistant Professor
Department of Internal Medicine
University of Nevada School of Medicine
Reno, Nevada

Sachiko T. St. Jeor, PhD, RD
Professor
Departments of Internal Medicine and
  Family and Community Medicine
Director
Nutrition Education and Research Program
University of Nevada School of Medicine
Reno, Nevada

Mary Story, PhD, RD
Associate Professor
Public Health Nutrition
Division of Epidemiology
University of Minnesota
School of Public Health
Minneapolis, Minnesota

Christy C. Tangney, PhD
Associate Professor
Rush Presbyterian St. Luke's Medical Center
Chicago, Illinois

Lesley Fels Tinker, PhD, RD
Nutrition Scientist
Women's Health Initiative Clinical Coordinating Center
Fred Hutchinson Cancer Research Center
Seattle, Washington

Linda Van Horn, PhD, RD
Professor
Department of Preventive Medicine
Northwestern University Medical School
Chicago, Illinois

Annie O. Wong, MS
Research Assistant
Department of Preventive Medicine
Northwestern University Medical School
Chicago, Illinois

Paula C. Zemel, PhD, RD
Assistant Professor
Department of Nutrition
The University of Tennessee
Knoxville, Tennessee

Foreword

To the casual observer, it may seem as if women's health suddenly burst on the national scene as a full-fledged social and political issue. In fact, the attention women's health now attracts is the result of years of advocacy by dedicated health professionals and congressional supporters. Today, programs such as the Women's Health Initiative (WHI), a $625 million National Institutes of Health (NIH) clinical and observational study, serve as testimony that women's health has finally assumed its rightful place on the nation's health agenda.

Complementing this long-overdue focus on women's health is The American Dietetic Association's (ADA) Nutrition and Health Campaign for Women, an ambitious consumer education and research advocacy effort. Although many organizations have taken up the banner for women's health, ADA's campaign is the only program exclusively focused on the vital link between nutrition and major diseases affecting women—such as heart disease, breast cancer, osteoporosis, diabetes, and obesity.

The ADA has long been a leader in working for the inclusion of medical nutrition therapy in our health care delivery system. The Nutrition and Health Campaign for Women strongly supports that objective, positioning registered dietitians as health professionals who can make a measurable difference—not only in women's well-being but also in the overall cost-effectiveness of health care. *Nutrition in Women's Health*, a collection of work from eminent researchers and practitioners, is an important resource for dietetics and other allied-health professionals. It clearly and concisely lays out the scientific underpinnings supporting the role of nutrition in women's health.

In the scientific and medical communities, in the halls of Congress, and in the media, women's health was once an invisible issue. For years, women were regularly excluded from clinical and preventive research for various reasons, such as the effect of variable menstrual cycles and potential risks to unborn fetuses. As a result, research into diseases that affect *both* men and women often included only male participants, but results from these studies were applied to women as well.

For example, the 1982 Multiple Risk Factor Intervention Trial (aptly called "Mr. Fit"), a long-term study of life-style factors related to cholesterol and heart disease, included 13,000 men and no women. The Physicians' Health Study, popularly known as the "aspirin study," is another typical example. This research concluded that taking an aspirin every other day may reduce the risk of heart disease, but the study sample included no females—even though heart disease is the number 1 killer of women.

Revelations about this research gap in women's health spurred a 1990 General Accounting Office (GAO) investigation that showed that, despite years of rhetoric to the contrary, the NIH had done little to implement research policies supportive of women's health. Laws passed in 1993 subsequently mandated an NIH Office of Women's Health with a $16.7 billion budget. These same laws specify that studies must not only include women (when appropriate) but also must be conducted so that gender differences can be analyzed.

The WHI, launched in 1993, grew out of NIH's renewed commitment to 52% of the population. The WHI is the largest intervention study ever undertaken in the United States. It will address three of the most common causes of death, disability, and impaired quality of life among postmenopausal women—heart disease, cancer, and osteoporosis. One portion of the WHI—a randomized, controlled clinical trial involving 60,000 women aged 50 to 79—will explore approaches to prevention, including the effects of a low-fat diet on heart disease and breast and colon cancer; the effect of estrogen-replacement therapy on heart disease, osteoporosis, and increased risk for breast cancer; and the effect of calcium and vitamin D supplementation on osteoporosis and colon cancer.

Of course, health experts have long agreed that nutrition can play a vital role in disease prevention. In 1989, the *Surgeon General's Report on Nutrition and Health* confirmed that dietary factors are associated with the leading causes of death in the United States—heart disease, some types of cancer, stroke, non–insulin-dependent diabetes, and atherosclerosis. In fact, for Americans who do not drink or smoke, eating patterns shape long-term health prospects more than any other personal choice. Nevertheless, as Bernadine Healey, MD, former NIH director and chief architect of the WHI, notes, nutrition research has not attracted the attention it merits. In fact, she says, the gaps in our knowledge of nutritional science rival only our enormous gaps in knowledge of women's health.

That women have been neglected in our present health care system is underscored by the fact that many of the diseases and disorders affecting adult women are preventable, or at a minimum, their toll on health and well-being can be diminished through early diagnosis and intervention. Although surveys indicate that most women are aware of the risk factors associated with these diseases, far fewer are actually *doing* something to reduce their personal risks. For example, nearly 80% of respondents in a Gallup survey sponsored by the ADA and Weight

Watchers International expressed concern about the effect of their food choices on their future health, but less than one-third described their diets as very healthy. And nearly half the women interviewed described themselves as overweight; even more said they were in poor physical shape.

The ADA launched its Nutrition and Health Campaign for Women to empower women to take charge of their health—to take that important step beyond knowledge and into action. The campaign is designed to help women who are not scientists or dietitians make good nutrition decisions, choices that will have a life-long effect on their health and their quality of life. By translating the very latest scientific findings about the role of nutrition in disease prevention, the campaign helps women make realistic changes in their diet and life style—simple changes that build confidence and self-esteem and improve health. The campaign also seeks to shift the focus of women's nutritional goals away from preoccupation with body image and toward an understanding of healthy body weight.

Behind this comprehensive public education agenda is the campaign's commitment to develop a clearly focused plan for continued research on women's health. Central to the total effort is the positioning of the registered dietitian as the health professional most qualified to assist women along a path toward preventive health through good nutrition.

Among the campaign's most important messages are the facts about major diseases afflicting women. We know, for example, that heart disease claims the lives of more than 400,000 women each year. It is, in fact, the single largest killer of women. We also know that nutrition intervention is proved to be effective in preventing and treating heart disease in women. We know that one in eight women can now expect to develop breast cancer in her lifetime; 20 years ago, that ratio was only 1 in 20. Although more research is needed, nutrition may be important in the prevention of this disease. Consequently, we are now urging women to follow a diet low in fat and high in fiber to promote overall health and lessen the likelihood of breast cancer.

We know that good nutrition practices over a lifetime—such as adequate calcium and vitamin D intake—can help prevent the onset and reduce severity of osteoporosis, a disorder resulting in loss of bone density that afflicts 25 million Americans, most of them women. Nearly one-third of all postmenopausal women will be afflicted by osteoporosis. And we know that half of the 13 million Americans who have diabetes are women, and that 60% of all new cases of diabetes are diagnosed in women. With its complications—heart disease, stroke, blindness, kidney disease, and nerve damage—diabetes is the fourth leading cause of death by disease in the United States.

Recently released research from the National Center for Health Statistics shows that obesity rates in the United States continue to increase despite a lower intake of fat and a growing awareness of negative health effects. In general, approximately 35% of adult women are estimated to be overweight, up from 27%

a decade earlier. Weight management is central to good health and disease prevention in women, especially because the propensity toward weight gain and obesity has placed women in higher-risk categories than men for five of the leading causes of death—heart disease, certain types of cancer, stroke, diabetes, and atherosclerosis.

The evolution of women's health from an obscure issue to a nationally recognized priority is destined to change the lives of individual women and their families. It will also have a profound impact on our total health care system as the influence of healthy women is felt across generations from prenatal care to the care of aging parents. In this new paradigm of women's health, registered dietitians occupy a unique and powerful position. With government support (WHI), public education programs (ADA's Nutrition and Health Campaign for Women), and books such as *Nutrition in Women's Health*, nutrition is now at the forefront of chronic disease prevention where it belongs.

—Susan Calvert Finn, PhD, RD
1992–1993 American Dietetic Association President
Co-chair, ADA Nutrition and Health Campaign for Women

Preface

During the past decade, interest in women's health has attained a level of prominence that was unimaginable as recently as 10 years ago. The American Dietetic Association and the National Institutes of Health (NIH) are supporting major efforts to improve women's health. Because of its central role in the ontogeny of the chronic diseases that affect women, nutrition is a major focus of these activities.

With the growing interest in women's health, *Nutrition in Women's Health* was written to provide a comprehensive reference that covers topics related to the health of women. This book was written for nutritionists and other allied health professionals who have an interest in women's health or have women as clients.

Nutrition in Women's Health is divided into 3 parts. Part I discusses Normal Nutrition Throughout the Life Cycle. Chapter 1 covers the myriad of factors affecting adolescent nutrition and growth. The complexity of nutrition and pregnancy in the growing adolescent is discussed in Chapter 2. Definitions, assessment, and the role of nutritionists in the treatment of eating disorders are covered in Chapter 3. Chapter 4 reviews general food consumption patterns in women, and Chapter 5 discusses the relationships between diet, sex steroids, and the menstrual cycle. Chapters 6 and 7 present practical guidelines for normal nutrition in the premenopausal woman and the pregnant or lactating woman. Chapter 8 discusses nutrition issues for vegetarian women and describes strategies for implementation. Information on how to manage optimal nutrition in female athletes is provided in Chapter 9. The last chapter in Part I describes the unique nutritional needs of elderly women.

Part II addresses Preventive Nutrition Throughout the Life Cycle. Chapter 11 provides insight into preventive nutrition in adolescent girls. Chapters 12–16 cover the chronic diseases of concern to women, i.e., obesity, cardiovascular disease, osteoporosis, diabetes, and cancer.

Part III focuses on Resources for Women's Health Research. It discusses such topics as the ongoing activities and efforts at NIH as found in Chapter 17. The nutrition components of the Women's Health Initiative are highlighted in Chapter 18. Lastly, in Chapter 19, sample menus that meet contemporary dietary recommendations for women are presented.

Our hope is that *Nutrition in Women's Health*, in some way, will make health professionals more knowledgeable about the role of nutrition in women's health. This awareness may inspire more readers to join in the pursuit of preventive nutrition efforts that will improve the health and well-being of women.

—Debra A. Krummel, PhD, RD
—Penny M. Kris-Etherton, PhD, RD

Acknowledgments

We would like to thank Aspen Publishers, Inc., for the opportunity to make *Nutrition in Women's Health* a reality, and our contributors for their commitment and patience with the process. We are grateful for the assistance of Cindy Nucciarone, Satya Jonnalagadda, Abir Farhat-Wood, and Kristin Moriarty.

Without our families' encouragement, support, and understanding, this book would not have been possible. Specifically, Debra would like to thank her husband, Dan Fox, for continuously supporting her career endeavors; her sons, Connor and Trevor Fox, for being the great little boys that they are; and her parents, Peggy and George Krummel, for the constant encouragement to "follow your dreams." Penny would like to thank her husband, Terry Etherton, for his wisdom and insight about professional endeavors; and her sons, Mark and Phillip Etherton, who define the essence of life.

Part I

Normal Nutrition Throughout the Life Cycle

1

❧

Becoming a Woman: Nutrition in Adolescence

Mary Story and Irene Alton

Adolescence (from the Latin word *adolescer,* to grow up) is the period of life between the onset of puberty and full maturity (i.e., 10 to 21 years of age) and is the process of maturing physically and developmentally from a child into an adult. Some of the most complex transitions of life occur during adolescence. No other 10-year period in life contains as many tasks and momentous changes as adolescence. The experiences of the child and the adolescent are the template from which the adult emerges. Thus, adolescence needs to be considered as both a unique part of the life cycle and an integral element of it.[1]

The biologic, social, psychological, and cognitive changes that occur during adolescence can significantly affect nutritional health. The rapid physical growth creates an increased demand for energy and nutrients. Also, growing independence and eating away from home, intense concern with appearance and weight, the need for peer acceptability, and an active life style, all impact on eating patterns and food choices. Good nutrition during adolescence is significant not only to achieve full growth potential and optimal health but also for the prevention of adult chronic diseases. There is also growing recognition of the importance of preconceptual nutrition and healthy pregnancy outcome. This pivotal developmental period offers special opportunities for working with adolescents to help them achieve healthy life styles. This chapter focuses on the adolescent female's physical and psychosocial development and its relationship to nutrient needs and eating patterns.

PHYSICAL GROWTH

The biologic process of puberty is characterized by rapid growth in height and weight, changes in body composition and tissues, and the acquisition of primary and secondary sex characteristics; Figure 1-1 diagrams the major events of

1

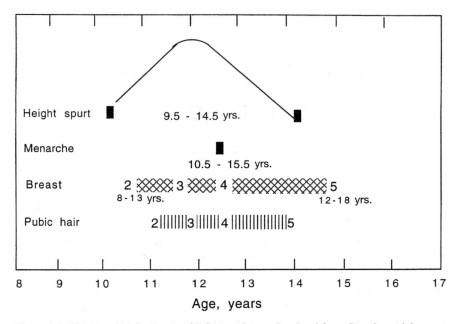

Figure 1-1 Diagram of Major Events of Puberty   *Source:* Reprinted from *Growth at Adolescence,* ed 2 by JM Tanner with permission of Blackwell Scientific Publications, © 1962.

puberty. Among adolescents, there is wide variability in the timing, intensity, and duration of the growth spurt. An individual, though, will follow an orderly sequence of maturational events. The average duration of puberty in girls is 4 years, with a range of 1.5 to 8 years.[2] Nutrient needs parallel the rate of growth, with the greatest nutrient demands occurring during the peak velocity of growth (the time when growth is maximal). Because of the high individual variability in maturation and growth, nutrient requirements are better correlated with physiologic development than with chronologic age.[3] For example, a 12-year-old girl who is prepubescent will have different nutrient needs than a 12-year-old girl who is in her growth spurt.

Developmental stage can be assessed using sexual maturation ratings (SMR) based on secondary sex characteristics of pubic hair growth and breast development.[4] The rating scales (Table 1-1) described by Tanner for grading stages of pubic hair and breast development in girls and pubic hair and genital development in boys are the most widely used means for recording pubertal development.[5] SMR or stage 1 is prepubertal before signs of development of secondary sex characteristics appear, and SMR 5 characterizes adulthood. Limited research has been conducted on nutrient assessments using sex maturity ratings. Daniel et al[3,6,7] found that plasma and/or serum concentrations of folate, iron, protein, and alkaline phosphatase had higher concordance with sex maturity ratings than with

Table 1-1 Sex Maturity Ratings for Girls

Stage	Pubic Hair	Breasts
1	Preadolescent	Preadolescent
2	Sparse, lightly pigmented, straight, medial border of labia	Breast and papilla elevated as small mound; areolar diameter increased
3	Darker, beginning to curl, increased amount	Breast and areola enlarged, no contour separation
4	Coarse, curly, abundant, but amount less than in adult	Areola and papilla form secondary mound
5	Adult femine triangle spread to medial surface of thighs	Mature; nipple projects, areola part of general breast contour

Source: Reprinted from *Growth at Adolescence,* ed 2 by JM Tanner with permission of Blackwell Scientific Publications, © 1962.

chronologic age. Further research is needed in this area. Nutritionists should be familiar with sex maturity ratings and use this information to judge nutritional needs and counseling.[3] Developmental correlation, not chronologic age, should be the basis of assessing nutritional needs in adolescents. Nutrient demands will be greatest during peak growth velocity. Daniel[3] found that girls had their highest calorie intake at SMR 2 (the time of peak height velocity). If menstruation has occurred, one can assume the girl is at SMR 4, that growth is decelerating, and that nutrient needs are nearing adult levels.[3]

Height

Approximately 15 to 20% of adult height is gained during adolescence, most of it during the growth spurt that lasts 24 to 36 months.[8] Before puberty, girls grow at a steady rate of about 5.5 cm/yr (ranging from 4.0 to 7.5 cm/yr). The onset of the growth spurt is quite variable (ranging from 9.5 to 14.5 years of age) but typically occurs by age 10.5 years in girls.[9] In general, this spurt occurs about 2 years earlier than in boys. Peak height velocity (PHV) occurs at a mean age of 11.5 years, with velocity rates averaging 8.3 cm/yr (ranging from 6.0 to 10.5 cm/yr).[9] PHV occurs most often between pubic hair rating 2 and breast rating 3. Ninety-five percent of the time, girls will grow most rapidly between 9.7 and 13.3 years of age. PHV is reached about 6 to 12 months before menarche (the first menses).

The height spurt occurs relatively early in female puberty, whereas menarche, often erroneously assumed to mark the onset of puberty, occurs relatively late in puberty.[10] Menarche occurs most often at SMR 4. The mean age of menarche in the United States is 12.5 years, with a normal range of 10 to 16.5 years.[3] Menarche occurs at the time of maximum deceleration of linear growth. By menarche, approximately 95% of adult height has been obtained.[2] Using longitudinal data, Roche and Davila[11] reported that increases in height between menarche and adulthood were 1.7 in., 2.9 in., and 4.2 in. at the 10th, 50th, and 90th percentiles, respectively. Although they have an earlier start, girls reach an average final adult height of 163.8 cm, compared with 176.8 cm for boys.[9] This difference is due to the lower PHV in girls and the earlier cessation of growth in girls (mean age, 16 years) compared with boys (mean age, 18 years).[10]

Velocity

During adolescence, serial measurements of height should be plotted on a height velocity chart (expressed in centimeters of growth per year) to document the acceleration of growth that marks the pubertal growth spurt[12] (Figure 1-2). These charts are useful because they accentuate modest changes in growth rate and make it possible to identify the onset of the pubertal growth spurt and the point of maximal height velocity.[13]

Weight

Pubertal weight gain in girls accounts for approximately 50% of adult ideal body weight.[8] Peak weight velocity (PWV) in girls occurs about 6 months after PHV and frequently coincides with menarche. During PWV, girls gain 5.5 to 10.6 kg/yr.[9] After PWV, girls continue to gain weight but at a sharply reduced rate. Girls typically gain 5 to 10 kg between menarche and the time they achieve their full adult weight.

Secular Trends in Growth

There has been a secular trend of increased weight and height among adolescents in industrialized countries during the past 100 years. Also, puberty (as judged by menarcheal age) is occurring at an earlier age, induced by improved nutrition and the decline of chronic infections.[14] In Norway, where there are rather complete records, the mean age of menarche decreased from 15.6 years for women born in 1860 to 13.3 years in women born after 1940.[15] In the United States, it is estimated that recent decreases in the average age of menarche have

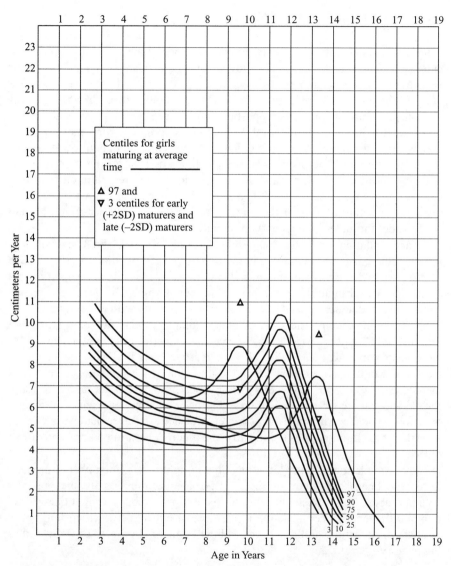

Figure 1-2 Growth Chart for Adolescent Girls   *Source:* Reprinted with permission from *Journal of Pediatrics* (1985;107:317), Copyright © 1985, Castlemead Publications.

occurred at about 3 months per decade. Thus, at the turn of the century, the average age of menarche would have been 14.6 years of age, approximately 2 years older than the current average of about 12.6 years.[16] Over the past three decades, the secular trend has reached a plateau in most of North America and Europe.

Body Composition

Distinct gender differences in body composition, which affect nutrient needs, emerge during adolescence. The body composition changes are mediated for females by the sex hormones estrogen and progesterone and for males testosterone and the anabolic adrenal androgens. During adolescence, girls deposit proportionately more fat and boys proportionately more lean body tissue and skeletal mass, so that by the time physical maturation is complete, girls have approximately twice the percentage of body fat as do boys but only about two-thirds as much lean tissue.[17] The changes in body composition have important implications for nutritional needs for adolescents, particularly in regard to energy, iron, and protein for tissue synthesis.[18] The greater lean body mass in males, which is the active metabolic mass of the body, explains the higher energy and protein requirement for males compared with females.[14]

Fat accumulation markedly changes during adolescence. In the 3 years preceding PHV, there is modest decrease in the rate of fat accumulation in girls.[19] Once PHV is reached, there is a dramatic and continuous increase in the velocity of fat accumulation, particularly in regions of the pelvis (hips and buttocks), breast, upper back, and upper arms. Although girls enter puberty with an average of 15% body fat, by the time physical maturation is complete, body fat comprises about 28% of body weight.[20] Frisch[21] has noted that pubertal girls experience a 44% increase in lean body mass and a 120% increase in body fat. Thus, the lean body mass-to-fat ratio changes from 5:1 at the initiation of the growth spurt to 3:1 at menarche. She also postulates that 17% of total body weight as fat is necessary for menarche to occur and 25% of body fat for onset and maintenance of regular ovulatory cycles.[22] Although the association of body fat to menarche is controversial,[20] it is commonly used clinically to explain delayed menarche and amenorrhea.

The accumulation of body fat, although a normal part of the pubertal process, is perceived negatively by most girls.[23,24] The ideal of thinness and the emphasis on a prepubertal body shape is believed to contribute to body weight dissatisfaction and the emergence of dieting at the time of puberty. Adolescent girls need awareness, education, and reassurance about the natural process of fat gain during puberty.

Pubertal Timing

The timing of maturation may affect the adolescent's transition. Early maturation appears to be a disadvantage for girls, in contrast to early maturing boys who are advantaged in many aspects of socio-emotional, academic functioning, and sports performance.[25] Early maturing girls have been found to have a poorer body image and more eating problems than on-time or late maturers.[25–27] Because early maturers are heavier and have more body fat compared with later maturers, it is not surprising that they may be more dissatisfied with their shape and more concerned about dieting. Early maturing girls may also experience poorer emotional health and depressive effect than late-maturing girls.[25,26] Early maturers have also been shown to engage in adult behaviors (such as smoking, drinking, and sexual intercourse) at an earlier age than later maturers.[26,28] Although their onset of puberty may well be within the normal range, early maturing adolescent girls will frequently need more reassurance about their development than do girls who mature later.

NUTRIENT NEEDS

The dramatic growth that occurs during adolescence, which is preceded only by the first year of life, creates increased demands for nutrients and energy. Total nutrient needs are higher during adolescence than at any other time during the lifespan.[17] Interestingly, data regarding specific nutrient requirements of adolescents are extremely limited. For many nutrients, estimates of requirements have been interpolated from studies of young children and adults or are recommended intakes associated with adequate growth.[8,18] The Recommended Dietary Allowances (RDAs)[29] established by the Food and Nutrition Board of the National Research Council are based on the best scientific knowledge available (Table 1-2). It should be noted that the RDAs are based on chronologic age rather than developmental age. In the future, it is hoped that the RDAs and the underlying nutrient requirement research will be based on SMR.

National surveys document inadequate dietary intakes of certain vitamins and minerals in subgroups of adolescents.[30–33] Adolescent girls are more likely than boys to have low intakes of essential vitamins and minerals. Analysis of national data sets have not found an association between diet quality of adolescents and income level. In analyzing dietary intake data of U.S. adolescents from the Nationwide Food Consumption Survey, Johnson et al[32] found that the two most significant predictors for consuming low intakes of several essential vitamins and minerals were race (black girls) and region (girls living in the South). According to national surveys, the minerals that adolescent girls most often consume in inadequate amounts are iron, calcium, zinc, magnesium, and phosphorus. Vitamins that are consumed at less than the recommended intake levels include folate, vitamin A, vitamin E, and vitamin B_6[30–33] (Table 1-3). Dietary fiber intake is also below recommended levels.[33] Inadequate protein is not a problem among most adolescent girls in the United States.[30–33] Dietary excesses of total fat, saturated fat, cholesterol, sodium, and sugar are common among adolescent girls and are found in all income and ethnic groups.[30–35] Overall, the average macronutri-

Table 1-2 Recommended Dietary Allowances of Nutrients for Females Aged 11 to 24 and Pregnant Adolescents

	Females			Pregnant Females
	11–14 yr	15–18 yr	19–24 yr	
Weight (kg)[a]	46	55	58	—
Height (cm)[a]	157	163	164	—
Energy (total kcal)	2200	2200	2200	+300
Energy (kcal/kg)	47	40	38	—
Protein (g)	46	44	46	60
Vitamin A (μg RE)	800	800	800	800
Vitamin D (μg)	10	10	10	10
Vitamin E (mg α-TE)	8	8	8	10
Vitamin K (μg)	45	55	60	65
Vitamin C (mg)	50	60	60	70
Thiamine (mg)	1.1	1.1	1.1	1.5
Riboflavin (mg)	1.3	1.3	1.3	1.6
Niacin (mg NE)	15	15	15	17
Vitamin B_6 (mg)	1.4	1.5	1.6	2.2
Folate (μg)	150	180	180	400
Vitamin B_{12} (μg)	2.0	2.0	2.0	2.2
Calcium (mg)	1200	1200	1200	1200
Phosphorus (mg)	1200	1200	1200	1200
Magnesium (mg)	280	300	280	320
Iron (mg)	15	15	15	30
Zinc (mg)	12	12	12	5
Iodine (μg)	150	150	150	175
Selenium (μg)	45	50	55	65

[a]Weights and heights represent actual median weights and heights for adolescents derived from national data collected by the National Center for Health Statistics.
RE, retinol equivalents; α-TE, α-tocopherol equivalents; NE, niacin equivalents.
Source: Reprinted with permission from *Recommended Dietary Allowances,* ed 10, 1989, by the National Academy of Sciences. Published by the National Academy Press.

---

ent distribution for adolescent girls is 52% of energy from carbohydrate, 14% of energy from protein, and 34% of energy from fat.[35]

Inadequate diets during adolescence can potentially retard growth or delay sexual maturation. Excessive intakes (fat and cholesterol) or inadequate intakes (e.g., calcium) of some nutrients can increase the risk for chronic diseases in adulthood. Also, inadequate dietary intakes before conception appear to influence the risk of fetal neural tube defects, certain fetal malformations, and spontaneous abortion. Key nutrients found to be problematic in the diets of adolescent girls are discussed below.

Table 1-3 Mean Nutrient Intakes among Adolescent Girls from Two National Surveys

	NHANES III 1988–1991		NFCS 1987–1988	
	mean	*SEM*	*mean*	*SD*
Energy (kcal)				
12–15 yr	1838	46	1744	532
16–19	1958	57	1618	606
Protein (g)				
12–15 yr	62	2.0	66	21
16–19	67	2.2	62	24
Fat (g)				
12–15 yr	72	2.6	71	24
16–19	77	3.1	66	28
Carbohydrates (g)				
12–15 yr	243	6.1	215	70
16–19	254	8.2	196	77
Vitamin A (IU)				
12–15 yr	4014	442	4308	3208
16–19	5179	713	4309	4007
Vitamin C (mg)				
12–15 yr	91	6.2	85	60
16–19	101	8.4	80	70
Thiamin (mg)				
12–15 yr	1.3	0.05	1.3	0.5
16–19	1.5	0.06	1.2	0.5
Riboflavin (mg)				
12–15 yr	1.7	0.06	1.8	0.7
16–19	1.7	0.07	1.6	0.8
Vitamin B_6 (mg)				
12–15 yr	1.4	0.06	1.4	0.7
16–19	1.4	0.07	1.2	0.6
Folate (µg)				
12–15 yr	220	11.8	211	114
16–19	234	12.9	189	121
Calcium (mg)				
12–15 yr	796	33	833	407
16–19	822	34	718	387
Iron (mg)				
12–15 yr	12.2	0.54	12.0	5.8
16–19	12.5	0.60	10.4	5.3
Zinc (mg)				
12–15 yr	9.5	0.52	9.4	3.7
16–19	9.6	0.43	8.9	4.5

Source: Data from Third National Health and Nutrition Examination Survey, Phase 1 (NHANES III), 1988–1991 and USDA Nationwide Food Consumption Survey (NFCS), 1987–1988.

Calcium

Calcium needs during adolescence are greater than they are in either childhood or adulthood because of the dramatic increase in skeletal growth and lean body mass. During adolescence, approximately 45% of adult skeletal mass is formed and 20% of adult height is obtained.[8] Because approximately 99% of total body calcium is found in the skeleton and teeth, calcium requirements closely parallel skeletal growth. Matkovic and Heaney[36] found that during adolescence, the average maximal calcium retention in girls is close to 400 mg/day at the intake threshold of about 1500 mg/day. However, more typical intakes of calcium (~ 900 mg/day) have led to lower peak rates of calcium absorption and retention. Abrams and Stuff[37] found that net calculated calcium retention for pre-, early, and late pubertal girls was 131, 161, and 44 mg/day, respectively. These findings indicate that peak calcium retention during early puberty in girls consuming typical U.S. diets is far below that previously reported and could have a substantial effect on bone mass development. If continued for 3 years, the low calcium retention could lead to a skeletal calcium deficit of 100 to 150 g, about 10 to 15% of total body calcium in an adult woman.[37]

The RDA for calcium increases from 800 mg/day during childhood to 1200 mg/day for females aged 11 to 24 years. The RDA for adolescents is based on average calcium retention rates of 140 to 165 mg/day and a relatively conservative estimate of absorption efficiency of 40%.[29] There exists, however, growing evidence that the current RDA for calcium may not be adequate to ensure peak bone mass (PBM) development in adolescents.[36] It has been suggested that the intake of calcium associated with maximal development of bone mass be considered an appropriate biomarker to evaluate the RDA for calcium.[36] A recent NIH Consensus Development Conference on Optimal Calcium Intake[38] called for an increase in calcium intake among adolescents and young adults (11 to 24 years) from 1200 to 1500 mg/day, stating that calcium intakes in this range may result in higher adult PBM.

The PBM represents the maximum size, weight, and density of the skeleton. Genetic factors play a major part in the determination of PBM, accounting for up to 80% of the variance. Still, 20% or more may be due to environmental factors, such as nutrition and exercise.[39] Among nutritive factors, calcium appears to be the most important determinant of PBM. The period between 9 and 20 years of age seems to be critical for achievement of PBM.[36,39–41] A maximal bone mass at skeletal maturity is considered the best protection against age-related bone loss and subsequent fracture risk.[29] It has been hypothesized that low PBM rather than excessive loss of bone may be the major contributor to osteoporosis.[40]

Given the importance of calcium in bone health and potential prevention of osteoporosis, it is of concern that calcium intake among adolescent girls starts to decline at puberty, the time of maximal requirements. The average calcium intake for teenage girls in the United States is considerably less than the RDA of 1200 mg/day[30-33] (Table 1-3). Adolescent girls consume only 66% of the RDA for calcium.[33] Slight ethnic/racial variations also exist. According to the NHANES II and Hispanic HANES data, the mean calcium intake for 11- to 17-year-old girls by ethnic group is 842 mg/day for whites, 700 mg/day for African-Americans, 853 mg/day for Mexican-Americans, 774 mg/day for Cubans, and 886 mg/day for Puerto Ricans.[42] Eck and Hackett-Renner[43] used NHANES data to assess calcium intake in youth, and using a multiple regression model found that socio-economic status was not a significant predictor of calcium intake. Studies have also found that adolescent boys have higher calcium intakes than girls, and specifically among white boys, their intake meets or exceeds the RDA.[42,43]

The decline in calcium intake parallels adolescent girls' decreasing consumption of milk and dairy products with age. Kenney et al[44] found this more noticeable among white girls, as black girls consumed less dairy products at all ages. Considering that milk and other dairy products contribute more than 55% of the calcium intake of the U.S. population,[29] the avoidance of dairy products is a significant factor influencing the calcium intake of adolescent girls. Evidence suggests that the low calcium intake of adolescent girls is caused, in part, by substitution of milk with soft drinks,[45] although this has not been found in all studies.[46] Another proposed reason is adolescent girls' preoccupation with their weight.[43] If high-calcium foods are perceived as fattening, they may not be consumed. Recently, Barr[46] assessed the association of social and demographic variables with calcium intakes of high school students. More than half of the 444 girls had calcium intakes below recommended levels. Multiple regression analysis found the following variables were positively associated with total calcium intake in females: taste enjoyment of dairy products, number of meals and snacks per day, behavioral modeling of milk consumption, perceptions of other's opinions, and soft drink consumption. The results of this study imply that nutrition education programs focusing on taste enjoyment of dairy products and building on the social influence of peers and family members may be beneficial in increasing calcium intake. More research is needed on factors influencing adolescents' calcium intakes and strategies to increase calcium-rich foods.

When adolescents find calcium-rich foods unacceptable or are lactose-intolerant, counseling regarding acceptable calcium sources is indicated. If the recommended calcium intake cannot be met by diet, a supplement may be warranted. Of the calcium supplements commercially available, calcium carbonate contains the highest proportion (40%) of elemental calcium by weight.[47,48] Also, it is the least expensive. Familiar brand names containing calcium carbonate are Tums, Os-cal, and Caltrate.[47] Calcium absorption can be enhanced by taking supplements in divided doses with no more than 400 to 500 mg at a time, taking supplements with a meal, and avoiding coingestion of large quantities of interfering substances such as oxalate (i.e., spinach, beet greens, rhubarb) and phytate (outer husks of cereal grains).[47]

Other dietary factors, such as unusually high consumption of phosphorus or protein, especially from animal foods, and sodium, may adversely affect calcium metabolism and thereby affect bone metabolism.[29] Therefore, a challenging task is to encourage adolescents to consume calcium-rich foods, but not too much protein, phosphorus, sodium, or fat.

Iron

Iron is a component of hemoglobin, myoglobin, and several heme-containing and iron-dependent enzymes.[29] Also, there is evidence that iron may be essential for skeletal growth.[49] Lean body tissue increments and rapid expansion of the red cell mass associated with adolescent growth result in iron requirements that are higher than during any other period of life. The onset of menarche approximately 1 year after peak growth (before mobilized iron stores may be replenished) further increases iron needs of adolescent girls.[49,50]

Absorbed iron needs of female adolescents have been estimated to be approximately 1.9 mg/day, based on average growth requirements and basal and menstrual losses (0.5 mg, 0.75 mg, and 0.6 mg/day, respectively).[51] The RDA of 15 mg iron per day, which assumes a dietary iron absorption rate of 10 to 15%, should result in absorbed iron intakes of 1.5 to 2.2 mg/day. This amount of dietary iron is thought to be sufficient to maintain positive iron balance and achieve a target iron storage level of 300 mg in most adolescents with mixed dietary intakes and average menstrual losses.[29,52] However, more recent calculations based on the variation of basal and menstrual losses suggest a significantly higher iron requirement of 3.2 mg/day for 95% of adolescent girls.[53] Assuming a bioavailability of 16% of dietary iron, Hallberg[53] suggests that an iron intake of 19 mg/day may be necessary to meet iron needs in this age group.

Average dietary iron intakes of U.S. adolescent girls in the NHANES III were 12.2 mg/day in 12- to 15-year-olds and 12.5 mg/day in 16- to 19-year-olds.[33] Approximately 7 to 10% of dietary iron in adolescent girls is in the form of heme iron from animal tissues sources. Highly bioavailable, heme iron is absorbed directly into the intestinal mucosal cells as an intact porphyrin complex and is thus not affected by meal composition. The greatest proportion of dietary iron is contributed by the less bioavailable inorganic or nonheme iron from vegetable and plant sources. Absorption of nonheme iron is dependent on physiologic need and, also, may vary nearly 15-fold as a result of interaction with other meal components.[54] Substances that enhance and those that bind or make nonheme iron insoluble (and thus prevent its uptake by the brush border) are listed in Exhibit 1-1.[42]

Exhibit 1-1 Substances That Enhance and Inhibit Iron Availability

---

Enhancers (increases nonheme iron absorption)
- ascorbic acid
- meat, fish, poultry, seafood

Inhibitors (decreases nonheme iron absorption)
- calcium
- phosphorus
- magnesium
- polyphenols (coffee, tea)
- phytates (cereals and legumes)
- bran
- antacids

Iron status may be especially critical in adolescents who may have lower than average dietary iron intakes or increased iron losses. Included are those who practice total vegetarianism or who consume little meat, fish, poultry, or ascorbic acid, or high amounts of iron absorption inhibitors, as well as those who engage in frequent meal skipping or chronic dieting. Above-average iron losses may occur in adolescents who have heavy or lengthy menstrual periods or those who chronically use analgesics, donate blood frequently, or participate in endurance sports or intensive physical training.[55]

Increased iron demands and marginal iron intakes make the female adolescent especially vulnerable to iron-deficiency anemia. The prevalence of iron-deficiency anemia is approximately 3.5% in girls 12 to 14 and 18 to 19 years of age. A higher rate of nearly 6% has been observed in girls between 15 and 17 years of age.[56,57] Anemia, characterized by hypochromic, microcytic erythrocytes and a lowered production of hemoglobin, is a late manifestation of iron deficiency. Normocytic iron-deficient erythropoiesis may be at least as prevalent in adolescents and appears to share some of the same potential consequences of frank anemia.[52] These may include fatigue, impaired physical performance, lowered endurance, reduced attention span, and decreased school performance. Adverse effects on the immune system and physical growth may also occur.[49,55] The age-specific criteria for anemia in young girls[58] is shown in Table 1-4.

There is little change in hematocrit percentages as adolescent girls mature. This is in direct contrast to adolescent boys, who have a striking rise in hematocrit percentages with increasing SMRs. This increase in boys is presumed to be related to increasing testosterone stimulus on the bone marrow.

Management of iron deficiency in the adolescent involves improvement of dietary habits and iron therapy. Regular consumption of lean meat, fish, or poultry, as well as fortified breakfast cereals, will improve dietary iron intake. Increased consumption of liver, although a rich iron source, may not be desirable

Table 1-4 Hemoglobin Values Diagnostic of Anemia in Adolescent Girls[a]

Age	Hemoglobin (g/dl)
10–11	11.6
12–14	11.8
15+	12.0

- Hemoglobin cutoffs for African-American adolescents may be 0.8–1.0 g/dl lower.[52]
- Cigarette smoking raises the anemia cutpoint 0.3 g/dl at 10–20/day; 0.5 g/dl at 21–40/day.
- Altitude raises the anemia cutpoint (e.g., 0.5 g/dl at 5000–5999 ft).

[a]Based on 5th percentile values from NHANES II.
Source: Adapted from Centers for Disease Control and Prevention. CDC Criteria for anemia in children and childbearing-aged women. Morbidity and Mortality Weekly Review. 1989;38:440–444.

because of its high cholesterol and potentially high carcinogen content. Inclusion of an ascorbic acid source with meals and snacks is recommended to enhance dietary iron absorption. Ferrous sulfate (e.g., 325 mg, supplying 65 mg elemental iron) is the most efficient and economical form of iron therapy. Resolution of anemia should occur approximately 6 to 8 weeks after iron supplementation. However, repletion of iron stores requires iron therapy for an additional 2 to 4 months. Adolescents with ongoing risk factors for anemia (e.g., hypermenorrhagia) may require long-term, low-dose iron supplementation. Adolescents who fail to respond to iron therapy should be evaluated for compliance with the prescribed regimen as well as for other causes of anemia (e.g., infection) if iron deficiency is confirmed by depleted iron stores (serum ferritin level ≤12 to 15 µg/ml).

Folate

The need for folate is increased during adolescent growth and sexual maturation because of its role in DNA and RNA synthesis and amino acid metabolism. The RDA for folate is 32 µg/kg body weight or 150 µg/day for girls 11 to 14 years of age and 180 µg/day for those between 15 and 19 years of age.[29] The richest dietary sources of folate are liver, super-fortified breakfast cereals, dried beans, asparagus, and spinach. However, the more frequent consumption of orange juice, enriched grains, dried beans, green salads, and regular or nonfortified breakfast cereals make these the highest contributors of folate in the U.S. diet.[59] Adolescents who skip breakfast or consume few fruits and vegetables are more likely to have low dietary folate intakes.

Although frank folate deficiency (manifested as megaloblastic anemia) is rare, several studies have indicated inadequate folate status among adolescents.[59–61] Low serum folate levels have been observed in 12% and low red cell folate levels (indicative of longer-term deficiency) in 8% of 11- to 19-year-old girls.[59] Another study of 103 healthy 12- to 16-year-old girls from different ethnic and economic backgrounds found that 12% were folate-deficient using serum levels and 48% by erythrocyte levels.[60] The data are inconsistent with the relationship of family income level and adolescent folate status. Results from some studies[61,62] have found that adolescent girls from low-income households are at increased risk for inadequate folate status whereas others[5,60] have reported no association. Adolescents who are heavy users of tobacco or alcohol, who take anticonvulsant drugs, or who are long-term oral contraceptive users are at increased risk for folate deficiency.[17,59]

Among adolescent girls, serum folate levels and dietary folate decrease with increasing age from early adolescence (12 years) through middle adolescence (16 years).[60] Bailey[61] and Daniel et al[5] found that folate status in adolescent girls was negatively correlated with an increase in sexual maturity. When assessing folate status of adolescents, it is recommended that biologic maturity be assessed through sexual maturity ratings.

Studies have recently confirmed that adequate folate intakes can reduce the risk of recurrent neural tube defects (NTDs) by 70% and first occurrences of these birth defects by 50%.[63–65] Approximately 95% of NTD cases occur in those with no previous history of spina bifida or anencephaly, and women of all ages, including adolescents, are at risk. Malformations of the neural tube occur early in gestation (i.e., by the 20th day after conception), before pregnancy is confirmed and prenatal care begun. The U.S. Public Health Service has thus recommended that all women of childbearing age who are capable of becoming pregnant should consume 0.4 mg of folate per day (more than twice that of the RDA).[66] Those who have had a previous pregnancy affected by spina bifida or other NTDs should consult their physician for higher doses (4.0 mg/day) during the periconceptional period if a subsequent pregnancy is planned.[66] Folate intakes of approximately 0.2 mg have been observed in adolescent girls.[60] However, those who consume a diet consistent with the daily food guide pyramid are likely to achieve the recommended daily intake of 0.4 mg/day. Nutrition education should be provided to achieve this goal.[66]

Energy

Energy is the primary dietary requirement because if energy needs are not met, available protein, vitamins, and minerals cannot be used effectively for various metabolic functions. The energy requirements of adolescents are based on basal metabolic rate (BMR), rates of growth, body composition, and physical activity level.[17] The BMR generally constitutes the largest component of total energy expenditure, unless physical activity is unusually high. The BMR correlates highly with lean body mass.[14] Thus, girls who have less lean body tissue than boys will have lower metabolic rates and total energy needs compared with boys. From birth to age 10 years, the energy needs of males and females are similar. After age 10 years, when differences in body composition and growth rates occur, there are separate RDAs for boys and girls. The RDA for energy for girls 11 to 18 years of age is 2200 kcal/day.[29]

In the national surveys, the mean energy intake for adolescent girls is substantially less than the RDA (Table 1-3). Data from NHANES I and NHANES II studies showed a 3 to 4% decrease in the energy intake of girls in both the 6- to 11-year and 12- to 17-year age groups. However, in NHANES III, mean energy intake was the same for 12- to 15-year-old girls as in NHANES II but 270 calories higher in 16- to 19-year-old girls.[35] Although little data exist for adolescents, Murphy et al[67] analyzed dietary data for adults from the 1987 to 1988 Nationwide Food Consumption Survey and found that the strongest predictor of diet quality was energy intake. Higher energy intakes were associated with higher levels of nutrients. Adolescent girls with low energy intakes will have a difficult time meeting the RDA for vitamins and minerals.

The adolescent growth spurt is extremely sensitive to energy and nutrient deprivation. Low energy intake can lead to delayed puberty or growth retardation.[68–70] Insufficient energy consumption may occur because of inadequate resources to purchase food, intentional dieting, or secondary to other factors such as substance abuse or chronic illness. Pugliese and colleagues[70] have documented poor growth and growth retardation in adolescent girls who were chronically restricting their energy intake. Of 503 adolescent girls studied, 25% were less than 90% of their ideal body weight-for-height, and 1.8% exhibited linear growth retardation associated with poor weight gain. In another study by the same research team,[68] deteriorating linear growth and nutritional dwarfing occurred in adolescents who did not meet the diagnostic criteria for anorexia nervosa but who had self-imposed caloric restriction due to a fear of becoming obese.

Fats

Recently, several authoritative groups and national agencies have reached consensus on dietary guidelines and recommend that all healthy children older than 2 years of age adopt a diet that reduces dietary fat to about 30% of total calories (33 g/1000 kcal), saturated fat to less than 10% of calories (11 g/1000 kcal), and daily cholesterol to less than 300 mg/day, for prevention of cardiovascular disease later in life.[71–73] The diets of American adolescents, both boys and girls, contain excessive amounts of total fat and saturated fat (Table 1-5). Recent national data have shown a positive trend of decreased fat intake over the past decade for adults as well as adolescents. For example, in NHANES III phase 1 (1988 to 1991), the percentage of energy from fat was 34% for girls aged 12 to 19 years compared with 37% in NHANES II.[35] There are some differences by race/ethnicity within both gender groups. In NHANES III, non-Hispanic black girls (12 to 19 years) had the highest percentage of energy from fat, approximately 37%, compared with 35% in Mexican-American girls and 33% in non-Hispanic white adolescent girls.[35] To help reduce excessive consumption of total fat, food choices should emphasize increased intakes of fruits, vegetables, and whole-grain products and cereals. Lower-fat dairy products, leaner cuts of meat, and reduction of other high-fat foods should also be encouraged. Interventions need to be targeted toward all race and ethnic groups.

PSYCHOSOCIAL DEVELOPMENT

The period of adolescence which extends over a decade can be subdivided into three substages: early adolescence (10 to 14 years); middle adolescence (15 to 17 years); and late adolescence (18 to 21 years). Looking at characteristics of these substages provides a useful context for understanding food behaviors and body image issues of youth, as well as a framework for developing nutrition education programs and providing clinical care. Nutrition interventions that do not incorporate the social, cognitive, and psychological needs of adolescents are likely to be ineffective. Table 1-6 summarizes the substages of adolescent development.

Table 1-5 Current[a] versus Recommended[b] Fat and Cholesterol Intakes in Adolescent Girls

	Current Intake		Recommended
	12–15 yr	*16–19 yr*	
Saturated fatty acids (% of calories)	12.0	12.3	<10
Total fat (% of calories)	33.7	34.4	Average no more than 30
Polyunsaturated	6.6	7.0	Up to 10
Monounsaturated	12.6	12.6	10–15
Cholesterol (mg/day)	202	210	<300

[a]*Source:* McDowell MA, et al. *Energy and Macronutrient Intakes of Persons Ages 2 Months and Over in the U.S.* Third National Health and Nutrition Examination Survey, Phase 1, 1988–91. Advance Data, U.S. Department of Health and Human Services, NCHS, No. 255, October 24, 1994.
[b]*Source:* National Cholesterol Education Program. *Report on the Expert Panel on Blood Cholesterol Levels in Children and Adolescents.* U.S. Department of Health and Human Services; 1991.

Table 1-6 Characteristics of Early, Mid, and Late Adolescence

Characteristics	Early Adolescence	Mid Adolescence	Late Adolescence
Growth	Secondary sexual characteristics have begun to appear Growth rapidly accelerating; reaches peak velocity	Secondary sexual characteristics well advanced Growth decelerating; stature reaches 95% of adult height	Physically mature; statural and reproductive growth virtually complete
Cognition	Concrete thought dominant Existential orientation Cannot perceive long-range implications of current decisions and acts	Rapidly gaining competence in abstract thought Capable of perceiving future implications of current acts and decisions but variably applied Reverts to concrete operations under stress	Established abstract thought processes Future oriented Capable of perceiving and acting on long-range options
Psychosocial self	Preoccupation with rapid body change Former body image disrupted	Re-establishes body image as growth decelerates and stabilizes Preoccupation with fantasy and idealism in exploring expanded cognition and figure options Development of a sense of omnipotence and invincibility	Emancipation completed Intellectual and functional identity established May experience "crisis of 21" when facing societal demands for autonomy
Family	Defining independence-dependence boundaries No major conflicts over parental control	Major conflicts over control Struggle for emancipation	Transposition of child–parent dependency relationship to the adult–adult model
Peer group	Seeks peer affiliation to counter instability generated by rapid change Compares own normality and acceptance with same sex/age mates	Strong need for identification to affirm self-image Looks to peer group to define behavioral code during emancipation process	Recedes in importance in favor of individual friendships
Sexuality	Self-exploration and evaluation Limited dating Limited intimacy	Multiple plural relationships Heightened sexual activity Testing ability to attract opposite sex and parameters of masculinity or femininity Preoccupation with romantic fantasy	Forms stable relationships Capable of mutuality and reciprocity rather than former narcissistic orientation Plans for future in thinking of marriage, family Intimacy involves commitment rather than exploration and romanticism
Age range	Initiates between ages 11 and 13 and merges with mid-adolescence at 14 to 15 years	Begins around 14 to 15 years and blends into late adolescence about age 17	Approximately 17 to 21 years; upper end particularly variable; dependent on cultural, economic, and educational factors

Source: Reprinted from *Adolescent Medicine*, ed 2 (p 13) by A Hofmann and D Greydanus, eds, with permission of Appleton & Lange, © 1989.

Early Adolescence

Early adolescence is characterized by the rapid acceleration of physical growth. Not surprisingly, young adolescents become intensely preoccupied with these physical changes. During this time, reassessment and restructuring of body image occurs. In general, early adolescence is dominated by the individual response to pubertal changes. There are frequent comparisons to peers and worry over any perceived abnormalities. Early adolescence also reflects the shift toward emerging independence and beginning the symbolic movement away from the home environment. At the same time, peer acceptance and conformity become increasingly important. Cognitions are limited primarily to concrete and present-oriented thinking; however, abstract thought is beginning to develop.

Middle Adolescence

By middle adolescence, girls have already experienced most of their physical growth and ideally should internalize and adjust to a new body image.[74] Given the societal emphasis and value placed on thinness and a certain body type, this is an exceedingly difficult task for many girls to accomplish. The middle adolescent years are characterized by developing a sense of identity and increasing autonomy. Middle adolescents spend less time with their family as friends and group activities assume greater importance. The developing capacity to think abstractly enhances adolescents' ability for problem solving, future-oriented thinking, understanding complexities and causality, and appreciating the perspectives of others. Many youth also become concerned about social and environmental issues and develop altruistic tendencies to help others. It is also a time for experimentation. Although this serves a positive developmental purpose, it also leads to an increase in health risk behaviors, the potential negative consequences of which are likely to be underestimated by the adolescent.

Late Adolescence

Late adolescence is marked by preparation for adult roles and focuses on future education or vocation, sexuality, and individuation. The emerging identity question at this stage is "Who am I in relation to other people and to the future?"[74] The late adolescent girl characteristically has become more comfortable with her own values and sense of identity, and peers have become less important. Important developmental tasks, for the establishment of self-identity and adult role responsibilities, need to be accomplished during the adolescent years. A successful passage through adolescence prepares youth for successful adult life styles.

ADOLESCENT EATING BEHAVIOR

Factors Influencing Eating Behaviors

Adolescent girls' eating habits and food choices are complex and are influenced by multiple interacting factors. These include physical, social, and cultural environments, family and peer influences, and psychological factors. Figure 1-3 depicts several influences on adolescent food behavior. These factors do not act directly on food behavior but are integrated by the individual and incorporated into one's life style, thus affecting food behavior.[75]

During childhood, the family has predominant influence on a child's food behavior. The family is not only the main provider of food but also the transmitter of attitudes toward food and weight, food preferences, and patterns that affect lifetime eating habits. As adolescents strive toward independence and autonomy, they begin to spend more time away from home and hence eating away from home. Food practices of adolescents reflect the changing influence of parents.

Peers exert a major influence on adolescent eating behavior. The peer group defines what is socially acceptable and sets behavioral standards and expectations. Adolescents spend a significant amount of time with friends, and eating is an important form of socialization and recreation. Because adolescents desperately want approval, particularly by their friends, peer influence and group conformity are important determinants in food acceptability and selection. In a group context, food selected usually needs to meet the social approval of the peer group.[75]

The "sociability" of foods and desirability for a certain body shape are influenced by the mass media through both explicit and implicit messages. Advertisers are keenly attuned to adolescent developmental stages and their need for peer approval, status, sexual attractiveness, and independence. Because of their buying power (in 1991, U.S. teenagers spent approximately $82 billion), youth are viewed as a lucrative market with specific ad campaigns targeted toward them.[76,77]

The advertising industry is also a powerful force in influencing cultural standards of beauty and ideal body type. The current emphasis on excessive thinness is a clear example of advertising's power to influence cultural standards and consequently individual behavior. Adolescents need to be educated to be critical viewers of advertising and the mass media. Another potent influence on adolescent girls' eating behavior is weight concerns. This issue is discussed under the section on nutrition-related issues.

Typical Eating Behaviors

The cognitive, physical, socio-emotional, and life-style changes can create profound effects on adolescent food habits. Recognizing the wide individual vari-

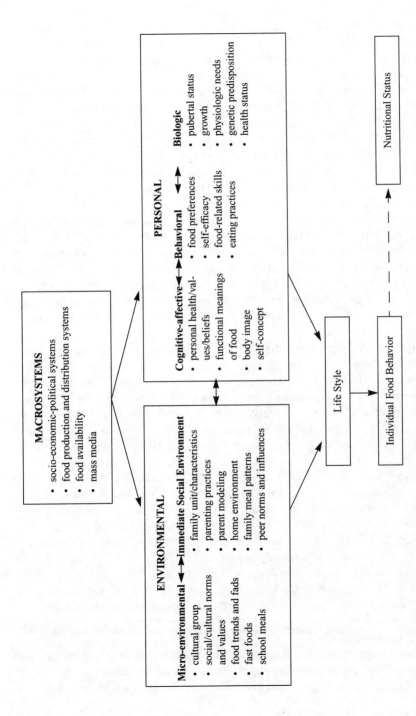

Figure 1-3 Conceptual Model for Factors Influencing Eating Behavior of Adolescents   *Source:* Copyright © 1995, Mary Story, PhD, RD.

ability that exists in eating patterns, as a group, teenagers tend to snack, miss meals, eat a larger proportion of meals away from home, consume fast foods, and try unconventional diets more often than other age groups.[75] Snacking is a major part of the adolescent life style. According to the National Adolescent Student Health (NASH) survey,[78] which surveyed more than 11,000 eighth and tenth graders nationwide, 88% of the girls ate at least one snack the previous day with almost one-fourth (24%) eating four or more snacks. Almost two-thirds of these snacks (62%) were categorized as high-fat or high-sugar foods (chips, soda, candy, ice cream, cake). Snacking or foods consumed outside of traditional meals provide between 20 and 35% of adolescents' total energy intakes.[79] Several studies have shown that the nutrient density is lower for snacks than for meals.[79,80]

Busy schedules or dieting may cause many adolescents to miss meals. The NASH survey[78] found that 29% of eighth and tenth grade girls ate breakfast daily (the survey period being "the previous week") and that 44% ate lunch and 62% ate dinner daily. By contrast, 18% never ate breakfast during the past week, 7% never ate lunch, and 1% never ate dinner. Girls ate fewer meals in a week than did boys, and tenth grade girls ate fewer meals than eighth grade girls. For example, 33% of eighth grade girls ate breakfast daily compared with only 24% of tenth grade girls. For many adolescent girls, the evening meal is the most regularly consumed meal of the day.

Adolescents, especially middle and late adolescents, consume much of their total energy intake eating away from home. Fast-food outlets represent 83% of the restaurant visits by youth younger than 17 years of age.[81] Fast-food outlets hold great appeal to adolescents for a number of reasons: (1) They provide a socially acceptable and casual place to hang-out with their friends; (2) the food served is what they like; (3) the food is relatively inexpensive and is convenient; and (4) fast-food outlets are a prime employer of adolescents. The most popular foods ordered by 6- to 17-year-olds are soft drinks (43%), french fries (30%), hamburgers/cheeseburgers (24%), pizza (21%), fried chicken (10%), ice cream (9%), and side-dish salads (6%). Although high-fat, high-calorie foods are still prevalent in fast-food outlets, within the past 5 years there have been healthy trends, with companies both improving existing foods and introducing healthier ones, such as grilled chicken sandwiches, fat-free muffins, lower-fat shakes, and vegetable salads with reduced-calorie dressings.[81] The nutritional impact of fast foods is dependent on the food choices made, the frequency that they are eaten, and the quality of the other food being consumed. Nutrition education of adolescents should address and identify the high-fat, high-calorie foods and focus on selecting lower-fat foods and healthier foods. Nutrient content of selected fast foods are shown in Table 1-7.

In addition to increasing autonomy, which causes more eating away from home, another central issue in adolescence is the establishment of identity, a sense of oneself as a unique individual. Because food is charged with symbolic

Table 1-7 Fast Foods: Higher and Lower Fat/Calorie Choices

Food	Calories	Fat (g)	Fat (% kcal)
Burger King double whopper with cheese	935	61	59
Burger King broiler chicken sandwich	267	8	27
Taco Bell taco salad, with shell	905	61	61
Fiesta tostado	167	7	38
Dairy Queen Heath blizzard, reg.	820	36	40
DQ vanilla cone, small	140	4	26
Pizza Hut pepperoni, personal pan pizza	675	29	39
Pizza Hut cheese pizza, med (2 sl)	492	18	33
Hardee's bacon cheeseburger	610	39	58
Hardee's roast beef sandwich	350	11	28
McDonald's Big Mac	500	26	47
French fries, med.	320	17	48
McDonald's hamburger	255	9	32
Garden salad, with lite vinaigrette dressing	98	4	37

Source: Data from *Fast-Food Guide,* ed 2 by MF Jacobson and S Fitschner, Workman Publishing, 1991.

meanings and emotional connotations, it may be used as a means of establishing individuation and of expressing one's identity and uniqueness. Food choices convey strong messages about the individual to family, friends, and the outside world. Experimentation and idealism are important developmental aspects of adolescence. Eating patterns such as vegetarianism and macrobiotic or organic diets may be adopted as a way of exploring new roles and life styles, testing adult restrictions, or showing genuine concern for environmental or ecologic issues.[75]

It is important to understand the intrinsic and functional meanings that food plays in the lives of adolescents. Chapman and Maclean[82] used qualitative research methods to explore the meanings of food among 93 Canadian adolescent girls aged 11 to 18. The girls participated in semistructured individual interviews or small group discussions in which they talked about what, where, and with whom they ate. The major food classification scheme that emerged from the data analysis was the dichotomization of foods into two groups; "healthy foods" and "junk foods." The girls thought that "junk food" was associated with pleasure, friends, weight gain, independence, and guilt, whereas eating "healthy food" was linked with family, meals, and being at home. Eating "junk food" was a way for teenagers to demonstrate increasing independence from the family and a growing loyalty to their peer group.

Most teenagers have an overriding orientation toward the present and little concern about the future in terms of their own health. Because of this, teenagers do not perceive much urgency to change their behavior, because the future is so ephemeral and far away. Also, the long-term benefits of good health and eating practices do not outweigh the short-term advantages of certain unhealthy activities. For example, as teenagers themselves explained in the Minnesota Youth Poll,[83] eating, smoking, drinking, and the use of leisure time involves much more than the choices of adopting healthy practices and discarding destructive ones. Many of the activities, which according to teenagers are unhealthy, are inextricably intertwined with issues of identity, self-concept, friendship, security, independence, and authority. Thus, to give up eating what teenagers call "junk foods" would be to give up much more than the activity itself. Nutrition interventions must address these deeper and more subtle social and developmental issues.

NUTRITION-RELATED ISSUES

Special nutrition-related concerns among adolescent girls include dieting, eating disorders, obesity, athletic activities, oral contraceptives, pregnancy, and substance use. Selected issues are briefly discussed below. Others such as adolescent pregnancy, eating disorders, and sports are discussed in subsequent chapters.

Dieting and Weight Concerns

During adolescence, girls become preoccupied with and sensitive about their changing size, shape, and physical appearance. This is part of normal adolescent development, but in our culture with the emphasis on excessive thinness in females, body dissatisfaction becomes inevitable. Weight concerns and restrictive eating have become so common among adolescents (particularly whites) that they are considered normative behavior. In the NASH survey,[78] 61% of adolescent eighth and tenth grade girls reported dieting during the past year (as compared with 28% of boys). The prevalence of weight control practices among high school girls in the national 1990 Youth Risk Behavior Survey[84] are shown in Table 1-8. As can be seen, 44% of the girls were trying to lose weight. More than one-fourth of the girls who considered themselves to be the right weight were trying to lose weight. The desire for thinness frequently leads to unhealthy weight loss methods. Of the girls who dieted during the past year in the NASH survey,[78] more than half (55%) reported they fasted to control their weight; 19% used diet pills, 13% induced vomiting, and 7% used laxatives.

Weight concerns and dieting practices are now occurring with greater frequency among older children and young teenagers. A recent study[85] found that 45% of 8- to 13-year-old girls wanted to be thinner and 37% had already tried to

Table 1-8 Prevalence and Reported Frequency of Specific Weight Control Practices among High School Girls from the Youth Risk Behavior Survey, 1991

	Female Students (n = 5882)			
	Trying to Lose Wt. (%)	*Trying to Maintain Wt. (%)*	*Trying to Gain Wt. (%)*	*Not Doing Anything (%)*
Participants	43.7	26.4	6.6	23.2
Grade				
9	42.5	25.0	7.9	24.6
10	45.3	24.9	7.0	22.8
11	43.4	27.3	5.9	23.4
12	43.7	28.7	5.6	22.1
Race				
White	47.4	27.3	3.6	21.7
Black	30.4	26.7	16.1	26.8
Hispanic	39.1	24.5	11.2	25.2
Other	45.6	18.7	8.1	27.6
Weight perception				
Underweight	3.7	3.3	65.7	27.4
Right Weight	27.5	35.5	3.2	33.8
Overweight	79.6	15.7	0.2	4.5

	Female Students (n = 2476)			
	Exercise (%)	*Diet Pills (%)*	*Vomiting (%)*	*Skipping Meals (%)*
Frequency				
In the past 7 days				
Never done this	5.0	67.2	78.1	—
None	22.7	26.5	16.4	27.9
1 or 2 times	21.7	2.3	2.9	27.0
3–6 times	31.7	2.4	1.2	28.1
7–14 times	13.7	1.2	0.7	14.9
15 or more times	5.2	0.3	0.8	2.1
Total	72.3	6.2	5.5	72.1

Source: Reprinted with permission from *Annals of Internal Medicine* (1993;119:667), Copyright © 1993, American College of Physicians.

lose weight. Fear of fatness and disordered eating behaviors occur regardless of weight status. Feldman et al[86] found that almost half of teenage girls thought they were too fat, although only 17% were actually overweight. Worrying about weight and feeling conflictive and guilty about food and eating are almost constant issues in the lives of many teenage girls.[87] Dieting, inappropriate eating, and body dissatisfaction are best understood as women's responses to the cultural emphasis on slimness and low body weight. Kilbourne[88] stresses we must speak out forcefully about the dangers of the obsession with thinness and advocate to change the societal norms about dieting and thinness. The societal norms for cigarette smoking have changed dramatically in the past 20 years. This is a result of many factors, including consistent messages, advertising restrictions, product liability suits, and increased health information. Some of these same measures could be used to change the norms about excessive thinness.

Overweight

Adolescent obesity is a significant public health issue with health and social implications. The prevalence of obesity among adolescents has increased markedly since 1964,[89] and recent data from NHANES III indicate that these trends have continued for adolescents, particularly for girls.[90] Prevalence estimates from NHANES II data indicate that 23% of adolescent girls (12 to 17 years of age) are obese, as defined by tricep skinfolds greater than the 85th percentile.[89] Adolescent girls are more likely to be overweight than boys, and this persists throughout adulthood.[90] The limited data available indicate that proportionately more overweight adolescents, principally girls, are found in Hispanic and American Indian groups.[90]

Adolescent girls who are overweight may be at an increased risk for immediate and long-term morbidity, including hypertension, hypercholesterolemia, and diabetes mellitus.[91] Overweight conditions during adolescence are likely to persist into adult years. Even if weight normalizes in later years, girls who are overweight as adolescents may be eight times more likely to have difficulty with daily living activities and twice as likely to suffer from arthritis as adults than leaner peers.[92] Psychosocial consequences of overweight that may persist into adulthood include feelings of isolation and rejection and low self-esteem.[93] Recently, overweight adolescents, particularly girls, have been shown to suffer adverse social and economic consequences in early adult life when compared with nonoverweight counterparts. These include completion of fewer years of school, failure to marry, lower household incomes, and higher poverty rates.[94]

The severe consequences of overweight in adolescents emphasize the need for management of this condition, focusing on the promotion of physical activity, healthful eating patterns, family involvement, and the use of behavioral change strategies and supportive counseling.[93] The complexity and difficulty of its management make evident the importance of primary prevention of overweight in youth.

Substance Use

Adolescent substance use and abuse is a major public health concern. Alcohol and tobacco are most likely to be used regularly or in large quantities by U.S. adolescents. With the exception of cigarettes and nonprescription diet pills, adolescent girls report lower levels of substance use compared with boys.[78] In the NASH survey,[78] 83% of adolescent girls reported at least one occasion in which they had an alcoholic beverage, 41% reported drinking alcohol in the past month, and 31% reported consuming five or more drinks on one occasion in the past 2 weeks. Almost one-fourth (23%) had smoked cigarettes in the past month, with 5% reporting smoking one to five packs and 4% smoking more than five packs in the past month. Adolescent drug use increases with age, and racial/ethnic differences exist. The Monitoring the Future project,[95] a nationally representative sample of high school seniors found that the following subgroups of adolescent girls reported half-pack or more daily use of cigarettes: whites (13%); African-Americans (2.2%); Mexican-Americans (2.5%); Puerto Ricans (4.2%); Asians (4.5%); Native Americans (23.4%). Among teenage girls, daily alcohol use was reported by whites (2.8%); African-Americans (0.7%); Mexican-Americans (2.6%); Puerto Ricans and Asians (0.9%); and Native Americans (5.4%).

Excessive use of alcohol or drugs may adversely affect nutritional health. High intakes of alcohol may suppress the appetite and compromise nutrient intakes. Also, heavy alcohol use may alter the absorption, metabolism, and use of several nutrients, including amino acids, zinc, folate, and vitamin B_6. Illicit drug use, particularly cocaine, as well as heavy cigarette smoking, can interfere with a balanced intake of nutrients. Cigarette smoking may interfere with energy use and increase the need for ascorbic acid, β-carotene, folate, and zinc.[96] Evaluation of chemical use should be an integral part of the nutrition assessment of all adolescents. If use or abuse is identified, referral for appropriate education, counseling, or treatment is indicated.

Contraceptive Use

Lower doses of estrogen and progestin appear to have reduced many of the biochemical and physiologic effects of oral contraceptive use that may affect nutritional status.[17,97] However, long-term oral contraceptive users with inferior-quality diets may be at an increased risk for compromised folate status.[17] Although weight gain is usually not a concern, some adolescents may experience mild-to-moderate weight increases. Adverse effects on serum lipid levels may be of concern for adolescents with strong family histories of hypercholesterolemia. This is particularly true if other risk factors, such as obesity, are present. Improvement of iron status related to decreased menstrual blood loss is a positive nutrition effect that may occur with oral contraceptive use.[98]

Both injectable progestin (Depo-provera) and Levonorgestrel implants (Norplant) may be associated with weight gain in some individuals.[99,100] Also, frequent or prolonged bleeding patterns that may occur during early use may compromise iron status. However, long-term use of these methods is usually associated with decreased total blood loss.[99,101]

Contraceptive users should receive ongoing nutrition education and counseling. Topics to address include the importance of a nutritionally adequate diet, including dietary sources of folate, a reduction of dietary fat and excess calories, and regular aerobic exercise.

FOOD GUIDANCE FOR ADOLESCENT GIRLS

The Dietary Guidelines for Americans[102] and the Food Guide Pyramid[103] provide a framework and foundation for a healthful diet for all healthy Americans 2 years of age and older. The Food Guide Pyramid provides recommendations for daily servings of food and is shown in Table 1-9. The number of servings in each

Table 1-9 Food Guide for Adolescents

Food Group	Servings/Day[a]	Serving Size
Bread, cereal, rice, pasta	6–11	• 1 slice bread • 1 oz (3/4 to 1 cup) dry cereal • 1/2 cup cooked rice, pasta, or cereal • 1/2 bun, bagel, or English muffin • 1 6 in. tortilla • 3 or 4 small plain crackers
Vegetables	3–5	• 1 cup raw leafy vegetables • 1/2 cup of other vegetables • 3/4 cup vegetable juice
Fruits	2–4	• 1 medium apple, banana, or orange • 1/2 cup of small or diced fruit • 3/4 cup of fruit juice
Milk, yogurt, cheese	3	• 1 cup of milk or yogurt • 1 1/2 oz of cheese • 2 oz of processed cheese
Meats, poultry, fish, dry beans and peas, eggs, nuts	2–3	• 2–3 oz of cooked lean meat, poultry, or fish[b] • 1/2 cup of cooked dry beans, 1 egg, or 2 Tbsp of peanut butter = 1 oz of lean meat
Fats, oils, sweets	Use sparingly	

[a]Note that the suggested number of servings is expressed as a range. The lower number of servings is the minimum needed by adolescent girls. Adolescents who are more physically active require a larger number of servings from each group.
[b]A handy guide to determine how much meat, chicken, fish, or cheese weigh: 1 ounce is the size of a match box; 3 ounces are the size of a deck of cards; 8 ounces are the size of a paperback book.
Source: U.S. Department of Agriculture. *The Food Guide Pyramid.* Hyattsville, Md: Human Nutrition Information Service; 1992. Home and Garden Bulletin no. 252 (HG-249).

food group depends on several factors including growth status, age, body size, and activity level.

What is not addressed in the U.S. Dietary Guidelines is the enjoyment and pleasure of eating. Adolescent girls, many of whom are in constant conflict with food, need to learn how to enjoy food, the pleasures attained from eating, and the value of sharing social meals. The Japanese have dietary guidelines similar to ours, but they have an added one, "Make all activities pertaining to food and eating pleasurable ones. Use the mealtime as an occasion for family communication. Treasure family taste and home-made cooking." A similar guideline should be considered for the United States.

The challenge of improving the nutritional health of adolescent girls will require the coordinated efforts of health care providers, teenagers, parents, educators, schools, communities, the food industry, and policy makers all working together to create more opportunities for healthful eating, promoting the same consistent messages, and advocating changing the norms against excessive thinness and more toward a range of healthy body weights.

References

1. Elliott GR, Feldman SS. Capturing the adolescent experience. In: Feldman SS, Elliott GR, eds. *At the Threshold: The Developing Adolescent.* Cambridge, Mass: Harvard University Press; 1990:1–13.

2. Marshall WA, Tanner JM. Variations in pattern of pubertal changes in girls. *Arch Dis Child.* 1969;44:291–303.

3. Daniel WA. Nutritional requirements of adolescents. In: Winick M, ed. *Adolescent Nutrition.* New York, NY: John Wiley & Sons; 1982:19–34.

4. Tanner JM. Issues and advances in adolescent growth and development. *J Adolesc Health Care.* 1987;8:470–478.

5. Tanner JM. *Growth at Adolescence.* 2nd ed. Oxford: Blackwell Scientific Publications; 1962.

6. Daniel WA, Gaines EG, Bennett DL. Dietary intakes and plasma concentrations of folate in healthy adolescents. *Am J Clin Nutr.* 1985;28:363–370.

7. Daniel WA. Hematowo: Maturity relationship in adolescence. *Pediatrics.* 1973;52:388–394.

8. Gong EJ, Heald FP. Diet, nutrition and adolescence. In: Shils ME, Olson JA, Shike M, eds. *Modern Nutrition in Health and Disease.* 8th ed. Philadelphia, Pa: Lea & Febiger; 1994:759–769.

9. Tanner JM, Davies PSW. Clinical longitudinal standards for height and weight velocity for North American children. *J Pediatr.* 1985;107:317–329.

10. Slap GB. Normal physiological and psychosocial growth in the adolescent. *J Adolesc Health Care.* 1986;7:13S–23S.

11. Roche AF, Davila GH. Late adolescent growth in stature. *Pediatrics.* 1972;50:874–880.

12. Vaughan VC, Litt IF. *Child and Adolescent Development: Clinical Implications.* Philadelphia, Pa: WB Saunders Co; 1990.

13. Underwood LE. Normal adolescent growth and development. *Nutr Today.* 1991;26:11–16.

14. Forbes GB. Nutrition and growth. In: McAnarney ER, Kreipe RE, Orr DP, Comerci GD, eds. *Textbook of Adolescent Medicine.* Philadelphia, Pa: WB Saunders Co; 1992:68–74.

15. Brudevoll JE, Liestol K, Walloe LW. Height, weight and menarcheal age of Oslo school children during the last 60 years. *Ann Hum Biol.* 1980;7:307–322.

16. US Congress, Office of Technology Assessment. What is adolescent health? In: *Adolescent Health—Volume II: Background and the Effectiveness of Selected Prevention and Treatment Services.* OTA-H-466. US Government Printing Office; November 1991: 16.

17. Story M. Nutritional requirements during adolescence. In: McAnarney ER, Kreipe RE, Orr DP, Comerci GD, eds. *Textbook of Adolescent Medicine.* Philadelphia, Pa: WB Saunders Co; 1992:75–84.

18. Gong EJ, Spear BA. Adolescent growth and development: implications for nutritional needs. *J Nutr Educ.* 1988;20:273–279.

19. Barnes HV. Physical growth and development during puberty. *Med Clin North Am.* 1975;59: 1305–1315.

20. Kreipe RE. Normal somatic adolescent growth and development. In: McAnarney ER, Kreipe RE, Orr DP, Comerci GD, eds. *Textbook of Adolescent Medicine.* Philadelphia, Pa: WB Saunders Co; 1992:44–67.

21. Frisch RE. Fatness, puberty and fertility: the effects of nutrition and physical training on menarche and ovulation. In: Brooks-Gunn J, Petersen AC, eds. *Girls at Puberty: Biological and Psychosocial Perspectives.* New York, NY: Plenum Press; 1983:29–49.

22. Frisch RE, McArthur J. Menstrual cycles: fatness as a determinant of minimum weight for height necessary for their maintenance or onset. *Science.* 1974;185:949–951.

23. Scott EC, Johnston FE. Critical fat, menarche, and the maintenance of menstrual cycles. *J Adolesc Health Care.* 1982;2:249–260.

24. Brooks-Gunn J. Antecedents and consequences of variations in girls' maturational timing. *J Adolesc Health Care.* 1988;9:365–373.

25. Brooks-Gunn J, Reiter EO. The role of pubertal processes. In: Feldman SS, Elliott GR, eds. *At the Threshold: The Developing Adolescent.* Cambridge, Mass: Harvard University Press; 1990:17–53.

26. Attie I, Brooks-Gunn J. The development of eating problems in adolescent girls: a longitudinal study. *Dev Psychol.* 1989;25:70–79.

27. Killen JD, Hayward C, Litt I, et al. Is puberty a risk factor for eating disorders? *Am J Dis Child.* 1992;146:323–325.

28. Wilson DM, Killen JD, Hayward C, et al. Timing and rate of sexual maturation and the onset of cigarette and alcohol use among teenage girls. *Arch Pediatr Adolesc Med.* 1994;148:789–795.

29. National Academy of Sciences, National Research Council. *Recommended Dietary Allowances.* 10th ed. Washington, DC: National Academy Press; 1989.

30. National Center for Health Statistics. *Dietary Intake Source Data, United States 1976-80.* Hyattsville, Md; US Department of Health & Human Services. 1983. Vital and Health Statistics, series 11, no. 231.

31. Wright HS, Guthrie HA, Wang MQ, Bernardo V. The 1987–88 nationwide food consumption survey: an update on the nutrient intake of respondents. *Nutr Today.* 1991;26:21–27.

32. Johnson RK, Johnson DG, Wang MQ, et al. Characterizing nutrient intakes of adolescents by sociodemographic factors. *J Adolesc Health.* 1994;15:149–154.

33. Alaimo K, McDowell MA, Briefel RR, et al. *Dietary Intakes of Vitamins, Minerals and Fiber of Persons Ages 2 Months and Over in the United States: Third National Health and Nutrition Examination Survey, Phase I, 1988–91.* Hyattsville, Md: National Center for Health Statistics; 1994. Advance data from Vital and Health Statistics; no. 258.

34. Kimm SY, Gergen P, Malloy M, et al. Dietary patterns of US children: implications for disease prevention. *Prev Med.* 1990;19:432–442.

35. McDowell MA, Briefel RR, Alaimo K, et al. *Energy and Macronutrient Intakes of Persons Ages 2 Months and Over in the United States: Third National Health and Nutrition Examination Survey, Phase I, 1988–91.* Hyattsville,Md; National Center for Health Statistics; 1994. Advance data from Vital and Health Statistics; no. 255.

36. Matkovic V, Heaney RP. Calcium balance during human growth: evidence for threshold behavior. *Am J Clin Nutr.* 1992;55:992–996.

37. Abrams SA, Stuff JE. Calcium metabolism in girls: current dietary intakes lead to low rates of calcium absorption and retention during puberty. *Am J Clin Nutr.* 1994;60:739–743.

38. Porter D. Washington update: NIH Consensus Development Conference statement. Optimal calcium intake. *Nutr Today.* 1994;29(5):37–40.

39. Matkovic V, Ilich JZ. Calcium requirements for growth: are current recommendations adequate? *Nutr Rev.* 1993;51:171–180.

40. Matkovic V. Calcium intake and peak bone mass. *N Engl J Med.* 1992;327:119–120.

41. Lloyd T, Andon MB, Rollings N, et al. Calcium supplementation and bone mineral density in adolescent girls. *JAMA.* 1992;270:841–844.

42. Looker AC, Loria CM, Carroll MD, et al. Calcium intakes of Mexican Americans, Cubans, Puerto Ricans, non-Hispanic whites and non-Hispanic blacks in the United States. *J Am Diet Assoc.* 1993;93:1274–1279.

43. Eck LH, Hackett-Renner C. Calcium intake in youth: sex, age, and racial differences in NHANES II. *Prev Med.* 1992;21:473–482.

44. Kenney MA, McCoy JH, Kirby AL, et al. Nutrients supplied by food groups in diets of teenaged girls. *J Am Diet Assoc.* 1986;86:1549–1555.

45. Guenther PM. Beverages in the diets of American teenagers. *J Am Diet Assoc.* 1986;86:493–499.

46. Barr S. Associations of social and demographic variables with calcium intakes of high school students. *J Am Diet Assoc.* 1994;94:260–266.

47. Levenson D, Bockman RS. A review of calcium preparations. *Nutr Rev.* 1994;52:221–232.

48. Whiting SJ. Safety of some calcium supplements questioned. *Nutr Rev.* 1994;52:95–97.

49. Brabin L, Brabin B. The cost of successful adolescent growth and development in girls in relation to iron and vitamin A status. *Am J Clin Nutr.* 1992;55:995–998.

50. Federation of American Societies for Experimental Biology. *Guidelines for the Assessment and Management of Iron Deficiency in Women of Childbearing Age.* Bethesda, Md: 1992.

51. Lanzikowsky P. Iron deficiency in adolescents. In: Winick M, ed. *Adolescent Nutrition.* New York, NY: John Wiley & Sons; 1982:73–96.

52. Herbert V. Recommended dietary intakes (RDI) of iron in humans. *Am J Clin Nutr.* 1987;45:679–686.

53. Hallberg L, Rossander-Hulten L. Iron requirements in menstruating women. *Am J Clin Nutr.* 1991;54:1047–1058.

54. Cook J. Adaptation in iron metabolism. *Am J Clin Nutr.* 1990;51:301–308.

55. Raunikar R, Sabio H. Anemia in the adolescent athlete. *Am J Dis Child.* 1992;146:1201–1205.

56. Dallman P, Yip R, Johnson C. Prevalence and causes of anemia in the United States, 1976–1980. *Am J Clin Nutr.* 1984;39:437–445.

57. Johnson-Spear MA, Yip R. Hemoglobin difference between black and white women with comparable iron status: justification for race-specific anemia criteria. *Am J Clin Nutr.* 1994;60:117–121.

58. Centers for Disease Control. CDC criteria for anemia in children and childbearing-aged women. *MMWR.* 1989;38:440–444.

59. Hine R. Folic acid: contemporary clinical perspective. *Perspect Appl Nutr.* 1993;1:3–14.

60. Clark A, Mossholder S, Gates R. Folacin status in adolescent females. *Am J Clin Nutr.* 1987;46:302–306.

61. Bailey LB. Folate status assessment. *J Nutr.* 1990;120:1508–1511.

62. Bailey LB, Wagner PA, Christakis GJ, et al. Folacin and iron status and hematological findings in black and Spanish-American adolescents from urban low-income households. *Am J Clin Nutr.* 1982;35:1023–1032.

63. MRC Vitamin Study Research Group. Prevention of neural tube defects: results of the Medical Research Council Vitamin Study. *Lancet.* 1991;338:131–137.

64. Czeizel A, Dudas I. Prevention of the first occurrence of neural-tube defects by periconceptional vitamin supplementation. *N Engl J Med.* 1992;327:1832–1835.

65. Werler M, Shapiro S, Mitchell A. Periconceptional folic acid exposure and risk of recurrent neural tube defects. *JAMA.* 1993;269:1257–1261.

66. Lin-Fu J, Anthony M. *Folic Acid and Neural Tube Defects: A Fact Sheet for Health Care Providers.* MCHB, HRSA, PHS; May 1993.

67. Murphy SP, Rose D, Hudes M, Viteri FE. Demographic and economic factors associated with dietary quality for adults in the 1987–88 Nationwide Food Consumption Survey. *J Am Diet Assoc.* 1992;92:1352–1357.

68. Pugliese MT, Lifshitz F, Grad G, et al. Fear of obesity: a cause of short stature and delayed puberty. *N Engl J Med.* 1983;309:513–518.

69. Lifshitz F, Moses N. Nutritional dwarfing: growth, dieting and fear of obesity. *J Am Coll Nutr.* 1988;7:367–376.

70. Pugliese M, Recker B, Lifshitz F. A survey to determine the prevalence of abnormal growth patterns in adolescents. *J Adolesc Health Care.* 1988;9:181–187.

71. National Research Council. *Diet and Health: Implications for Reducing Chronic Disease Risk.* Washington, DC: National Academy Press; 1989.

72. American Academy of Pediatrics, Committee on Nutrition. Statement on cholesterol. *Pediatrics.* 1992;90:469–473.

73. Expert Panel on Blood Cholesterol Levels in Children and Adolescents. *Report of the Expert Panel on Blood Cholesterol Levels in Children and Adolescents.* Bethesda, Md. US Department of Health & Human Services.1991. NIH Publ No. 91-2732.

74. Ingersoll GM. Psychological and social development. In: McAnarney ER, Kreipe RE, Orr DP, Comerci GD, eds. *Textbook of Adolescent Medicine.* Philadelphia, Pa: WB Saunders Co; 1992: 91–98.

75. Story M. Adolescent life-style and eating behavior. In: Mahan LK, Rees JM, eds. *Nutrition in Adolescence.* St Louis, Mo: Times Mirror/Mosby; 1984:77–103.

76. O'Neill B. Youth, money and financial planning. *J Home Econ.* 1992;84:12–16.

77. Bailey AW. Teenagers' employment, earnings and spending. *J Home Econ.* 1992;84:20–24.

78. American School Health Association. Association for the Advancement of Health Education, Society for Public Health Education. The National Adolescent Student Health Survey. *A Report on the Health of America's Youth.* Oakland, Calif: Third Party Publication Co; 1988:1–178.

79. Bigler-Doughten S, Jenkins RM. Adolescent snacks. Nutrient density and nutritional contribution to total intake. *J Am Diet Assoc.* 1987;87:1678–1684.

80. Ezell JM, Skinner JD, Penfield MP. Appalachian adolescents' snack patterns: morning, afternoon, and evening snacks. *J Am Diet Assoc.* 1985;85:1450–1456.

81. Jacobson MF, Fritschner S. *Fast-Food Guide.* 2nd ed. New York, NY: Workman Publications; 1991.

82. Chapman G, Maclean H. "Junk food" and "healthy food": meanings of food in adolescent women's culture. *J Nutr Educ.* 1993;25:108–113.

83. Hedin D, Resnick M, Blum R. *Minnesota Youth Poll: Youth's Views on Health, Illness and Medical Care.* Minneapolis, Mn: Agricultural Experiment Station, University of Minnesota; 1980. Report 174.

84. Serdula MK, Collins ME, Williamson DF, et al. Weight control practices of US adolescents and adults. *Ann Intern Med.* 1993;119:667–671.

85. Maloney MJ, McGuire J, Daniels SR, Specker B. Dieting behavior and eating attitudes in children. *Pediatrics.* 1989;84:482–489.

86. Feldman W, Feldman E, Goodman JT. Culture versus biology: children's attitudes toward thinness and fatness. *Pediatrics.* 1988;81:190–194.

87. Olsen L. *Food Fight: A Report on Teenager's Eating Habits and Nutritional Status.* Oakland, Calif: Citizen's Policy Center; 1984.

88. Kilbourne J. Still killing us softly: advertising and the obsession with thinness. In: Fallon P, Katzman MA, Wooley SC, eds. *Feminist Perspectives on Eating Disorders.* New York, NY: The Guilford Press; 1994:395–418.

89. Gortmaker SL, Dietz WH, Jr, Sobal AM, Wehler CA. Increasing pediatric obesity in the United States. *Am J Dis Child.* 1987;141:535–540.

90. Harlan WR. Epidemiology of childhood obesity: a national perspective. *Ann NY Acad Sci.* 1993;699:1–5.

91. Rocchini A. Adolescent obesity and cardiovascular risk. *Pediatr Ann.* 1992;21:235–240.

92. Must A, Jacques P, Dallal G, et al. Long-term morbidity and mortality of overweight adolescents: a follow-up of the Harvard Growth Study of 1992–1995. *N Engl J Med.* 1992;327:1350–1355.

93. Story M, Alton I. Current perspectives on adolescent obesity. *Top Clin Nutr.* 1991;6:51–60.

94. Gortmaker S, Must A, Perrin J, et al. Social and economic consequences of overweight in adolescence and young adulthood. *N Engl J Med.* 1993;329:1008–1012.

95. Bachman JG, Wallace JM, O'Malley PM, et al. Racial/ethnic differences in smoking, drinking, and illicit drug use among American high school seniors. *Am J Public Health.* 1991;81:372–377.

96. Preston A. Cigarette smoking—nutritional implications. *Prog Food Nutr Sci.* 1991;15:183–217.

97. Liukko P, Erkkola P, Pakarinen P, et al. Trace elements during 2 years' oral contraception with low-estrogen preparations. *Gynecol Obstet Invest.* 1988;25:113–117.

98. Larsson G, Milsom I, Linkstedt G, Rybo G. The influence of a low-dose combined oral contraceptive on menstrual blood loss and iron status. *Contraception.* 1992;46:327–334.

99. Speroff L, Darney P. *A Clinical Guide for Contraception.* Baltimore, Md: Williams & Wilkins; 1992.

100. Berenson A, Wiemann C. Patient satisfaction and side effects with levonorgestrel implant (Norplant) use in adolescents 18 years of age and younger. *Pediatrics.* 1993;92:257–260.

101. Faundes A, Tejada A, Brache V, Alvarez F. Subjective perception of bleeding and serum ferritin concentration in long-term users of Norplant. *Contraception.* 1987;35:189–196.

102. US Department of Agriculture. *Dietary Guidelines for Americans.* 3rd ed. Washington, DC: US Department of Health & Human Services; 1990. Home and Garden Bulletin no. 232.

103. US Department of Agriculture. *The Food Guide Pyramid.* Hyattsville, Md: Human Nutrition Information Service; 1992. Home and Garden Bulletin no. 252 (HG-249).

2

ॐ

Adolescent Pregnancy: Implications for Nutritional Care

Paula C. Zemel and Barbara Levin

ADOLESCENCE IN THE 1990s

In 1985, 20% of the children in the United States were living in poverty; thus, an increasing number of youth will enter adolescence already impoverished. Six percent of adolescents do not live in a "family" unit. Thirty-one percent of the adolescent population will consist of minorities by the year 2000, as compared with 25% of the entire population. States in the South, Southwest, and West will experience the greatest increase in numbers of adolescents.

Substance use remains high during adolescence with lifetime prevalence rates as follows: 91% for alcohol, 66% for cigarettes, 44% for marijuana, 19% for stimulants, 19% for inhalants, 9% for cocaine, 5% for crack, and 1% for heroin. One-third of high school seniors report having drunk at least four alcoholic beverages during the past 2 weeks. One in 10 high school seniors smoke at least half a pack of cigarettes per day. Black and Hispanic youth report lower levels of substance use than whites.

Sexual activity rates have dramatically increased in the adolescent population from 1972 to 1982; 62% of adolescent girls and 72% of adolescent boys report having at least one experience with sexual intercourse by their 19th birthday. Sexually transmitted disease rates have dramatically increased from 1960 to 1988 with a 325% increase in the prevalence of gonorrhea among 10- through 14-year-olds and a 170% increase among 15- through 19-year-olds. Consistent use of some form of contraception remains low during adolescence. Although birth rates for unmarried adolescents remained constant in the 1970s and 1980s, there has recently been an increase in the incidence of pregnancy among adolescents.[1]

The issues regarding sexual activity and decision making is key to the discussion of teenage pregnancy. The cascade of lack of information, misinformation, or indecision flows from unclear awareness of sexuality to inadequate use of contraception to consideration regarding abortion to lack of appreciation of personal

35

skills needed for childbirth and motherhood. The state of adolescent pregnancy is perhaps best described by Emans and Goldstein:[2]

> The maturation process during adolescence involves the formation of a stable self-image, a sexual identity, and a concept of self as separate from parents. This process does not occur in an orderly fashion; and thus, the adolescent does not always see herself as a woman capable of fertility at the same time that she is in fact able to bear children and has become sexually mature. During early adolescence, girls are particularly prone to impulsive action and have difficulty with long-range goals; part of the adolescent developmental process involves swings between irresponsibility and constraint, thoughtfulness and indulgence. Unfortunately, the consistence, responsibility, and planning necessary for effective contraceptive use is not always compatible with the stage of adolescent development in which the adolescent may have chosen to become sexually active. (p. 260–261)

Although each society develops its own comfort level with adolescent experimentation in the area of sexual behavior, the negative impact of unwanted childbirth is not well tolerated in most cultures. Many European countries have high levels of teen sexual activity; however, their teen pregnancy rate is much lower. These outcomes relate to culturally accepted sexual education, availability of contraceptives, and negative stigma on adolescent parenthood.[3] The period of transition labeled as adolescence invokes a "series of crises for which each individual must develop coping and adaptation responses. These responses demand of the individual active involvement in decision making and exploration of options, and thus may be empowering or enabling" (p. ii).[4]

DEFINITIONS

Although adolescence is usually described chronologically as the second decade of life, the physiologic and psychological definitions vary greatly. Physically, puberty heralds the onset of adolescence and occurs at a mean age of 12.3 years for girls and 13.3 years for boys.[5] However, the psychological changes that begin with Piaget's abstract thinking stages usually begins around age 12.[4] These variables are individually occurring, so some teenagers mature both physically and/or emotionally and psychologically at exceedingly different rates.[3] A chronologic description of adolescence (early, middle, and late phases) is often used. Early adolescence (ages 12 to 14) is characterized by major physical changes. Middle adolescence (ages 15 to 17) is the prime time for emotional development and growth; self-image issues are most relevant at this point. The last phase of adolescence (ages 18 to 21) blends easily into young adulthood. The developmental tasks are psychological and social and relate to achievement of mature goals and implementation plans. The overall tasks characterizing the development of the adolescent are fourfold:

1. achieving independence from parents
2. adapting peer codes and life styles
3. assigning importance to body image and accepting one's own body image
4. establishing sexual, ego, vocational, and moral identity[4]

For this chapter, the first two stages of adolescence are used as a background for discussing adolescent pregnancy. In many cultures, childbirth at ages 18 or 19 is wholly accepted and well within the norm. Very few societies support childbirth to mothers younger than age 15. In the United States, this is the group with the greatest increase in pregnancy rates and represents the largest proportion of problem pregnancies.[1]

PREVALENCE

Each year, 1 in 10 teenagers aged 15 to 19 becomes pregnant in the United States. About half of these adolescents choose to continue their pregnancies. In 1991, 519,577 babies were born to adolescent mothers, an increase of almost 9% from the 477,710 teenagers giving birth in 1985.[6,7] Infants born to adolescent mothers are more likely to be born preterm (<38 weeks' gestation), be of low birth weight (<2500 g), require intensive care, or die at birth than infants of adult mothers.[8] The nutritional status of adolescents who become pregnant and choose to continue their pregnancies is a concern among health professionals because of the role of weight gain and intake of other nutrients on pregnancy outcome.[9] The overall costs of poor pregnancies for adolescents in the United States is approximately $8.5 billion per year.[10]

ADOLESCENT NUTRITION

The goal of providing optimal nutrient intake and appropriate weight gain in the adolescent who becomes pregnant actually is a juxtaposition of adolescent developmental tasks and desirable health behaviors. The adolescent is at a stage when learning occurs by trial-and-error, and immediate rewards are favored.[3] While adolescents in some studies have identified with positive health promoting messages, the primary health concerns of adolescent girls are immediate (beauty and appearance) rather than long-term health issues.[11,12] Thus, the developmental tasks of adolescence do not mesh with the expectations that the pregnant adolescent will understand that weight gain and optimal nutrient intake now will be associated with a healthy baby later. The multiple dyadic relationship between adolescence, nutrition, and pregnancy form the basis of a triangle of concern regarding adolescent pregnancy (Figure 2-1). The decisions that the adolescent does or does not make concerning adolescent development (sexual behavior, birth control), pregnancy (continuing pregnancy, seeking prenatal care), and nutrition (dietary habits before and during pregnancy, weight gain) are key to the outcome of the pregnancy.

Because of its characteristic rapid physical and psychological changes, adolescence is often considered a nutritionally vulnerable period. Nutrient needs for the adolescent are based on the needs for growth and development; total energy needs are greater during adolescence than at any other time in life (see Chapter 1). The major influences on nutrient needs during adolescence relate to genetic potential, to normal patterns of growth and development, and to physical activities that increase energy and nutrient needs.[2] Nutritional risks for both undernutrition and overnutrition are present and may be further increased during periods of physiologic stress such as pregnancy.[13]

Certain adolescent behaviors place girls at risk of inadequate nutrition. Many teenage young women will restrict their food intake in an attempt to control their weight. Others will depend mostly on fast-food restaurants and convenience stores for their meals and may eat erratically. Adolescents also commonly skip meals, eat on the run, and may give low priority to healthful dietary habits.[14]

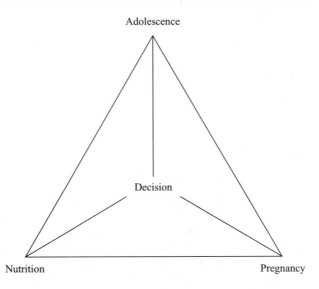

Figure 2-1 Interrelationships between Adolescence, Nutrition, and Pregnancy and Decisions Made by the Pregnant Teenager.

Energy intakes may primarily come from snacks and fast foods (influenced by peers) that include high-fat, low-fiber foods consumed away from home.[15] Calcium, iron, zinc, vitamins A, D, and B_6, riboflavin, folic acid, and total energy are most likely to be deficient in the diets of female adolescents based on surveys of dietary intake.[16]

Young women may also restrict their caloric intake to alter their physical appearance; some may exhibit eating disorders. The two most common eating disorders (see Chapter 3), bulimia nervosa and anorexia nervosa, are seen more in adolescence than at any other time in life, especially in females.[17,18] One study found that 13% of 15-year-old girls reported some form of purging behavior (vomiting, laxative, or diuretic use) to lose weight.[16]

Identifying short-term results of good nutrition may provide messages that will appeal to adolescents. The role of peer influences is also an important factor and may provide an opportunity for intervention. Nutrition education and other intervention programs need to consider the relevance of health information from the adolescent's perspective, because their perception of problems does not always correspond to how adults view the same problems.[11,19] Adolescents generally consider proper nutrition, maintaining a healthy weight, and taking vitamins as health-promoting behaviors, so these positive messages may be able to serve as a basis for developing programs that reach adolescents in their stage of development.[19,20]

The dietary needs of teenagers are best met through the recommendations of the Food Guide Pyramid, choosing at the high end of the range of serving recommendations to meet energy needs.[21] However, understanding the interaction of dietary intake and social interactions of adolescents is important for health care professionals.

ADOLESCENT PREGNANCY

Overall, adolescents generally visit physicians only for acute conditions and consequently have the lowest rates of outpatient visits of any age group. Healthy adolescent development must consider the factors that influence the process: demography, socioeconomics, cultural background, biology, previous health history, and historical factors.[1] Thus, ensuring adequate prenatal care may be problematic due to the adolescent's discomfort with traditional health care settings, inadequate resources to pay for care, parental consent requirements for some services, and physicians who may be uncomfortable or unskilled in dealing with adolescent patients.[22] Because of poorer outcomes, the pregnant adolescent has a special need for early and adequate prenatal care.

Pregnancy concerns do not differ in type for adolescents, only in magnitude. The issues of awareness of prenatal health needs, access to prenatal care, and acceptance of the pregnancy are vital for all pregnant women.[22] For the teenager, these factors are further complicated by denial, societal disapproval, and lack of relevant services. The three A's of teen pregnancy—awareness, access, and acceptance—describe a shaky relationship between individual and societal misunderstanding and denial. Although many teenagers have difficulty confronting the issues of their sexuality and preventing an unwanted pregnancy, the U.S. health environment also tends not to deal with these issues.[2,23] By denying or at least discouraging care to young adolescents, the basis for poor pregnancy outcomes is established. Acceptance, both by the individual teenager and the culture at large, of the magnitude of this problem must be the basis for adequate and appropriate intervention and management. Moreover, because 80% of teenagers report that their pregnancies were unintended, the difficulties that many teenagers have deciding on and obtaining family planning services has a further effect on their access to prenatal care.[23] Their ambivalent feelings about being pregnant make it much less likely that teenagers will begin prenatal care during the first trimester and to receive an adequate amount of prenatal care.[1,4] Malloy and coworkers[24] identified that early entry into prenatal care was associated with better outcomes in women who delivered at 37 through 42 weeks of gestation, although they identified problems associated with the use of vital statistics data for evaluating the effect of prenatal care due to possible misclassification of gestational age.[24]

Early adolescents (younger than 15 years) who are pregnant receive the least adequate prenatal care, have the greatest chance of having a low-birth-weight infant, and have the highest infant mortality rates. In 1986 to 1988, the percentage of low-birth-weight babies (<2500 g) born to adolescent mothers was 14% for early adolescents (younger than 15 years) and 9% for 15 to 19-year-olds (Table 2-1). By race, the percentage of low-birth-weight babies ranged from 8% for whites (15 to 19 years) to 16% for black adolescents (15 years or younger). Compared with mothers in their 20s, the risk of low-birth-weight babies is increased two times among youngest mothers (younger than 15 years); 1.5 times among mothers aged 15 to 17 years; and 1.3 times among mothers 18 to 19 years old.[4]

Low birth weights are strongly associated with survival rates.[25] And because younger adolescent mothers are more likely to have low-birth-weight infants, infant mortality is highest in this age group. Specifically, infant death rates (the number of infants newborn to 1 year who die per 1000 live births) was 31.5 for mothers 10 to 14 years old and 15.8 for mothers 15 to 19 years old. The lowest infant mortality rate for adolescent mothers was in white, older adolescents (13.6 per 1000), and the highest rate was in black younger adolescents (36 per 1000). The average infant death rate for all mothers was 11.0 per 1000 live births.[1]

The risk of delivering a small-for-gestational age (SGA) baby is associated with several factors related to adolescent pregnancy—inadequate prenatal care,

Table 2-1 Low Birth Weight as a Percentage of Total Live Births, by Age of Mother and Race of Infant, 1986–1988

Age of Mother	All Races(%)	White (%)	Black (%)	American Indian and Alaska Native (%)
Younger than 15 years	13.7	10.4	16.2	7.7
15–19 years	9.3	7.7	13.1	6.0
20–24 years	7.1	5.8	12.3	5.2
25–29 years	6.1	5.1	12.5	5.6
30–34 years	6.2	5.2	13.0	6.5
35–39 years	6.9	6.0	13.4	7.2
40 years and older	7.9	7.1	12.9	8.7

Source: Interagency Board for Nutrition Monitoring and Related Research, Ervin B and Reed D, eds. *Nutrition Monitoring in the United States. Chartbook I: Selected Findings from the National Nutrition Monitoring and Related Research Program.* Hyattsville, Md: Public Health Service; 1993.

insufficient weight gain, and African-American descent.[26–28] Younger adolescent mothers (<16 years old) are at increased risk of having a SGA infant compared with older adolescents.[27] Further, smoking adolescents have more SGA infants than nonsmoking adolescents (10.7% versus 5.6%).[29]

NUTRITION AND THE PREGNANT ADOLESCENT

Pregnancy places adolescent girls, who are already at risk for nutritional problems, at even greater risk because of the increased energy and nutrient demands of pregnancy, particularly in adolescents (younger than 14 years) who have not completed the growth phase.[30] Because many adolescents have chronically poor dietary habits, they may enter their pregnancies in marginal nutritional status.[31]

Weight Gain

Maternal weight gain is influenced by many factors. Data on weight gain show that more black mothers had inadequate weight gain than white mothers[32] (Table 2-2). Also, surveys of married women in 1980 and 1988 showed married black women were nearly three times as likely in 1988 to report being advised to gain less than the minimum guideline (Table 2-3). These surveys were completed when medical guidelines recommended a 22- to 27-lb weight gain, regardless of

Table 2-2 Percentage of Live Births of 40 Weeks' Gestation or Longer, by Maternal Weight Gain and Race of Mother, 1989

Maternal Weight Gain (lb)	White (%)	Black (%)
<16	7.0	13.0
16–20	9.7	13.5
21–25	15.3	14.8
26–30	21.4	18.5
31–35	16.1	12.0
36–40	13.5	11.3
≥41	17.0	17.0

Source: Interagency Board for Nutrition Monitoring and Related Research, Ervin B and Reed D, eds. *Nutrition Monitoring in the United States. Chartbook I: Selected Findings from the National Nutrition Monitoring and Related Research Program.* Hyattsville, Md: Public Health Service; 1993.

Table 2-3 Weight Gain Advice for Married Mothers, by Race, 1980 and 1988

	Percentage of Mothers			
	White		Black	
Weight Gain Advice (lb)	1980	1988	1980	1988
<22	27	11	34	27
22–27	49	37	40	37
28–34	22	38	24	25
≥35	3	14	2	11

Source: Interagency Board for Nutrition Monitoring and Related Research, Ervin B and Reed D, eds. *Nutrition Monitoring in the United States. Chartbook I: Selected Findings from the National Nutrition Monitoring and Related Research Program.* Hyattsville, Md: Public Health Service; 1993.

prenatal body mass index.[9] Unfortunately, adolescents are even less likely to receive medical advice about weight gain because many do not get prenatal care.

Maternal weight gain during pregnancy has been consistently associated with infant birth weight.[9] Low weight gain is one of the strongest predictors of low birth weight, including both preterm and SGA births, whereas large gains are associated with increased fetal size. Overall, adolescents deliver a higher percentage of low-birth-weight babies than older women.[32] The burden of low-birth-weight infants is especially seen in black women who gain less than 20 lb (Table 2-4).

Weight gain is particularly important during adolescent pregnancy, when total gains above the recommendation for mature women may help decrease the risk of poor pregnancy outcome.[25,29] By 24 weeks' gestation, inadequate weight gain among adolescents (based on prepregnancy weight status and gestational age) is

Table 2-4 Low Birth Weight as a Percentage of Total Live Births of 40 Weeks' Gestation or Longer, by Maternal Weight Gain and Race of Mother, 1989

Maternal Weight Gain (lb)	White (%)	Black (%)
<16	2.8	6.8
16–20	2.2	5.4
21–25	1.5	3.7
26–30	1.1	3.0
31–35	0.9	2.4
36–40	0.9	2.3
≥41	0.8	1.8

Source: Interagency Board for Nutrition Monitoring and Related Research, Ervin B and Reed D, eds. *Nutrition Monitoring in the United States. Chartbook I: Selected Findings from the National Nutrition Monitoring and Related Research Program.* Hyattsville, Md: Public Health Service; 1993.

associated with an increased risk of low birth weight, even when gains later in pregnancy result in adequate total weight gain.[33]

In a prospective study of weight gain, Scholl and coworkers[34] found that as early as 12 weeks' gestation, there was a significant association between the amount of weight gained and infant birth weight measured at the time of delivery. For every kilogram of weight that the mother gained by 12 weeks gestation, the birth weight increased by 12.89 g ($p < 0.005$). Rees and coworkers[35] also reported that adolescents with higher amounts of weight gain had better pregnancy outcomes, with 6% of infants weighing 3000 to 4000 g versus 15% of infants weighing less than 300 g needing intensive care at birth. After the 15th week of gestation, these mothers gained at a rate of 0.588 kg/wk, which is at the highest amount recommended by the Institute of Medicine. Thus, the need for early prenatal care that includes weight gain monitoring and intervention is important.

Continued maternal growth during pregnancy has been hypothesized to be an underlying cause of the increased incidence of poor outcomes that characterize adolescent pregnancy. Hickey and colleagues[36] conducted a retrospective analysis of adolescent weight status and term birth weight in first and second pregnancies. They showed that there was a positive relationship between second- and third-trimester rate of maternal weight gain and birth weight for adolescents 15 years and younger during the second pregnancy and for adolescents 16 years and older during their first pregnancy. Both groups showed a relationship between maternal weight for height (W/H) increase during pregnancy and increased birth weight, but this was only significant among older adolescents. Scholl and coworkers[37] measured stature and knee height to follow maternal growth during adolescent pregnancy. Compared with controls, maternal growth during pregnancy was associated with significantly decreased birth weight for infants during a subsequent adolescent pregnancy. Thus, preconceptual weight status and weight gain throughout pregnancy are important for fetal development and for continued maternal growth, especially in the youngest adolescents who are pregnant.

In an obstetric clinic for teenagers, there was no significant difference in the mean weight gain of white, black, and Hispanic mothers, but Hispanic mothers tended to gain the most weight. In assessment of the determinants of weight gain in pregnant adolescents, Stevens-Simon and McAnarney[38] found that two predictors of slow weight gain among 141 black adolescents included the consumption of fewer than three snacks per day and delayed (third trimester) enrollment in the Supplemental Food Program for Women, Infants and Children (WIC). Rapid weight gainers were more compliant with prenatal visits and reported more depressive symptoms and alcohol consumption than did other study subjects. Slow gainers gained 6.5 ± 2.3 kg during gestation and rapid gainers had a 22.7 ± 4.6-kg weight increase. These authors suggest that young women who are at highest risk for inadequate weight gain during pregnancy are apt to lose or gain little or no weight before the first prenatal visit.[38] These young women may benefit from prenatal interventions designed to promote more frequent eating and enrollment in WIC for eligible adolescents. In 1992, almost 12% of the almost 800,000 WIC participants were younger than age 18.[39]

The overall impact of smoking on nutrient status and weight gain must also be considered in adolescent pregnancy. Pregnant women who smoke reported diets that were lower in iron and other nutrients compared with diets of pregnant non-smokers.[40] The prevalence of pregnant women who smoke before and during pregnancy is higher among younger, unmarried women with less education and ranges from 37% to 54%.[41] A disproportionate share of these young women also have poor outcomes. Babies born to women who smoke are, on average, 200 g lighter than babies born to comparable nonsmokers.[42] The addictive effect of smoking increases the woman's risk of vascular problems and multiplies the fetus's potential risks.[43]

Nutrient Intake

Less is known about the overall nutrient intake of pregnant adolescents and its relation to birth outcome. Pregnant adolescents have been found to have poor dietary habits compared with recommended intakes, although others have found that adolescents change their dietary practices during pregnancy and eat better than nonpregnant peers.[6,31,44] A wide range in mean nutrient intake has been reported; most are based on convenience samples of varying sizes (18 to 500+ adolescents) and geographic areas in the United States. Dietary intake methods varied but included some version of 24-hour dietary recall and recall plus records of dietary intake.

Overall, available studies report inadequate intakes (less than two-thirds of the recommended dietary allowance [RDA]) of selected nutrients—vitamin D, folate, vitamin B_6, vitamin C, iron, calcium, zinc, and magnesium (Table 2-5). However, two studies did show adequate intakes in pregnant adolescents. Endres and coworkers[45] found that the quantity and quality of the diet consumed by pregnant adolescents was similar to that consumed by pregnant adults. Loris et al[46] observed higher intakes of energy and most other nutrients among adolescents as well as a greater weight gain than is typical for adults. Adolescents receiving more nutrition education consumed greater amounts of energy (400 kcal/day) than did those with little formal nutrition education. The pregnant adolescents who had more nutrition education ($n = 22$) gained 40.3 ± 16.2 lb compared with a 35.0 ± 14.2 lb-weight gain for adolescents who received less nutrition education. Total weight gain and weight gain in the last trimester were correlated with infant birth weight ($r = .26; p < 0.001$; and $r = .30; p < .006$, respectively). There was no difference in infant birth weight for those who received more or less nutrition education.[46]

By contrast, the National WIC Evaluation[47] found that younger women consumed less energy, protein, and calcium. Zinc supplementation was found to improve pregnancy outcome of pregnant adolescents.[48] An assessment of dietary intake of 99 low-income adolescents indicated that 48% of the teenagers consumed adequate amounts of dairy products; 70% ate sufficient amounts of meats; 39% had adequate amounts of fruits and vegetables; and 76% met the daily grain group recommendations.[49] Thus, in this group, dietary intake was not adequate to meet nutrient and energy needs of pregnancy. The need for more information about the nutrient intakes of pregnant teenagers in specific age and economic groups has been identified by the Institute of Medicine as necessary to understand the relationship between food consumption and weight gain patterns of pregnant adolescents and their impact on pregnancy outcome.[9] Further, there are few reports of ingestion of non-nutritive substances by pregnant adolescents, and more information is needed about the prevalence of pica and its contribution to nutritional status, although one report suggested the prevalence was 5 to 10% in an urban clinic population of adolescent pregnant teenagers.[49]

Table 2-5 Adequacy of Nutrient Intake of Pregnant Adolescents

<67% RDA	67–100% RDA	>100% RDA
Vitamin D	Niacin	Energy
Folate	Riboflavin	Protein
Vitamin B_6		Vitamin A
Iron		Thiamin
Calcium		
Zinc		
Magnesium		

Nutrient Needs and Recommended Intakes

The need for energy, protein, and most vitamins and minerals is increased by the metabolic demands of pregnancy, especially in adolescents younger than 15 years of age who still may be experiencing growth. Energy promotes fetal growth and allows for use of protein, vitamins, and minerals. Adequacy of energy is best indicated by an appropriate weight gain. The RDA for protein for adolescent girls is approximately 45 g/day. An additional 10 g of protein is recommended throughout pregnancy to support fetal growth and maternal tissue increase.[50] Calcium intakes of 1200 to 1600 mg/day will promote an increase in bone mineralization associated with adolescence while supporting fetal skeletal growth.[51] Calcium may also be protective against gestational hypertension in pregnancy.[52,53] Iron needs are increased during pregnancy due to fetal and placental growth and the expansion of maternal blood volume. Iron supplementation is necessary to achieve this recommended intake. The absorption of dietary iron can be enhanced by the inclusion of foods containing heme iron such as meat, fish, and poultry, as well as foods high in vitamin C such as citrus fruits and juices and vitamin C-rich vegetables.[54]

Adequate folate intake, both before and during the first trimester of pregnancy, appears to reduce the incidence of congenital anomalies such as neural tube defects.[55] Also, folate adequacy may improve fetal growth.[56] The recommended intake of 400 μg folate per day during pregnancy is more than twice the amount recommended for the nonpregnant adolescent girl.[50,55]

Nutrient intakes that meet with these recommended levels can be achieved by selecting foods consistent with the U.S. Dietary Guidelines and the Food Guide Pyramid, with the exception of iron. Recommended servings appropriate for pregnant adolescents are

- 2–4 servings of fruits/juices, including a vitamin C source
- 3–5 servings of vegetables, including a dark green or deep orange vegetable
- 4–5 servings of low-fat dairy products
- 3 servings of meat or meat alternatives
- 6–11 servings of whole or enriched grain products to enhance iron and folate intake[21]

Supplements

Supplemental iron intake (30 mg elemental iron) is recommended, and calcium or folate supplementation may be indicated in pregnant adolescents. Iron-deficiency anemia has been associated with higher rates of preterm delivery, low birth weight, and decreased maternal and fetal iron stores.[57–59] Low-income adolescents, those who use substances, and young adolescents are at greatest risk for anemia. The Institute of Medicine recommends a supplement of 30 mg elemental iron per day during the second and third trimesters for adolescents with normal hemoglobin. When anemia is present (<11.0 g hemoglobin/dl during the first and third trimester and <10.0 g hemoglobin/dl during the second trimester), the recommended iron dosage is increased to 60 to 120 mg elemental iron per day until normal hemoglobin levels are attained. To ensure adequate zinc and copper status, which can be compromised when taking a therapeutic dose of iron, a vitamin-mineral supplement that contains 15 mg zinc and 2 mg copper is also recommended.[9]

Because calcium needs are greatest during adolescence, a supplement of approximately 1000 mg calcium per day may be appropriate for adolescents with dietary intakes of less than 1200 mg calcium per day. Calcium supplements would be taken at mealtime to enhance absorption and limit interaction with iron supplements. Also, a folate supplement of 40 mg per day during the first trimester is recommended for adolescents who have had a previous infant with neural tube defects (NTD). For women without a NTD history, .4 mg per day is recommended.[55]

Pregnant adolescents who drink milk that is not fortified with vitamin D or who are complete vegetarians should consume 10 µg of vitamin D daily. Complete vegetarians should also receive 1 µg of vitamin B_{12} daily.[9]

The Institute of Medicine recommends a low-dose, balanced vitamin-mineral supplement when, despite nutrition counseling, a nutritionally adequate diet is not regularly consumed. This level of supplementation is also indicated for adolescents who smoke heavily, use alcohol or drugs, are strict vegetarians, or are carrying multiple fetuses.[9]

NUTRITION ASSESSMENT

The assessment of prepregnancy weight for height status, continued assessment of weight gain patterns during pregnancy, individual counseling, and referral to food assistance programs may improve weight gain and thus reduce low birth weight among pregnant adolescents.

Throughout their pregnancies, adolescents require nutrition care provided by dietetics professionals in interdisciplinary programs specializing in serving this age group. The components of nutrition care for pregnant adolescents were recently outlined.[14] Dietetic professionals can integrate the recommendations of the American Dietetic Association into targeted nutrition assessment, care plan development, and nutrition counseling and evaluation.

Story and Alton[60] identified four components to evaluate in the nutrition assessment of pregnant adolescents:

- dietary assessment
- relevant history assessment
- height/weight assessment
- laboratory assessment

Diet

Dietary practices and patterns as well as food resources and management issues need investigation, and inadequacies warrant further evaluation and intervention. If adequate calcium intake is unattainable by diet and a calcium intake of less than 1200 mg/day is consumed, a 1000-mg/day calcium supplement may be appropriate. If a nutritionally adequate diet is not being regularly consumed, a low-dose, balanced vitamin-mineral supplement should be recommended. If the adolescent is a complete vegetarian, then vitamin D and vitamin B_{12} should be recommended. If access to food and risk of hunger are issues, referral to programs that provide access to food is critical.[61]

Previous History

Previous medical, obstetric, and psychosocioeconomic histories relevant to pregnancy need consideration, and issues such as chronic disease, substance use, or stress suggest the need for further attention. If the adolescent has a past obstetric history of a previous pregnancy affected by neural tube defects, then a folate supplement of 4.0 mg/day is recommended during the first trimester of pregnancy. Thus, the need for early entry into prenatal care is especially important for pregnant adolescents.

Height and Weight

Measurement of height and weight, consideration of prepregnancy weight status, and evaluation of body mass index and weight gain pattern are important components of nutrition assessment and intervention, particularly if the adolescent was under- or overweight at conception or if gestational weight gain pattern is inadequate or excessive. Weight gain ranges are shown in Table 2-6. Young adolescents and all black women should strive for gains at the upper end of the range (for the appropriate pregnancy-for-target category). Gestational weight gain can be best monitored when plotted on a weight gain grid (Figure 2-2). Prepregnancy weight status and weight gain goals should be identified, and progress should be shared with the adolescent. Inadequate weight gain should be evaluated and managed.

Table 2-6 Recommended Total Weight Gain Ranges for Pregnant Women[a]

| | Recommended Total Gain | |
Pregnancy Weight-for-Height Category	lb	kg
Low (BMI <19.8)	28–40	12.5–18
Normal (BMI 19.8–26)	25–35	11.5–16
High (BMI >26.0–29.0)	15–25	7.0–11.5
Obese (BMI > 29)	≥15	≥7.0

[a]For singleton pregnancies. The range for women carrying twins is 35–45 lb (16–20 kg). Young adolescents (<2 years after menarche) and black women should strive for gains at the upper end of the range. Short women (<62 in. or <157 cm) should strive for gains at the lower end of the range. BMI = body mass index.
Source: Reprinted with permission from *Nutrition During Pregnancy and Lactation.* Copyright © 1992 by the National Academy of Sciences. Courtesy of the National Academy Press, Washington, DC.

Laboratory Tests

Hemoglobin and other laboratory tests, such as an oral glucose tolerance test, are indicators of nutritional status and can warrant subsequent dietary interventions. Iron supplementation is used in normal pregnancy and to correct anemia. Nutrition counseling would include recommendations for alleviating gastrointestinal discomfort related to iron supplementation and ways to enhance iron absorption. Abnormal glucose tolerance tests should be followed up with appropriate dietary counseling.[9]

PROFESSIONAL SKILLS AND COUNSELING

The basic question for the dietetics professional regarding adolescent pregnancy may be the impact of the growing fetus on the potential physical and physiologic growth of the individual. The overall concern for the culture is the effect on the eventual maturation, both social and physical, of the individual. Thus, the implications for intervention must stem from the adolescent decision-making process (or rather, lack thereof). Awareness of adolescent self-image and motivational issues are the keys to successful counseling endeavors.

Story and Pontius[62] reported that dietitians who are involved with adolescents perceived skill deficits, especially in the areas of communication, counseling, and applications of adolescent development theory. Understanding theories of adolescence, including biologic, psychosocial, cognitive-developmental, social-learning, and historical orientations, helps frame the adolescent experience and understand the role of adolescence in their culture.[3]

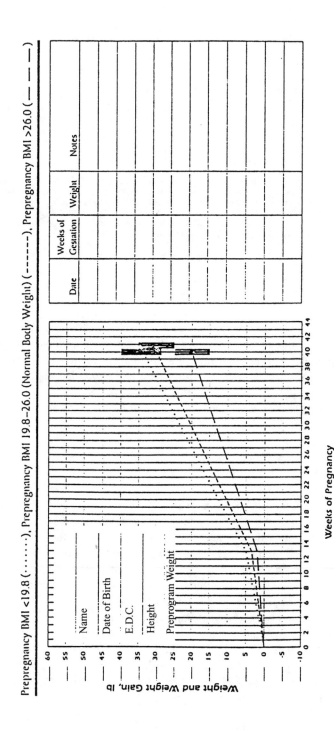

Figure 2-2 Prenatal Weight Gain Chart

Health care professionals must understand the concerns of adolescents to address the needs of the pregnant adolescent. The primary health concerns identified by adolescent girls included body weight, their future, their hair, their figure, and condition of their skin.[12] Fortunately, adolescents generally consider proper nutrition, maintaining a healthy weight, and taking vitamins as health-promoting behaviors, whether or not they are part of the adolescents' behavioral repertoire. These positive messages may be able to serve as a basis for developing counseling strategies for pregnant adolescents.[19,20] Further, Lee and Grubbs[63] conducted interviews with adolescents who had recently delivered and found that teenagers had an adequate knowledge level regarding diet and other self-care topics during pregnancy, regardless of whether they entered prenatal care during the first or third trimester. If that knowledge, however, was a result of health education received during prenatal care and was practiced by the teenager, then there would be a better net benefit for teenagers who began receiving prenatal care in the first trimester. Knowledge also needs to be acted on by healthy behaviors that may have a long-term impact on pregnancy outcome. Recently, teenagers who participated in focus groups contributed their perceptions about needs during pregnancy to form the basis for development of a film that can provide nutrition education.[64] This approach to the development of educational materials for pregnant teenagers may help to focus the nutrition content from an adolescent perspective.

Prenatal care also needs to address the problems of acceptance because the decisions the adolescent makes about infant care during the postpartum period will have an effect on the outcome of pregnancy. These decisions depend on social, environmental, and biologic risk factors, including mother–infant interactions, feeding practices, relationships with significant others, and health professional intervention. Church[65] outlined a postpartum assessment tool developed for use with adolescent mothers. Nutritional care of the pregnant adolescent must include assessment, counseling, and education regarding postpartum nutrition and infant feeding issues. The adolescent's inability to clarify self-image issues makes breastfeeding more problematic. The acceptance of the pregnancy and the mothering role is crucial for good breastfeeding practices. Although limited data are available on the problem, young mothers usually do not choose to breast-feed.[49] In a WIC population of 207,586 participants, only 3.8% of breastfeeders were younger than 18 years.[39] Barriers to the decision to breast-feed include lack of social support and lack of support on the part of the father.[66] Community outreach programs targeted for adolescent fathers may provide an opportunity to help reduce this barrier to breastfeeding among adolescents who become parents.[67]

New Approaches to Providing Care

The overall concern for universal access, which is the hallmark of health care reform in the mid-1990s, may or may not have an effect on young pregnant adolescents.[22] The lack of access is compounded by lack of acceptance and awareness on the part of adolescents. The need for outreach and easily accessible services makes school-based clinics and community-based programs imperative. Additional funding for Head Start and WIC as well as active support for school-based child care are essential to comprehensive services for the pregnant teenager.[68]

A developmental approach to services needs to be implemented that integrates the adolescents' psychological, emotional, and physical maturation with the provision of health services and education. In all instances, programming needs to deal positively with matters of body image, peer relationships, independence, identity, and sexuality to educate the teenager both to parent successfully and to prevent a subsequent pregnancy.[4]

Services and other training materials developed specifically to address the needs of the pregnant adolescent have been compiled by agencies such as the National Center for Education in Maternal and Child Health and organizations such as the March of Dimes and provide a resource for dietetics professionals.[16] Positions of professional health organizations on prenatal and nutritional care of the pregnant adolescent can also set standards of care for health care professionals. For example, the American Dietetic Association recently underscored the importance of nutrition care provided by dietetics professionals in interdisciplinary management of the pregnant adolescent.[14]

Exhibit 2-1 National Maternal and Child Health Objectives for the Year 2000 Related to the Needs of the Pregnant Adolescent

1. Reduce pregnancies among girls aged 17 and younger to no more than 50 per 1000 adolescents.

2. Reduce by at least 50% the use of tobacco, alcohol, marijuana, and/or cocaine among adolescents ages 12 through 17.

3. Establish comprehensive, community-based health care systems that ensure family-centered, culturally competent, coordinated services.

4. Reduce low birth weight (<2500 g) to an incidence of no more than 5% of live births and very low birth weight (<1500 g) to an incidence of no more than 1% of live births.

5. Reduce the infant mortality rate (deaths of infants younger than 1 year) to no more than 7 per 1000 live births.

6. Increase the proportion of youth who complete high school by age 19 to at least 90 percent.

7. Decrease the proportion of children and youth younger than age 18 living in poverty by at least 50%.

Source: Reprinted from *Call to Action: Better Nutrition for Mothers, Children and Families* by CO Sharbaugh, ed, with permission of the National Center for Education in Maternal and Child Health, ©1990.

Exhibit 2-2 Maternal and Child Health Interagency Nutrition Group Recommendations Related to the Pregnant Adolescent

1. Improve the nutrition component of health services for adolescents, including pregnant adolescents.
2. Increase access to food assistance services (e.g., school feeding and the WIC program) for pregnant adolescents.
3. Provide intensive nutrition counseling for pregnant adolescents.
4. Establish or review nutrition standards for food service in maternity homes or other facilities serving pregnant adolescents and initiate action needed to improve standards.
5. Improve the nutrition knowledge base and skills of providers and educators who service the pregnant adolescent through training.
6. Expand the research base in adolescent nutrition, including the pregnant adolescent, to include market research data at local, state, and national levels to access and monitor the growth and nutrition status, knowledge, attitudes, concerns, and issues related to adolescents, including pregnant adolescents.
7. Establish baseline data and surveillance systems to assess growth and nutrition status of all adolescents, including pregnant adolescents.
8. Build coalitions to address the needs of pregnant adolescents.

Source: Reprinted from *Call to Action: Better Nutrition for Mothers, Children and Families* by CO Sharbaugh, ed, with permission of the National Center for Education in Maternal and Child Health, ©1990

Also, federal agencies have identified health goals for the year 2000 that address maternal and child health.[69] Those goals that specifically address the needs of the pregnant adolescent are shown in Exhibit 2-1. To further delineate the nutrition needs of the maternal and child health population, a group of agencies and associations concerned with nutrition and mothers and families, the Maternal and Child Health Interorganizational Nutrition Group made nutrition-related recommendations.[65] Recommendations that specifically relate to pregnant adolescents are shown in Exhibit 2-2.

SUMMARY

Ideally, comprehensive adolescent primary health care would provide preconceptual nutrition education to all teenagers, including those who may become pregnant. However, developing programs that address the needs of pregnant teenagers and empower them to make decisions about their food intake, meet weight gain goals, and make decisions about other aspects of their health may improve pregnancy outcome and enable teenagers to take responsibility for becoming parents. Health care professionals need to use current nutritional guidelines to help teenagers learn about their needs and advocate for health care programs that provide nutrition and other services to teenagers.

References

1. Irwin CE, Brindis, Brodt SE, et al. *The Health of America's Youth: Current Trends in Health Status and Utilization of Health Services.* San Francisco, Calif: University of California; 1991.

2. Emans SJH, Goldstein DP. *Pediatric and Adolescent Gynecology.* 2nd ed. Boston, Mass: Little, Brown; 1982.

3. Dusek JB. *Adolescent Development and Behavior.* 2nd ed. Englewood Cliffs, NJ: Prentice Hall; 1991.

4. Neinstein LS. *Adolescent Health Care—A Practical Guide.* 2nd ed. Baltimore, Md: Urban & Schwarzenberg; 1991.

5. Tanner JM, Davies PSW. Clinical longitudinal standards for height and height velocity for North American children. *J Pediatr.* 1985;107:317–329.

6. U.S. Department of Health & Human Services. *Surgeon General's Report on Nutrition and Health*: Washington, DC: Government Printing Office; 1988. DHHS(PHS) Publ. no. 88-50210.

7. Office of Maternal & Child Health, Public Health Service, US Department of Health & Human Services. *Child Health USA '89.* Washington, DC: US Department of Health & Human Services; 1989.

8. Meredith CN, Dwyer JT. Nutrition and exercise: effects on adolescent health. *Annu Rev Public Health.* 1991;12:309–333.

9. Institute of Medicine. *Nutrition during Pregnancy: Weight Gain and Nutrient Supplements.* Washington, DC: National Academy Press; 1990.

10. Miaoulis G. Preadolescent pregnancy: a market segmentation perspective. *J Health Care Marketing.* 1989;9(2);42–51.

11. Elster A, Panzarine S, Holt K. *Adolescent Health Promotion. Proceedings of an American Medical Association State-of-the-Art Conference.* Arlington, Va: National Center for Education in Maternal and Child Health; 1992.

12. Smith KLD, Turner JG, Jacobsen RB. Health concerns of adolescents. *Pediat Nurs.* 1987;13(5): 311–315.

13. Lifshitz F, Tarim O, Smith MM. Nutrition in adolescence. *Endocrinol Metab Clin North Am.* 1993;22(3):673–683.

14. The American Dietetic Association. Nutrition care for pregnant adolescents. *J Am Diet Assoc.* 1994;94(4):449–450.

15. Bull NL. Dietary habits, food consumption and nutrient intake during adolescence. *J Adolesc Health.* 1992;13:284–288.

16. Story M. Nutrient needs during adolescence and pregnancy. In: Story M, ed. *Nutrition Management of the Pregnant Adolescent: Practical Reference Guide.* Washington, DC: MCH National Clearinghouse; 1990.

17. Fisher M, Schneider M, Pegler C, Napolitano B. Eating attitudes, health-risk behaviors, self-esteem, and anxiety among adolescent females in a suburban high school. *J Adolesc Health.* 1991;12:377–384.

18. Lucas AR, Huse DM. Behavioral disorders affecting food intake: anorexia nervosa and bulimia nervosa. In: Shills ME, Olson JA, Shike M, eds. *Modern Nutrition in Health and Disease.* 8th ed. Philadelphia, Pa: Lea & Febiger; 1994:977–983.

19. Altman DG, Revenson TA. Children's understanding of health and illness concepts: a preventive health perspective. *J Prim Prev.* 1985;6(1):53–67.

20. Korblin JE, Zahorik P. Childhood, health and illness: beliefs and behaviors of urban American schoolchildren. *Med Anthropol.* 1985;9(4):337–353.

21. U.S. Department of Agriculture, Human Nutrition Information Service. *The Food Guide Pyramid.* Hyattsville, Md: 1992. Home and Garden Bulletin no. 252.

22. Wiener JM, Engle J. *Improving Access to Health Services for Children and Pregnant Women.* Washington, DC: The Brookings Institution; 1991.

23. Lewit EM. Teenage childbearing. In: Behrman RD, ed. *The Future of Children.* 1992;2(2):186–191.

24. Malloy MH, Kao T, Lee YJ. Analyzing the effect of prenatal care on pregnancy outcome: a conditional approach. *Am J Public Health.* 1992;82(3):448–450.

25. Wilcox AJ, Skjoerven R. Birth weight and perinatal mortality: the effect of gestational age. *Am J Public Health.* 1992;82(3):378–382.

26. Lang JM, Cohen A, Lieberman E. Risk factors for small for gestational age birth in a preterm population. *Am J Obstet Gynecol.* 1992;166(5):1374–1378.

27. Kondamudi VK, Bhattacharyya A, Noah PK, et al. Adolescent pregnancy in Grenada. *Ann Trop Paediatr.* 1993;13(4):379–383.

28. Parker JD, Abrams B. Prenatal weight gain advice: an examination of the recent prenatal weight gain recommendations of the Institute of Medicine. *Obstet Gynecol.* 1992;79:664–669.

29. Scholl TO, Salmon RW, Miller LK, et al. Weight gain during adolescent pregnancy. *J Adolesc Health Care.* 1988;9:286–290.

30. Rees JM, Lederman SA. Nutrition for the pregnant adolescent. In Nussbaum LMP, Dwyer JT, eds. *Adolescent Nutrition and Eating Disorders. Vol 3. Adolescent Medicine: State of the Art Reviews.* Philadelphia, Pa: Hanley & Belfus; 1992:439–457.

31. McAnarney ER. Young maternal age and adverse neonatal outcome. *Am J Dis Child.* 1987;141:1053–1059.

32. Interagency Board for Nutrition Monitoring and Related Research, Ervin B and Reed D, eds. *Nutrition Monitoring in the United States. Chartbook 1: Selected Findings from the National Nutrition Monitoring and Related Research Program.* Hyattsville, Md: Public Health Service: 1993.

33. Lederman SA: Recent issues related to nutrition and pregnancy. *J Am Coll Nutr.* 1993;12(2):91–100.

34. Scholl TO, Hediger ML, Ances IG, et al. Weight gain during pregnancy in adolescents: predictive ability of early weight gain. *Obstet Gynecol.* 1990;75(6):948–953.

35. Rees JM, Engelbert-Fenton KA, Gong EJ, Bach CM. Weight gain in adolescents during pregnancy: rate related to birth-weight outcome. *Am J Clin Nutr.* 1992;56:868–873.

36. Hickey CA, Cliver SP, Goldenberg RL, Blankson ML. Maternal weight status and term birth weight in first and second adolescent pregnancies. *J Adolesc Health Care.* 1990;75(6):948–953.

37. Scholl TO, Hediger MC, Ances IG. Maternal growth during pregnancy and decreased infant birth weight. *Am J Clin Nutr.* 1990;51:790–793.

38. Stevens-Simon C, McAnarney, ER. Adolescent maternal weight gain and low birth weight: a multifactorial model. *Am J Clin Nutr.* 1988;47:948–953.

39. Randall B, Boast L. *Study of WIC Participants and Program Characteristics.* Cambridge, Mass: Ab + Associates; 1994.

40. Haste FM, Brooke OG, Anderson HR, et al. Nutrient intake during pregnancy: observations on the influence of smoking and social class. *Am J Clin Nutr.* 1990;51(1):29–36.

41. Fingerhut LA, Kleinman JC, Kendrick JS. Smoking before, during, and after pregnancy. *Am J Public Health.* 1990;80(5):541–544.

42. Scholl TO, Salmon RW, Miller LK. Smoking and adolescent pregnant outcome. *J Adolesc Health Care.* 1986;7:390–394.

43. U.S. Department of Health & Human Services. *The Health Consequences of Smoking for Women. A Report of the Surgeon General.* Washington, DC: U.S. Government Printing Office; 1980.

44. Skinner JD, Carruth BR. Dietary quality of pregnant and nonpregnant adolescents. *J Am Diet Assoc.* 1991;91:718–720.

45. Endres JM, Poell-Odenwald K, Sawicki M, Welch P. Dietary assessment of pregnant adolescents participating in a supplemental-food program. *J Reprod Med.* 1985;30(1):10–17.

46. Loris P, Dewey KG, Poirier-Brode K. Weight gain and dietary intake of pregnant teenagers. *J Am Diet Assoc.* 1985;85(10):1296–1305.

47. Abrams B. Preventing low birth weight: does WIC work? A review of evaluations of the special supplemental food program for women, infants and children. *Ann NY Acad Sci.* 1993;678:306–316.

48. Cherry FF, Sanstead HH, Rojas P, et al. Adolescent pregnancy: associations among body weight, zinc nutriture and pregnancy outcome. *Am J Clin Nutr.* 1989;50:945–954.

49. Schneck ME, Sideras KD, Fox RA, Dupuis L. Low-income pregnant adolescents and their infants: dietary findings and health outcomes. *J Am Diet Assoc.* 1990;90(4):555–558.

50. National Research Council, Food and Nutrition Board. *Recommended Dietary Allowances.* 10th ed. Washington, DC: National Academy Press; 1989.

51. Matkovic V. Calcium and peak bone mass. *J Intern Med.* 1992;231(2):151–160.

52. Belizan JM, Villar J, Gonzalez L, et al. Calcium supplementation to prevent hypertensive disorders of pregnancy. *N Engl J Med* 1991;325(20):1399–1405.

53. Zemel MB, Zemel PC, Berry S, et al. Altered platelet calcium metabolism as an early production of increased peripheral vascular resistance and preeclampsia in urban black women. *N Engl J Med.* 1990;323(7):434–438.

54. Institute of Medicine. *Nutrition During Pregnancy and Lactation—An Implementation Guide.* Washington, DC: National Academy Press; 1992.

55. Use of folate acid for prevention of spina bifida and other neural tube defects—1983–1991. *MMWR.* 1991;40:(30):513–516.

56. Blankson ML, Goldenberger RL, Cutter G, Cliver SP. The relationship between maternal hematocrit and pregnancy outcome: black-white differences. *J Natl Med Assoc.* 1993;85(2):130–134.

57. Fairbanks VF. Iron in medicine and nutrition. In: Shills ME, Olson JA, Shike M, eds. *Modern Nutrition in Health and Disease.* 8th ed. Philadelphia, Pa: Lea & Febiger; 1994:185–213.

58. Scholl TO, Hediger ML. Anemia and iron-deficiency anemia: compilation of data on pregnancy outcome. *Am J Clin Nutr.* 1994;59(Suppl):492S–500S.

59. Rosso P. *Nutrition and Metabolism in Pregnancy—Mother and Fetus.* New York, NY: Oxford University Press; 1990.

60. Story M, Alton I. Nutrition and the pregnant adolescent. *Contemp Nutr.* 1992;17(5):1–2.

61. *Nutrition: Eating for Good Health.* Washington, DC: US Department of Agriculture; 1993. Agricultural Information Bulletin no. 685.

62. Story M, Pontius S. Service providers' perceptions of their knowledge and skill levels in the nutrition management of pregnant adolescents. *J Nutr Educ.* 1988;20(6):303–306.

63. Lee SH, Grubbs LM. A comparison of self-reported, self-care practices of pregnant adolescents. *Nurs Pract.* 1993;198(9):25–29.

64. Skinner JD, Carruth BR, Ezell JM, Shaw AM. Adolescents' reactions to a prototype videotape on nutrition during pregnancy. In: Society for Nutrition Education 26th Annual Meeting Abstracts of Presentations; July 17–21,1993, St, Paul, MN: 30. Abstract 18.

65. Church J. Neonatal implications of adolescent pregnancy. *NAACOGS Clin Issu Perinat Womens Health Nurs.* 1991;2 (2):245–253.

66. Bryant CA, Coreil J, D'Angelo SL, et al. A strategy for promoting breastfeeding among economically disadvantaged women and adolescents. *NAACOGS Clin Issu Perinat Womens Health Nurs.* 1992;3(4):723–730.

67. Association of Maternal and Child Health Programs. *Adolescent Fathers: Directory of Services.* Washington, DC: National Center for Education in Maternal and Child Health; 1993.

68. Sharbaugh, CO. *Vision for America's Future: An Agenda for the 1990s—A Children's Defense Budget.* Washington, DC: Children's Defense Fund; 1989.

69. Sharbaugh CO, ed. *Call to Action: Better Nutrition for Mothers, Children and Families.* Washington, DC: National Center for Education in Maternal and Child Health; 1990.

3

&

Eating Disorders

Jennifer R. McDuffie and Betty G. Kirkley

Eating disorders are psychiatric syndromes that manifest themselves in nutrition-related symptoms. Anorexia and bulimia nervosa are not distinct disorders; rather, the symptoms appear in several combinations along a continuum of disordered eating. The latest edition of the *Diagnostic and Statistical Manual for Mental Disorders* (DSM-IV) acknowledges the existence of this now-blurred picture, designating "subtypes" of anorexia and bulimia. A new provisional category called *binge eating disorder* has also been established.[1] Because these disorders have multifactorial etiologies, they are best addressed by a team approach, which should include a nutritionist.

DEFINITION AND PREVALENCE

Anorexia Nervosa

First described in the late 1800s, anorexia nervosa, or voluntary self-starvation, remained a rare disorder until the 1960s when the incidence began to increase steadily. Bruch's now classic observational paper[2] delineated the basic problem of young women fighting for personal control in a stifling family environment. These young women were "perfect," according to the standards of their high society families, but had never been given the freedom to develop a sense of self. They were subconsciously rebelling the only way they could—by not eating. Originally thought to be a disease limited to white, upper-class women in western societies, it is now spreading into other races, socioeconomic classes, and throughout the developed world.[3] The prevalence in the United States is now estimated to be 0.7 to 1% of young women. Onset has a bimodal distribution; the first peak occurring at 13 to 14 years and the second at 17 to 18 years.[4]

Four characteristics must be present for the diagnosis of anorexia nervosa (Exhibit 3-1). If only some of the characteristics are present, but the disordered eating is severe enough to warrant treatment, the diagnosis of eating disorder, not otherwise specified, is given. These criteria are symptom-oriented and do not speak to the complex, multifaceted etiology of the disease.

Bulimia Nervosa

Bulimia, the ingestion and subsequent purging of copious amounts of food, has been part of human society, sporadically, since the Roman orgies. In the 1960s, it re-emerged as a dissolution of primary anorexia. When an anorexic patient could no longer sustain her rigid self-denial, she gave in to her desire to eat but then vomited to maintain her low body weight.[5] By 1980, bulimia had appeared singularly with enough frequency to warrant a separate classification in DSM-III. Now, bulimia is estimated to affect 4 to 10% of adolescent and college-aged women, with some estimates rising as high as 19 to 20%.[3,6,7] It is also on the rise in men.[8] However, it is a disease based in feelings of shame, insecurity, and inadequacy, so

---

Exhibit 3-1 Diagnostic Criteria for Anorexia Nervosa

1. Refusal to maintain body weight at or above a minimally normal weight for age and height (e.g., weight loss leading to maintenance of body weight less than 85% of that expected; or failure to make expected weight gain during periods of growth, leading to body weight less than 85% of that expected).
2. Intense fear of gaining weight or becoming fat, even though underweight.
3. Disturbance in the way in which one's body weight or shape is experienced, undue influence of body weight or shape on self-evaluation, or denial of the seriousness of the current low body weight.
4. In postmenarcheal females, amenorrhea [i.e., the absence of at least three consecutive menstrual cycles]. (A woman is considered to have amenorrhea if her periods occur only following hormone [e.g., estrogen] administration.)

Specify type:

Restricting type: during the current episode of anorexia nervosa, the person has not regularly engaged in binge-eating or purging behavior (i.e., self-induced vomiting or the misuse of laxatives, diuretics, or enemas)

Binge eating/purging type: during the current episode of anorexia nervosa, the person has regularly engaged in binge eating or purging behavior (i.e., self-induced vomiting or the misuse of laxatives, diuretics, or enemas)

Source: Reprinted with permission from the *Diagnostic and Statistical Manual of Mental Disorders,* ed 4, American Psychiatric Association, © 1994.

the best estimates probably fall short of the true magnitude of the problem.[9] Sub-clinical bulimia is much more prevalent. Binge eating was reported by 65 to 69% of female undergraduates in surveys[6,10] but is estimated to affect up to 80% of collegiate women.[11]

Bulimia nervosa is defined by five characteristics (Exhibit 3-2), all of which must be present for the diagnosis. If only the bingeing behavior is present, in the absence of purging, the provisional diagnosis of binge-eating disorder may be given. The validity of this classification as a completely separate entity is still under investigation and hotly debated.[12,13]

ETIOLOGY

The complex etiology of the eating-disordered patient is multifactorial, involving biologic, psychological, and environmental factors. Environment contributes to these disorders at both the familial and sociocultural levels.

Exhibit 3-2 Diagnostic Criteria for Bulimia Nervosa

1. Recurrent episodes of binge eating. An episode of binge eating is characterized by both of the following:
    - eating, in a discrete period of time (e.g., within any 2-hour period), an amount of food that is definitely larger than most people would eat during a similar period of time and under similar circumstances
    - a sense of lack of control over eating during the episode (e.g., a feeling that one cannot stop eating or control what or how much one is eating)
2. Recurrent inappropriate compensatory behavior in order to prevent weight gain, such as self-induced vomiting; misuse of laxatives, diuretics, enemas, or other medications; fasting; or excessive exercise.
3. The binge eating and inappropriate compensatory behaviors both occur, on average, at least twice a week for 3 months.
4. Self-evaluation is unduly influenced by body shape and weight.
5. The disturbance does not occur exclusively during episodes of anorexia nervosa.

Specify type:

Purging type: during the current episode of bulimia nervosa, the person has regularly engaged in self-induced vomiting or the misuse of laxatives, diuretics, or enemas
Nonpurging type: during the current episode of bulimia nervosa, the person has used other inappropriate compensatory behaviors, such as fasting or excessive exercise, but has not regularly engaged in self-induced vomiting or the misuse of laxatives, diuretics, or enemas

Source: Reprinted with permission from the *Diagnostic and Statistical Manual of Mental Disorders,* ed 4, American Psychiatric Association, © 1994.

Biologic Factors

The clinician will often find that a sister, aunt, or even the mother of the patient has abnormal issues with and around food and body image. Anorexia and bulimia are both more common among first-degree relatives than would be expected by chance.[14–16] Twin studies have shown a heritability value of 41 to 56% for anorexia nervosa.[17,18]

Eating disorders are positively correlated with other psychiatric disorders being present in a family—depression, obsessive-compulsive disease, bipolar disorder, seasonal affective disorder, post-traumatic stress disorder, and substance abuse.[15,16,19,20] Some of these affective disorders also exhibit a neurotransmitter imbalance in common with anorexia and bulimia—a dysregulation of the serotoninergic system.[21–23] Whether this is a premorbid condition or an imbalance that occurs as a result of the disease state is unknown.

The incidence of eating disorders is higher among children of mothers who have eating disorders themselves.[24,25] In one study, 28% of children whose mothers had a history of anorexia nervosa were classified as having eating and weight problems beyond the first year of life. Nine percent of these children had emotional, social, or behavioral problems.[25] It has not been determined whether these statistics are the result of inherited tendencies or due to environmental factors.

Psychological Factors

At the base of anorexia is a fear of losing control or being out of control. In the "classic case," the young woman has grown up in an environment where everything was decided for her, if not overtly, then by expectation. Consequently, her personality constellation includes a need to control, a rigid pattern of thinking and behavior (black-and-white thinking; extreme self-discipline), low self-esteem, perfectionism, and social withdrawal.[26,27] This is a lethal combination as it does not allow for failure but also does not provide the self-confidence and realistic expectations that produce success. Often, the young woman was chubby as a child and losing weight was her first independent success. As the pressures and decisions demanded in adolescence increase, the young woman developing anorexia retreats into the safe world of dieting, where it is just herself and food. Her world retracts into what she eats, what she does not eat, and what she weighs— things she can continue to control—instead of expanding into what career she will choose, whether she will marry and have children, and what she will believe spiritually, socially, politically, and economically.

Bulimia nervosa is characterized by a drive for acceptance, looking to external sources for approval because basic self-esteem is lacking. Many of the personality traits are the same as in anorexia—perfectionism, low self-esteem, and a need to be in control. However, the bulimic patient is more socially developed, partially due to the later age of onset. The rigidity and social isolation are replaced by impulsivity and emotional lability.[19] In the "classic case," the young woman is trying to please everyone else yet does not know how to please herself. The family and others often had high expectations for her so the young woman learned to live up to these rather than create her own. Consequently, when finally on her own in college, her "facade" collapses because it has no substance, only the external trappings of the perfect co-ed. Without an internal guide for making choices or coping mechanisms to deal with all the pressure, she literally tries to have her cake and eat it too. Food is used to keep her awake, calm her down, help her study, or avoid studying. Then it is purged so that she will keep her figure and stay popular.

Environmental Factors

Familial

Minuchin et al[26] described the interaction patterns that characterize the anorexic family. There is enmeshment, overprotectiveness, rigidity, lack of conflict resolution, and patient involvement in parental conflict. These patterns are all the result of inappropriate hierarchies and boundaries within the family unit. A mother and daughter may be "best friends," with the mother using the child as a confidante, preventing the child from developing normal peer relationships. Problems in the family are not discussed and solved. Either a decision is dictated by the dominant parent, often a father who is otherwise uninvolved, or the problem is "swept under the carpet" and ignored. The parents cannot solve problems between themselves effectively either. The child is pulled into a triangulation as "referee" where each parent attempts an alliance with the child rather than with each other. Anorexia is seen as a reaction to the psychosomatic family environment—making it physically evident that there are problems yet distracting the parents from their basic conflict. Thus, the "sick child" keeps the family together.

All the inappropriate interaction patterns of the anorexic family occur also in the bulimic family, with the addition of isolation and secretiveness, consciousness of appearances, and a special meaning attached to food and eating.[28] These are "all-American" families that exhibit the picture of happiness to society but are, in reality, torn apart by competitiveness and ambition. Thus, on the one hand, everyone in the family is very enmeshed in the maintenance of the "front," but on the other hand, they are very alone and unsupported in their attempts. According to Johnson and Connors,[19] bulimic families are "chaotic," with alcoholism and other impulse disorders very prevalent. Food becomes a means to communicate love and anger between family members who do not know how to talk to each other.

Studies of women with bulimia and their children reported some disturbing results.[24,29] These women were overconcerned about their children's sizes. Furthermore, 70% had problems breastfeeding, mostly because of the deleterious effect they thought it would have on their figures. Thirty-five percent reported bingeing and purging in front of their children or ignoring their children during a binge-purge cycle. Some reported not having sufficient food in the house to feed their children because of their own lack of control over having food in the house. One can only assume that this overconcern will increase the incidence of eating disorders developing in the children.

Sociocultural

Women today are caught between the average weight of an adult American woman, which has increased more than 5 lb over the past 20 years,[30] and the current "ideal" female form, which has become thin to the point of androgyny. A retrospective study of "Miss Americas" illustrates that desired proportions are moving in the direction of the unattainable "Barbie doll."[31,32] The net result has been body size dissatisfaction, which starts young and increases with age. In one survey, 50% of 14-year-old females wanted to lose weight. By age 18, this percentage has increased to approximately 75%.[33] Several other studies have found 50 to 70% of adolescent females discontented with their body weight or shape.[34,35] This desire to be thin, taken to the extreme, is a major factor contributing to the group of illnesses termed *eating disorders*.

Theoretical Framework

Many experts cite dietary restraint as the common etiologic factor in the vicious cycle of eating disorders[16,36–38] (Figure 3-1). A proposed etiologic model for eating disorders is based on the current cultural emphasis on thinness combined with a predisposition toward a stockier build and a greater tendency toward emotional reactivity resulting in consequent dietary restraint.[38] It is this initial dietary restraint with its lack of satiety or satisfaction that seems to initiate the vicious cycle of eating disorders.

Supporting this conclusion, most eating disorders can be traced to a "first" diet in response to body size dissatisfaction.[27] Initially, the patient may be "chubby" for a variety of reasons. Genetic make-up predisposes some individuals to obesity.[39] Environmental influences such as the type of food available, the opportunity to become involved in athletics, and the examples set by parents and other significant adults have an effect on the diet and exercise patterns developed.[15,40] A family that is dysfunctional due to alcohol or some other type of abuse is one cause for a young woman to seek comfort or safety in food.[26,41] Unfortunately, the

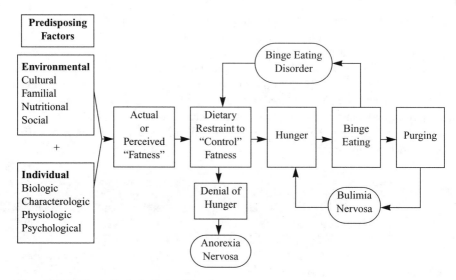

Figure 3-1 Etiologic Cycle for Eating Disorders

"thin ideal" of western society places the chubby child in a position to be teased, ridiculed, and excluded, all of which can be very damaging to self-esteem. As the child enters puberty and adolescence, the desire to be thin overrides common sense and spurs adherence to whatever fad diet is "in" and promises quick results.

Excessive dietary restraint leads to energy deprivation and hunger. This hunger, if combined with added stress, depression, anxiety, or just impatience with a diet that is not working fast enough, leads to frustration and overeating. In the person who will develop an eating disorder, this overeating is rapidly followed by guilt and worry over potential weight gain. Reaction to this guilt may include giving up on dieting and becoming obese, chronic dieting, subsequent fasting, or purging of food. Ironically, the reactions aimed at maintaining a low body weight cause a reduction in metabolic rate in adaptation to what the body interprets as starvation.[42,43] This makes it even harder for the individual to lose weight. The extent to which dietary restraint is broken and the method used to assuage the guilt determine the type of eating disorder that develops.

NUTRITIONAL IMPLICATIONS

Weight, Body Composition, and Basal Metabolic Rate

Epidemiologically, young women who develop eating disorders tend to be slightly overweight and of an endomorphic body type before disease onset.[44] This observation makes the profound weight loss of the anorexic even more striking and helps one understand how the bulimic may be biologically starved even though they are at a normal weight for height.[45] In anorexic patients, the weight at menarche serves as a useful guide for when menstruation may reoccur.[27] It is often helpful to plot weight against a standard growth chart or height and weight tables so the patient can be shown how her present status compares with her previous or usual status.

In anorexia nervosa, depending on the severity of the disorder, virtually all the body fat and somatic protein stores are depleted. Skeletal muscle is severely affected, and visceral proteins may also be affected.[18,45] In bulimia nervosa, the body compartment most affected is fluid. Plasma volume shifts occur with all types of purgation, making dehydration a real danger. Body fat stores and muscle mass are much more variable in bulimia. However, eating-disordered athletes often have the lowest level of body fat and less muscle mass than one would expect, given their level of fitness.[46]

The highest and lowest weight since achieving adult height and the rate of weight change give an indication of the effect of the weight loss on the basal metabolic rate (BMR).[43,47] Individuals with a personal or family history of obesity (higher premorbid weight) tend to have lower BMRs than those without such a history.[48] If the rate of weight loss was rapid and of recent onset (acute weight loss), the BMR may not be as depressed as with chronic low body weight. In chronic weight loss or chronic low body weight, adaption to starvation metabolism occurs and the BMR may be decreased by as much as 50%.[49]

Medical Management

Because eating disorders per se are not consistent in their presentation but vary between individuals depending on subtype, medical considerations have been presented in terms of the presence or absence of starvation or purgation. These two conditions are consistent, and medical signs, symptoms, and consequences can be delineated (Exhibit 3-3). The medical effects of chronic starvation were studied during and after World War II and are thoroughly addressed in the classic work by Keys et al.[49] The medical effects of purging are dependent on the type—vomiting, laxative or diuretic abuse, and/or excessive exercise. The most serious consequences are often the result of chronic repeated vomiting to the point that the muscles of the thoracic cavity are no longer responsive. The bulimic patient may then use emetine (Ipecac) to induce vomiting. Extensive use of this over-the-counter emetic can result in cardiomyopathy and heart failure.[45] Whatever medical or metabolic change is noted in an eating-disordered patient, it is as yet unknown which, if any, are premorbid or if all are the results of the disease.

Exhibit 3-3 Medical Complications of Eating Disorders

Starvation

Physical signs and symptoms: cachexia, emaciation, hyperactivity, early satiety, sleep disturbances, social isolation or withdrawal, dehydration (dry skin, peripheral edema), hypercar-
otenosis of the skin, cyanosis in the extremities, muscular weakness, loss of scalp, pubic
hair, and/or presence of lanugo hair, brittle broken nails (due to protein deficiency), gingi-
vitis and periodontal disease

Medical complications: hypothermia, constipation, delayed gastric emptying, slowed intestinal motility, hypotension, bradycardia, arrhythmias, anemia, neutropenia, thrombocytope-
nia, petechiae, metabolic alkalosis (increased bicarbonate), hypophosphatemia,
oligomenorrhea, muscle weakness

Severe complications: pancreatic insufficiency, cardiac atrophy, mitral valve prolapse or con-
gestive heart failure, pancytopenia, pneumonia and sepsis, hypokalemic nephropathy,
renal calculi, seizures, amenorrhea, osteoporosis, reduced stature and bone fractures, muscle atrophy

Laboratory indicators: elevated serum amylase, liver function tests (due to fatty liver), serum
cholesterol (due to faulty lipid metabolism) and blood-urea-nitrogen (due to dehydration),
increased insulin resistance and elevated ketone bodies, decreased glomerular filtration
rate, erratic vasopressin release, decreased estrogen and testosterone, prepubertal levels of
luteinizing hormone and follicle-stimulating hormone, "sick" euthyroid syndrome
(decreased T_3 and low normal T_4), depressed norepinephrine levels, increased cortisol,
dopamine and growth hormone, abnormal blood cell counts and differential.

Purging (vomiting, laxative or diuretic abuse)

Physical signs and symptoms: hypertrophy of the parotid glands, Russell's sign (bruises or lac-
erations of hands, fingers), cracked split nails, petechiae in and around the eyes, dehydration (dry skin) combined with complaints of bloating, especially in the abdominal area,
and pedal edema, polyuria and polydipsia (due to renal response to electrolyte imbalance),
dental caries, discoloration, dysplasia, perimolysis or pyorrhea

Medical complications: hypothermia, delayed gastric emptying, nausea, hematemesis, consti-
pation/diarrhea, steatorrhea, bloody stool or urine, transient hypovolemia with compensatory renal retention of sodium and water causing peripheral edema, transient electrolyte
imbalance, oligomenorrhea, muscle weakness, cramping

Severe complications: esophagitis, esophageal or gastric rupture, flaccid unresponsive bowel,
chronic electrolyte imbalance and metabolic acidosis (decreased potassium bicarbonate
due to laxative use) *or* metabolic alkalosis (hypochloremia due to loss of HCl in vomitus),
hyponatremia, hypophosphatemia, hypomagnesemia, cardiac arrhythmias, tachycardia,
hypotension, decreased cardiac output and muscle weakness (due to hypokalemia), secondary hyperaldosteronism, renal calculi, seizures (if bulimia is associated with alcohol
ingestion), hiatal hernia, osteoporosis

Laboratory indicators: increased serum amylase (due to salivary amylase entering blood
through esophageal tears), electrolyte imbalance (as above), elevated blood-urea-nitrogen,
creatinine (due to dehydration, tissue damage), decreased estrogen, serotonin

Eating disorders also affect pregnancy outcome. The rate of prematurity was twice that of the general population, and the rate of perinatal mortality was six times that of the general population. Therefore, if a woman presents with a chronic history of anorexia nervosa and expresses the desire to gain weight to conceive a child, it is of the utmost importance to emphasize to her the need to completely replenish herself nutritionally before conception.

Dietary Intake

The most striking thread of continuity within the eating habits of people with eating disorders is the extreme secretiveness and shame associated with food intake. For this reason, there is not a large amount of valid empirical data available on the dietary intakes of this population. There is, however, a large amount of observational and anecdotal evidence that is very consistent.

Anorexia is essentially an energy deficiency. Studies find that the energy intake of anorexic patients is approximately 50 to 65% of normal controls, and food aversions are largely based on caloric content of the foods.[52,53] Some studies have found an increased proportion of intake from protein.[54–56] Others have found the caloric distribution is the same as in normal controls.[53] Approximately half of anorexia nervosa patients are vegetarians.[56] This and other practices may increase their risk of protein, vitamins B_6 and B_{12}, iron, and zinc deficiencies. The general intake pattern of an anorexic often includes rigidly prescribed rituals in which specific foods are always eaten at specific times while other foods are always avoided—the "good and bad food lists." Therefore, virtually any nutrient could be inadequate in these diets, depending on the specific foods avoided. Other nutrients that have been found to be deficient in the anorexic patient's diet are calcium, thiamin, riboflavin, niacin, and ascorbic acid.[55] Therefore, a multivitamin supplement is almost always prescribed.

Whereas anorexic patients have good and bad days but total energy intake is always abnormally low, bulimic patients have good and bad days where total energy intake is highly variable. Bulimic patients have been found to have lower than normal intakes on "good days,"[57] with energy intakes in the range of 800 to 1200 kcal/day. However, compensation occurs on "binge days," with intakes ranging anywhere from 1800 to 5500 kcal/day. The definition of a "binge" is highly variable. In one study, binges were characterized by a high caloric content, a rapid rate of eating, a feeling of lack of control, but a typical distribution (50% carbohydrate, 40% fat, and 10% protein).[58] This general increase in overall meal size without a change in composition does not support the idea that bulimic patients have carbohydrate "cravings."[59] Alternatively, these results suggest that the essential abnormality in bulimia may be lack of control over the amount of food consumed. Perhaps bulimic patients are less responsive to the signals that terminate meals.[58] The eating patterns of the subtypes have also been explored.[60] It was found that there was no difference in the average binge or purging frequency between the three subgroups with bulimic behaviors.

NUTRITION ASSESSMENT

The goals for nutritional assessment of the eating-disordered patient are to determine the degree of cachexia and muscle wasting, to elucidate the patient's typical eating pattern if one exists, to identify the degree of restriction, bingeing and/or purgative usage in the patient's food habits, and to learn the weight, diet, and exercise histories of the patient as well as any pertinent family information. There are four primary tools used in a thorough nutrition assessment: a questionnaire, a clinical interview, a self-monitoring assignment, and anthropometric measurement. The use of both a questionnaire and an interview allows the clinician to assess the consistency of the patient's self-report.

The Questionnaire

The purpose of the questionnaire is to obtain a comprehensive, standardized symptom index. The questionnaire used in our clinic is the Diagnostic Survey of Eating Disorders.[61] Other potentially useful instruments are the Eating Attitudes Test,[62] the Eating Disorders Inventory,[63] and the Eating Disorders Examination.[64] Adolescents should be able to complete these surveys without excessive difficulty. However, if the child is younger than 13 to 14 years of age, the aid of a parent may be required or select sections may be completed verbally. Although these instruments provide helpful information to any professional working with eating-disordered patients, they are psychological questionnaires. Therefore, in an ideal situation, they would be administered and interpreted by a psychology professional.

The Clinical Interview

The interview includes a general history, a weight and body image history, a diet history, a history of the eating disorder itself, and an exploration of the pertinent environmental factors (Exhibit 3-4). It should be geared more to the attitudes of the individual patient and less toward factual information gathering. The interviewer can use the patient's answers to the just-completed questionnaire or the tables of example questions that follow in this section as a guideline.

Exhibit 3-4 Assessment Form

ASSESSMENT SHEET

DEMOGRAPHICS

Patient Name:_____   DOB:_____

Address:_____   Dx:_____

_____   Hosp:_____

Phone: (home)_____ (work)_____

Referred by:_____

Reason for referral:_____

_____

NUTRITION ASSESSMENT

Height:_____cm   Current Wt:_____kg (_____#)
Wrist circumference:_____cm   Usual Weight:_____kg (_____#)
Elbow breadth:_____cm   Preferred Weight:_____kg (___#)
Frame size: S   M   L   % Wt loss/gain:_____
TSF:_____mm _____% ile   _____chronic _____acute
SSF:_____mm _____% ile   Min. Wt.:_____Max. Wt.:_____
MAC:_____cm _____% ile   Recommended Weight Range (RBW):
MAMC:_____mm _____% ile   % RBW (midpoint):_____

CALCULATIONS

BEE:_____

Adjustments:_____

Activity Factor:_____

EEN:_____

EPR:_____

PRESENT HABITS

Bingeing:_____   Exercise:_____

Cigarettes:_____   Vomiting:_____

Alcohol:_____   Laxatives:_____

Drug Use:_____   Diuretics:_____

Rest/Relaxation:_____   Appetite Suppressants:_____

Vitamins/Supplements:_____

Prescribed Medications:_____

FAMILY Hx

	Occupation	Age	Ht.	Wt.	Exercise	Cig.	EthOH	Food Habits
Father:								
Mother:								
Sig. Other:								
Siblings:								

        WEIGHT Hx   EATING PATTERNS

   Age: Past   Present

  0 - 5:

  6 - 12:

 13 - 18:

 19 - 25:

                        What is the role of food in health?

IMPRESSIONS:

RECOMMENDATIONS:

Opening

The clinical interview provides an opportunity to establish rapport with the patient and to begin to understand the motivations and fears around the issues of weight and food. Good opening questions are "Why did you seek treatment at this time? How do you define your problem with food? What is your greatest concern about your health? What is your goal in examining your eating habits? How do you perceive the role of food in your body, in society?" The answers to these questions give information as to how to set the tone of the rest of the interview. Active listening lets the patient know that you want to understand. These patients will often respond favorably to a nonjudgmental, factual yet gentle approach. Questions that imply an understanding of the behaviors and feelings will elicit greater honesty and enhance the therapeutic relationship.

General History

The general history includes information on medical condition, health habits, socioeconomic data, family, and home environment. Other complicating medical conditions that affect diet, such as diabetes, should be ascertained at the beginning of the interview. Their presence may explain subsequent answers to questions and give an indication of the severity of the eating disorder.

Information on current health habits gives an overview of present self-care. This has an enormous effect on nutritional status. Items that need to be addressed are the amount and quality of sleep, the present exercise regime, current prescription medications, vitamins, or other supplements taken, the amounts of alcohol or caffeine usually ingested, and the use of cigarettes, appetite suppressants, laxatives, diuretics, or recreational drugs that may affect appetite.

Weight and Body Image History

Ideally, the weight history includes both numerical values and attitudes (Exhibit 3-5). This gives a comparison between the objective side of the individual and how big she feels. Many people cannot tell you how tall they were or what they weighed in grammar school, although they may be able to give you their birth weight. What they will remember is their size in relation to other classmates. If the patient is very young, a parent may be asked to provide the pertinent values. Important numerical values to obtain are self-estimated current weight, actual current weight, desired weight, premorbid (usual) weight, highest and lowest weights since achieving adult height, rate of weight change, and weight at menarche, if applicable. The answers to these questions give insight as to the source of the overconcern about weight and how to set realistic weight goals with the patient.

Exhibit 3-5 Attitudinal Weight History Questions

- In elementary school, were you taller, shorter, or the same height as the other girls? Were you thinner, chubbier, or the same weight?
- Were you teased about your weight or your size? In what way?
- Did you wear "chubby" or "extra"-size clothing when you were small?
- Could you perform adequately in gym class or was your size prohibitive?
- When did menarche occur? Do you remember any complications, uncomfortableness, or significant weight gain around menarche?
- What do you remember about your size in relation to the other girls in junior high school? In high school?
- When did you achieve your adult height?
- When did you first become aware of your weight?
- How often did you weigh yourself growing up?
- How did you feel about your size when you graduated from high school?

The weight history gives an indication of body size distortion, preference for thinness, and body size dissatisfaction—the three components of body image distortion.[38] The difference between self-estimated current weight and actual weight gives an estimation of the degree of body size distortion in a patient who does not know her weight.[65] The difference between the recommended normal weight and the desired weight gives an idea of the intensity of the "drive for thinness." The difference between self-estimated current weight and desired weight gives an indication of body size dissatisfaction.[66]

In addition to these comparisons, the use of body size silhouettes (Figure 3-2) provides valuable information concerning general body image.[67] The patient is asked to choose a silhouette that represents her present view of herself and a second silhouette that represents how she would ideally like to look. The difference between present and ideal values is the body size dissatisfaction score. A normal-weight individual without an eating disorder will select a present view that is accurate or slightly over her true weight and an ideal view that is slightly under her true weight, producing a small (5 to 10%) body size dissatisfaction score. An eating-disordered patient's choices will produce a much higher body size dissatisfaction score. The patient's degree of satisfaction with her current size and the estimation of the difference in appearance caused by attainment of her desired weight indicate the amount of value the patient places on her weight. Satisfaction scores indicate the extent of the patient's fear of gaining weight. For greater discussion of these and other techniques, see Williamson's chapter on body image assessment.[38]

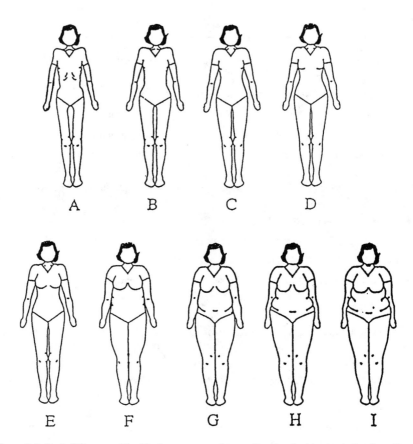

Figure 3-2 Body Silhouettes Used in Assessment   *Source:* Reprinted with permission from *Journal of General Psychology* (1966;108:19–33), Copyright © 1966, Heldref Publications, Inc.

Eating Behaviors and Exercise History

The nutrition history should explore both present and past habits. Present habits are addressed by taking both a 24-hour recall and a food frequency (targeted to the last 3 to 6 months). If the patient cannot remember what she ate the day before (and the patient may not want to remember what she ate), ask her to describe a "typical day." Depending on the problem, it may be necessary to get a recall of both a "good" day, one on which she is pleased with her intake, and a "bad" day, one on which she is disappointed with her intake.

It is often helpful to "set the stage" for the patient to obtain a truthful account of intake. Individuals with an eating disorder are very ashamed of their malady and often think that their eating habits are bizarre. In introducing the topic of a dietary recall, you may ask an anorexic patient, "Did you eat anything yesterday?" rather than "What did you eat yesterday?" intimating that it is not unusual for people to go without eating. Conversely, a bulimic patient will often tell you what she ate but not how much. Probing questions such as "How much ice cream, half a gallon?" convey that it is not unusual to consume large amounts of food at once. This type of questioning will help put the patient at ease, which should ensure a more accurate assessment of eating habits.

It is also helpful to ascertain what the patient believes is a healthful or perfect diet. Often, these patients are extremely knowledgeable about calories but know very little about good nutrition, the physiology of digestion, or the body's handling of nutrients.[51,68] To some eating-disordered patients, a healthful diet is 800 calories worth of nonfat "diet foods." Adequate protein is not considered. Some patients go so far in their "all-or-none" thinking about food that they categorize all foods as "allowed" or "not allowed." The food frequency will provide information about which foods the patient considers "safe" and which foods are "forbidden." It will also give information as to what nutritional deficits may be present if some food groups are absent or poorly represented.

Past eating habits must also be examined. At critical phases of the patient's life, with regard to her weight history, try to ascertain how balanced a diet was being consumed and how much control the patient had and/or wanted over her diet. Typically, the interviewer may want to ask about usual intake during (1) elementary and/or secondary school; (2) college or first job; and (3) just before the onset of the eating disorder. Questions used to obtain the patient's eating pattern are given in Exhibit 3-6.

With both bulimia or anorexia, the nutrition history questions include an exploration of dieting and binge/purge behaviors. In asking these questions, be aware that there is a difference between the technical term *binge* and what the word *binge* means to a patient. To bulimic subjects in one study, the four important characteristics defining the word *binge* were (1) consumption of a large amount of food; (2) extreme fullness; (3) the sense of loss of control; and (4) a subsequent dysphoric mood.[69] In the new DSM-IV, the criteria defining *binge* are both (1) eating, in a discrete period of time, an amount larger than most people would eat during a similar period of time; and (2) a sense of lack of control over eating during the episode.[70]

Excessive, obsessive exercise to expend binge calories is one of the accepted definitions of purging. Exercise can take many forms in daily life, so activity level must be determined carefully (Exhibit 3-7). Usually, solitary exercise regimens are preferred. Besides obvious physical activities such as jogging, intramurals, cheerleading or school sports, ask about lessons (i.e., dance, gymnastics, etc.), chores, or a part-time job that requires physical exertion. How often are each of these activities engaged in each week? What is the duration and intensity of each activity? Why is the activity pursued; is it required, enjoyed, or for the

Exhibit 3-6 Eating Pattern Questions

Present

- Where is food usually consumed?
- How many different places is food often consumed?
- Is there a regular frequency of meals and snacks (meal pattern)?
- If not, what are the frequency ranges for meals and snacks/day?
- Are one or more meals often "skipped"?
- Are meals eaten alone or with others? Is this helpful or harmful?
- Do you recognize "hunger"? Do you eat for reasons other than hunger that you are aware of?
- Do you have dietary "rules" that you think you must follow?
- Do you have any food rituals that are associated with your disorder?
- If a dietary rule is broken, what are the consequences?

Past

- What were family meals like when you lived at home?
- How did eating patterns change when you left home?
- Who do you think most influenced your eating habits?

Exhibit 3-7 Diet, Binge/Purge Behavior Questions

- What is the definition of a "diet" for you?
- What constitutes success on a diet for you?
- What is your definition of the term *binge*?
- How often does a binge occur?
- Are there specific "trigger" foods that inevitably start binges?
- Have you ever been successful in limiting or preventing a binge? How were you successful in this?
- How often do you purge?
- What method of purging do you use—vomiting, laxatives, subsequent fasting, or exercising?
- If vomiting, do you need to help yourself or is it spontaneous?
- If laxatives, what brand do you use? How many do you take at a time—half a box, a whole box?
- If exercise, how often is each activity engaged in per week? What is the duration and intensity of each activity? Is there any enjoyment or is the activity pursued for the sole purpose of burning kilocalories?
- How long a fast or how much exercise is adequate to make up for a binge for you?
- When did dieting, bingeing, or purging start?
- What were the specific circumstances around this event?
- How has the frequency or intensity changed over time?

sole purpose of burning calories? The clinician should also be observant of restless movement. Many severe eating-disordered patients will not sit when they can stand or sit still when they can fidget. Over a 16-hour period, on a daily basis, nervous activity can add up to be an additional 10% of basal energy expenditure (BEE), which is a significant calorie expenditure when compared with the marginal intakes of an anorexic patient.

Familial Factors

The last area of exploration for the interview is familial factors. Socioeconomic data and the family members' behavior patterns may shed light on the etiology of the eating disorder and therefore be useful for planning treatment strategies.[26,71] Is this a success-oriented family? Are performance expectations for the patient unreasonably high? For each member of the immediate family and other significant figures, determine age, height, weight, build, use of cigarettes and alcohol, and eating and exercise habits. Is any of this information out of the ordinary? More important, what does the patient think of her family's appearance and habits? Particular attention should be given to the presence of other family members with eating disorders, especially in the immediate family.

Self-monitoring

The self-monitoring instrument given to most patients after their first visit clarifies and corroborates the information gathered in the interview (Figure 3-3). The instrument is a log of eating behaviors, feelings, and activity to be kept by the patient for 1 week (to encompass most routine events and one weekend). Ideally, the log is a record of each eating episode—time of day, location, amount and type of food eaten, rate of ingestion, degree of hunger, mood before and after the episode, and any other activities pursued while eating. It can also record the amount, type, and intensity of daily physical activities. If filled out correctly, this record will give a clear picture of what traps the patient sets for herself, how motivated she is to change, and where to begin in therapy. Again, for a child younger than 13 to 14 years of age, parental aid may be required, and the mood sections may be completed verbally in a subsequent interview.

Analysis of Dietary Data

To determine the quality of the present diet, analysis of the 24-hour recall, the food frequency, and the self-monitoring log should assess the variables listed in Exhibit 3-8. Daily caloric intake of restrictive anorexic patients will generally be inadequate. However, for binge–purging anorexic patients and restricting bulimic patients, low caloric intakes may be seen only on "good" days. Caloric intakes on

Figure 3-3 Self–monitoring Instrument

DAILY FOOD RECORD

Date/ Time	Location	With Whom?	Hunger before Eating (0–10)	Binge? Mark (Y/N)	Food/Amount Eaten	Activity while Eating	Fullness after Eating (0–10)	Purged? Vomiting (V) Laxatives (L) Exercise (E)	Sensation/Feelings after Purging

Exhibit 3-8 Assessment of Dietary Data

- Variety or monotony in food selections
- Representation from each of the food groups
- Preferred consumption of only low-fat and diet-type foods
- Avoidance of starches except as components of a binge
- Over-consumption of fluids, gum, ice, etc., to maintain denial of hunger
- Presence or absence of adequate sources of vitamins and minerals
- Estimation of the macronutrient content of the diet
- Distribution of calories between carbohydrate, protein, and fat

"bad" days are difficult to calculate. Patients often lose track of what they consume during a binge, and caloric loss due to purging is variable, depending on the composition and size of the binge and how much time elapsed before purging. The current estimates of calories lost by vomiting range from 25 to 66%[72–74] and 10 to 15% for laxative use.[75]

Anorexic patients often shun dairy products and many protein foods because they contain fat. Consequently, diets may be deficient in protein, vitamin B_{12}, iron, and calcium, depending on how many nonfat products are eaten. Carbohydrate, although minimally present, usually comes from vegetables and fruits, with starches being meager or absent. Most bulimic patients consume adequate amounts of protein and variable amounts of fat, depending on whether it is a binge day. As with anorexic patients, they consume inadequate amounts of carbohydrate (when not bingeing) but not to the same severe degree. With the exception of restrictive anorexic patients, who may eat fruits and vegetables almost exclusively, most eating-disordered patients lack adequate amounts of fiber in their diets. Decreased fat and fiber in a meal reduces its satiety value, which may lead to bingeing or overeating. Because most eating-disordered patients subsist on low-calorie "healthy" foods and often take a vitamin supplement, specific vitamin deficiencies are not as common as would be expected. If an anorexic patient has restricted intake to a limited number of "safe" foods, additional deficiencies are more probable, often vitamins B_2, B_6, and E and zinc.

Anthropometrics

Anthropometric measurements provide an indicator of the patient's nutritional status by estimating protein and calorie reserves. This information is useful, both in determining nutrition goals and in illustrating nutrition education topics such as why the body needs protein and the value of fat stores in health. Measurements usually taken are height, weight, frame size by wrist circumference (Table 3-1),[76]

Table 3-1 Interpretation of Frame Size Factor[a]

	Small	Medium	Large
Male	>10.4	10.4–9.6	<9.6
Female	>10.9	10.9–9.9	<9.9

[a]Factor for estimation of frame size = height (cm)/wrist circumference (cm).
Source: Reprinted from Nutritional Assessment and Support by A Grant and S DeHoog with permission of Grant-DeHoog Publishers, © 1985.

skinfold thickness (triceps [TSF] for a female and subscapular [SSF] for a male) and mid-upper-arm circumference (MAC), from which mid-upper-arm muscle circumference (MAMC) is derived. Stated height and frame size should not be trusted. An anorexic patient may underestimate her height and frame size so that the weight loss does not seem so severe. A bulimic patient, who is heavier than recommended body weight, may say she is taller or big-boned because she is embarrassed about the number.

Weight

Weight is best measured in a hospital gown, first thing in the morning after voiding, due to variability in clothing, normal weight fluctuations, and the fact that eating-disordered patients may attempt to be deceptive about their weight. However, except on an inpatient unit, this is usually not feasible. A compromise is to ask patients to remove shoes and outer clothing and to try to void before weighing. Weight should always be measured on the same scale and at a regularly appointed time once or twice a week. The scale should be routinely calibrated.

Be aware that there is a great deal of fear associated with being weighed for an eating-disordered patient. This fear can go in either direction, weighing too much or too little. Always be aware that a severe anorexic patient could be water-loading, drinking 16 to 64 oz of water before coming to the clinic on weigh-in day, or dehydrating herself by taking diuretics. She could also wear several layers of heavy clothing, heavy jewelry, or actually hide small weights on her body to weigh heavier and meet her contracted weight gain goal. Therefore, periodically check for other indicators of true weight gain: improved hair, skin, and nail quality; lessening of edema; better percentile ratings in other anthropometric measurements such as TSF, SSF, MAC, and MAMC; or improved laboratory values such as higher albumin and total protein or disappearance of anemia without evidence of dehydration.

Ideal Body Weight

In adults, ideal body weight (IBW) can be determined using the Metropolitan Height and Weight Tables (1983) according to frame size.[77] The tables were constructed with subjects in street clothes wearing 1-in. heels. This discrepancy needs to be adjusted for when using the tables. If the patient measures 64-in. tall barefoot, they should be compared with the weights for 65 in. in the tables.

For individuals younger than age 18, comparison is made with standard growth charts. A combination of height for age, weight for age, and weight for height plotted on National Center for Health Statistics (NCHS) longitudinal charts is appropriate.[78] However, for adolescents aged 12 to 18 years, it is important to keep the variation in timing of the pubertal growth spurt between individuals in mind. If an adolescent is on the borderline of being underweight but does not exhibit the psychological symptoms, the professional may be dealing with over-anxious parents who just need to be reassured that their child is within the range of normal. For young girls whose normal maturation may have been interrupted (i.e., by anorexia), a chart that predicts pubertal onset and therefore adolescent growth tempo, has been devised.[79]

Body Composition

A general indicator of obesity or cachexia for adults is easily calculated with the Body Mass Index (BMI) (Table 3-2).[80] The skinfold is an estimate of the body's energy (or fat) stores. The TSF is perhaps the best single indicator of total skinfold thickness in young women.[81] The MAMC, which is derived from the TSF and the MAC, is an estimate of the body's protein stores.[82] These measurements, for assessment purposes, are taken on the nondominant side. Gender- and age-specific percentiles from the first National Health and Nutrition Examination Survey (NHANES I) are available.[83] These percentiles are used for a quick estimate of the severity of depletion (Table 3-3). If below the 5th percentile, the patient is considered severely depleted in body fat or protein stores.[84] Between the 5th and 15th percentile, the patient is considered moderately depleted, and between the 15th and 30th percentile, the patient is considered mildly depleted.

Table 3-2 Interpretation of Body Mass Index (BMI)[a]

<18	Severe underweight
18–20	Low body weight
20–25	Normal body weight
25–30	Overweight
30–40	Mild-moderate obesity
>40	Gross obesity

[a]BMI = weight (kg)/height^2 (m).
Source: Reprinted from *Principles of Nutrition Assessment* by R Gibson with permission of Oxford University Press, © 1990.

Table 3-3 Interpretation of TSF, MAMC^a Percentiles

>30th %ile	Within normal limits
15–30th %ile	Mildly depleted
5–15th %ile	Moderately depleted
<5th %ile	Severely depleted

^{a}MAMC (mm) = MAC (mm) − (p × TSF (mm)).
Source: Data from *Principles of Nutrition Assessment* by R Gibson with permission of Oxford University Press,1990.

Both of these measurements, the TSF and the MAMC, are often depressed below the 5th percentile in anorexic patients. A bulimic patient will have less depressed measurements, but the muscle mass is often less than expected for the level of physical exercise. This indicates either caloric and/or protein intakes are insufficient. Essentially, the patient is using muscle tissue for fuel.

The percentiles are also useful in helping the eating-disordered patient understand the reality of her size in relation to other American women. For the patient with anorexia, this means understanding that body stores are severely depleted. For the bulimic patient, this means understanding that she is "normal." Today, the in-vogue measure is percentage body fat. Many eating-disordered patients are anxious to know this value. The sum of three or four skinfolds is used to estimate body density,[85,86] which can then be translated into percentage body fat.[87,88] However, the measurement error is very large in depleted, very lean, and very obese populations.[87–90] Also, placing too much emphasis on body fat can cause the patient to be even more obsessed with the measurement. Therefore, it is advised to discourage the patient from trying to obtain this value.

Estimation of Energy and Protein Needs

Energy needs are lowered among eating-disordered patients due to their hypometabolic state.[27,49,91,92] However, setting calorie and protein goals is also influenced by what can realistically be expected from a patient who is afraid of food. Specific examples of this type of adjusted calculation are provided in the discussion of treatment.

Energy

As with any individual older than the age of 18, energy needs are assessed by calculating the BEE. The equation most commonly used is the Harris-Benedict equation. The metabolic response to underfeeding varies in different individuals, even at the same percentage below IBW. An anorexic patient's metabolism may be depressed as much as 25 to 30%, depending on severity of weight loss.[49,93] However, anorexia nervosa patients require more energy for activity than age-matched women. Therefore, the adjustment needed may not be as great as would be indicated by the hypometabolic state.[94]

A bulimic patient's metabolism may be depressed as much as 10 to 15%,[51,60] although this may be more due to a higher premorbid weight and/or a genetically lower BMR than to caloric restriction.[27,44,57,95] There is no consensus on the best method of correcting the BEE for hypometabolism in bulimic patients.

There are several proposed methods for determining the energy needs of the eating-disordered patient. First, the Harris-Benedict equation is calculated based on the actual reduced body weight of the patient. This method often overestimates energy needs[48]; therefore, the activity factor suggested for an anorexic patient is 1.1 instead of the standard sedentary factor of 1.2. The second method calculates the Harris-Benedict equation based on the patient's premorbid weight and multiplies the result by the actual percentage below recommended weight. This method uses a normal activity factor and may give a better estimate. It allows for the higher energy of activity observed in anorexic patients.[94] An exception to this adjustment is the acute weight-loss patient. In these patients, the BMR is not yet depressed and the multiplication by the actual percentage below recommended weight is not done. The above two methods are used for initial determinations and generally agree within 10%. Calories for weight gain are gradually added to these initial values. A large degree of individuation and readjustment of these calculations occurs during treatment. Once weight has been regained, one study[60] suggests that the best method of estimating caloric needs for both anorexic and bulimic patients may be the body surface area (BSA). The BSA is determined from the height and weight using a nomogram.[96] This method recommends 1575 kcal/BSA/day for patients with recent weight loss and 925 kcal/BSA/day for weight-stable patients.

Protein

The protein needs in starvation have been determined by Nitrogen Balance Studies.[49] Needs are influenced by activity level, degree of depletion (as indicated by MAMC, serum albumin, and transferrin levels), and degree of stress caused by any medical complication. Commonly used values are 1.2 to 1.5 g/kg for muscle mass repletion. An anorexic patient may also have depressed levels of some gastrointestinal enzymes (i.e., pepsin) due to the restrictive nature of the diet and the body's compensatory mechanisms in starvation. Consequently, reintroduction of protein into the diet may need to start at a much lower level, such as 0.8 to 0.9 g/kg actual weight or 0.5 to 0.6 g/kg ideal weight, and then increase gradually to the recommended levels over the course of a few weeks.[97] Protein recommendations are 0.8 to 1.0 g/kg for normal-weight bulimic patients unless they are very physically active. The "overexerciser" requires 1.0 to 1.5 g/kg body weight to avoid muscle being burned as fuel during nonbingeing periods.

TREATMENT

Successful treatment of an eating disorder requires that the patient learn to think of long-term instead of short-term gains and replace dietary restraint with commitment to eating and exercising in moderation. This is a slow, frightening process. There are often weight fluctuations or plateaus and fluid retention associated with recovering from anorexia and bulimia. The patient's body did its best to adapt to the lowered substrate availability and dehydration that accompanied the eating disorder. In recovery, it must readapt to normal substrate concentrations and adequate hydration. The patient needs education and support to help her understand and "wait out" these periods. With the help of the psychiatrist or psychologist, the patient will come to understand the factors that caused the eating disorder and deal with these issues in a more adaptive way. The nutritionist aids this process by helping the patient incrementally control her symptoms through realistic goal-setting, self-monitoring, and behavior change.

Nutritional therapy serves as an adjunct to psychotherapy for eating disorders. The universal goals of nutritional therapy of eating disorders are weight stabilization at a healthy but realistic weight range and normalization of eating habits. The information collected during the interview contributes to the accurate assessment of the patient's metabolic status, her dietary excesses and deficiencies, and the derivation of a treatment plan to gradually correct the problems identified. The strategies used to achieve incrementally closer approximations to ideal body weight include restructuring caloric intake closer and closer to maintenance needs, sequentially reformulating the diet closer to the recommended composition and implementing a regular but practical exercise program. To succeed with these strategies, food must be placed back in its original role of providing nutrients to the body. The patient must gradually master "non-food-related" alternative coping mechanisms to deal with her feelings to aid recovery and help prevent relapse.

Importance of the Therapy "Team"

Effective treatment demands a multidisciplinary treatment team. Garner and Garfinkel[27] emphasize the remarkable consensus between all the experts assembled for "integrating group, family and individual" therapy while "normalizing food intake through structured eating, meal plans, and diaries." The group therapist helps the patients learn interpersonal skills to end their isolation. The family therapist aids in restructuring the environment from one that helped to spawn the disorder to one that will promote recovery. The individual therapist explores the etiology of the disorder with the patient and confronts the thought distortions that contribute to its protraction. The physician monitors physical status and/or medication if the primary therapist is not qualified for these particular tasks. The registered dietitian conducts the nutritional assessment, monitors nutritional status, and provides dietary counseling for the patient or functions as the dietitian on an inpatient team where the therapy is handled by psychology professionals.

In this type of team situation, it is tempting to step into another's role, especially when encouraged by the patient. It is of the utmost importance to resist this temptation. Most people with an eating disorder have limited capacity to deal with negative emotions. They usually find a way to avoid dealing with them, often by obsessing about food instead. Another avoidance tactic is to talk about nutrition in the therapy session and therapy in the nutrition session. The nutritionist must recognize this when it happens and redirect the patient's focus. Because this population's eating problems are rooted in psychological conflict, attempts to help them change their eating behaviors will usually be met with resistance and psychological ploys far exceeding those found in most other patients. Hence, any nutrition professional who wants to work with this population needs additional training in psychology and, specifically, in treatment modalities used with eating disorders such as cognitive-behavioral therapy. Others should limit their involvement to nutritional assessment and monitoring intake.

Anorexia Nervosa

Restoration of a safe weight is the first goal for patients with anorexia nervosa. If weight is less than 70% of IBW, serum electrolytes are imbalanced, or the patient is orthostatic, the situation is very serious and hospitalization should be considered[40] (Figure 3-4). Concomitant presence of a personality disorder, as is the case with a substantial minority of this population, may also justify hospitalization if it is interfering with the patient's ability to function.[61] Orchestrating this type of admission can be difficult. The patient is already cognitively compromised due to weight loss and does not believe anything is wrong. The family often minimizes the problem, hoping that things will improve. Inpatient treatment is most effective if the patient is admitted voluntarily. The nutritionist can help the team effort to attain compliance with treatment recommendations by explaining to the patient and her family just how grave the situation is: A loss of 40% of body weight is life-threatening; continued weight loss in an already compromised person can be very rapid; continued subnormal weight in an adolescent can affect her optimal development of secondary sex characteristics, bone density, and normal hormone level fluctuations.[51,98] In this situation, you cannot be too firm.

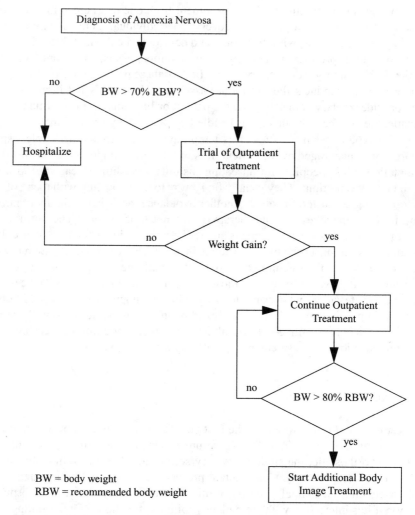

Figure 3-4 Flowchart for the Nutritional Treatment of Anorexia

---

Inpatient Treatment

Only a few years ago, long-term psychiatric hospitalization was the treatment of choice for anorexia nervosa. However, studies have shown that force-feeding the patient either through a tube or by means of supervised meals until the goal weight is obtained, even in conjunction with the best psychiatric care, often results in the immediate reloss of the weight gained and noncompliance with follow-up recommendations.[60,99,100] Increasingly, the recommendation is to hospitalize the patient for stabilization and attainment of at least 70% of recommended body weight but then to discharge the patient to outpatient follow-up, where the patient can have more control over recovery and learn to deal with a normal environment.

The primary nutritional danger with inpatient treatment of the severely emaciated anorexic patient is refeeding syndrome. This syndrome is characterized by severe hypophosphatemia, hypokalemia, hypomagnesemia, hyperglycemia, and marked fluid shifts.[93,97,101] Refeeding syndrome occurs when the rate of feeding is too fast for the compromised metabolism and gastrointestinal system. In anorexia, gastric motility, gastric emptying, intestinal surface area, and the levels of brushborder enzymes are all decreased.[101] Therefore, repletion should begin at a kilocalorie level that is 10 to 20% below the calculated Harris-Benedict estimation of BEE using the patient's actual body weight.[93] This value is usually 800 to 1000 kcal/day. The initial protein recommendation is 0.8 to 0.9 g/kg actual body weight. Repletion should also begin with less than full fluid and electrolyte needs. The intestinal tract, pancreas, and liver are restored within several days.[101] After this, circulatory volume, calories, and protein can be advanced slowly. Fluid status is best monitored through the blood pressure and pulse. Pulse should remain under 80 bpm in a previously dehydrated, bradycardic patient until fluids and electrolytes are stable. Kilocalories can be increased 100 to 200 kcal/day. Protein can be slowly increased to 1.2 to 1.5 g/kg, depending on serum albumin and total protein measurements. Electrolytes must be monitored daily. A vitamin and mineral supplement with additional thiamin and pyridoxal phosphate is recommended.

Outpatient Treatment

Because the energy cost of activity for an anorexic patient is higher than normal, all activity must be curtailed until a safer weight is reached.[94] Permitting an anorexic patient to exercise while attempting to gain weight only makes the process longer and, therefore, more painful. Given the anorexic patient's fear of food, if the calculated BEE is much more than their current intake, it is unlikely that the patient will be able to voluntarily ingest this basal amount initially. In this case, the nutritionist should set a starting calorie goal that is between current estimated intake and the BEE. Calorie levels can then be increased gradually in increments of 200 to 300 kcal every 4 to 7 days, depending on the patient's ability to tolerate increases, until a desirable initial level is reached.[27,84] Then, the rate of incremental increase can be slowed, recognizing that these patients are hypometabolic. Be aware that, in the beginning, weight gain is usually very rapid and primarily consists of retained fluid.[102]

It is necessary to remind the horrified patient (and yourself) that initial weight gain is a distorted reflection of intake and that a steady increase in intake really is necessary. Once safely above basal calories and past the initial gross weight fluctuation, weight gain goals of 0.5 to 1.0 lb/wk and kilocalorie increase increments of 100 kcal/wk are realistic. More rapid weight gain can rarely be tolerated and may be dangerous on an outpatient basis.[48] As weight gain progresses, weight maintenance will require higher than expected intakes until the metabolic rate normalizes.[60] Even though the BMR is depressed when a starving individual is resting, the energy cost of movement is above normal. The thermic effect of activity (TEA) increases because of the extra strain of activity by a compromised system.[94] The thermic effect of food (TEF) is also increased for the same reasons.[103] It is important that the patient understand that her body is in the process of readjustment. Unfortunately, recent research has shown that the metabolism of a person who has suffered from anorexia nervosa may never fully recover the last 3 to 5% of normal that was lost.[91,92,104]

Phase One. Realistically, increasing caloric intake may not be that easy. The patient may not be able to tolerate an increase of 300 kcal/wk. As long as weight is being gained consistently, smaller weekly increases are not contraindicated. To facilitate compliance, target a specific medical consequence of starvation such as amenorrhea, hypothermia, hair loss, or lack of concentration as a goal for correction through weight gain.[51] Choose the change that the patient is most concerned about. Often, a contract is needed. In the contract, an increase in activity level or some other desired outcome is made contingent on sufficient daily caloric intake assessed by a slow, steady weight gain. This contract may be revised at each appointment to reflect progress. If outpatient treatment continues one month without a satisfactory increase in weight or intake, hospitalization should again be considered.

During treatment, it is very important to have the patient record intake. This self-monitoring serves many purposes. For the patient, it encourages compliance and discourages back-sliding. For the clinician, it provides a concrete record that can aid with assessing progress, targeting problems, and directing treatment. However, the clinician must be aware that the patient may "lie" on their food record to please persons in authority positions. If this is suspected, bring up the observation that most people with an eating disorder do feel this way. Encourage the patient to talk about whether accurate food records can be kept.

Formulation of the diet prescription is individualized for patients. Some patients need rigorous prescriptions where foods are measured because of the sense of concreteness and control it gives them. In this case, a primary focus of subsequent prescriptions will be increasing variety and amount of acceptable foods. Other individuals require more freedom of choice for compliance. The diabetic exchange system works well with these patients.[105] Some common problems to be addressed include increasing numbers of exchanges, expanding variety, allowance of forbidden foods, consumption of regularly spaced meals including breakfast, and adequate intake of complex carbohydrate and fat. A multivitamin supplement should always be taken.

Phase Two. When the patient has achieved a safer weight (at least 80% of recommended weight), the issues of body image, nutrition education, and physical fitness must be addressed. Cognitive distortions about body image need to be challenged, emphasizing what is healthy for the patient as a unique individual in relation to height, weight, frame size, muscle mass, etc., rather than arbitrary numbers and comparison to peers. Nutrition education should focus on the variety of ways available to achieve a basic balanced diet and then how to make intelligent extra food choices to satisfy energy requirements. The benefits of moderate, consistent exercise should be discussed and encouraged for normalization of metabolic rate, better weight distribution, and improved muscle, pulmonary, and cardiac function. However, the contract can allow this only in relation to adequate caloric intake and continued weight gain. Be aware that there are universal "milestones"—points in recovery at which all patients seem to have an especially hard time.[106] These are at the 10-lb marks and at 100 lb in particular. Be patient at these times, and let the patient know that you understand. A final caution is to watch for signs of the onset of bulimia as weight increases, a phenomenon that occurs in approximately 50% of recovering anorexic patients.[99,100,107]

Bulimia Nervosa

Normalization of eating habits and cessation of purging behavior are the main goals in the nutritional management of bulimia. Bulimic patients are usually in a safer weight range, so weight is a secondary issue—at least to the clinician. Weight and appearance are very important issues to the patient. Even though the young woman is almost without fail very attractive and well proportioned, she sees herself as fat and unattractive.[27,108] Remaining sensitive to this low self-esteem when the patient looks perfectly normal is a challenge.

Hospitalization

Most bulimic patients should be treated on an outpatient basis. There is usually no medical reason for inpatient treatment, and removing her from the environmental stressors that trigger the binge/purge cycles only helps temporarily. When she is returned to this stressful environment, bulimia reappears.[19] However, self-harm, vomiting many times every day (e.g., more than 30 times a week), extreme laxative abuse (e.g., 20 to 30 tablets every day), and concomitant ethanol or drug abuse are all reasons for an initial hospitalization for tapering or withdrawal so that only one main diagnosis needs to be addressed on an outpatient basis. The presence of a severe personality disorder is also a reason for initial hospitalization as, unrestrained, the manipulation and splitting that are characteristic of these personality disorders can sabotage outpatient treatment. Electrolyte imbalance can occur repeatedly in up to 50% of bulimic patients.[109] Whether this is cause for hospitalization depends on the severity of the imbalance. These imbalances can be so slight as to go undetected, or they can cause dizziness, arrhythmias, or seizures.[51,110,111] If dizziness, unexplained rapid pulse, heart palpitations, or fainting occurs, the patient needs to be evaluated by a physician to determine if hospitalization to stabilize the electrolytes is necessary. A bulimic patient is often self-referred and very disturbed about her illness, so she is more amenable to admission if it is deemed necessary.

Motivation

Because bulimia is often associated with impulsiveness, which is played out in constantly considering but never committing to treatment, it is important to capitalize on the crisis that led the individual to seek help. What is her motivation to change? Was electrolyte imbalance so profound that the added dehydration from exercise caused her to pass out? Is needing to stay near a bathroom due to laxative use interfering with her ability to function? Are her teeth going to cost a fortune to repair due to the constant contact with stomach acid from vomiting? It is important to have these details right because you may need to remind the patient of this situation to keep her in treatment 2 weeks later.

Weaning from Purgative Behaviors

The underlying fear of fatness, body image distortion, and preoccupation with body size also found in bulimia make refocusing the patient's concern onto her health difficult. Remember that the patient is bingeing and, if normal weight, is rarely at risk for malnutrition. It is the purging behavior that can be medically compromising. Try to control this first even though bingeing may be more upsetting to the patient. Constantly but gently remind the patient of the adverse effects and lack of effectiveness of purging. Vomiting causes loss of dental enamel and consequent caries, esophageal tears, and bleeding due to contact with stomach acid, gastric inflammation and swelling, electrolyte imbalance that may lead to cardiac arrhythmia or seizure, and occasional death due to myocardial infarction or aspiration of vomitus.[112] Furthermore, most calories are usually absorbed during the binge, with the absorption dependent on the composition of the binge. Carbohydrates are rapidly metabolized by the body, and depending on the length of time before the patient purges, all these calories may be absorbed.[113] Gently point out to the patient that she is not achieving her purpose.

Laxatives cause electrolyte imbalance, dehydration, constipation, abdominal cramping, bloating, and a flaccid bowel.[112] There are many types of laxatives: bulk-forming, stimulants, saline-based, hyperosmotics, stool softeners, lubricants, and carbon dioxide-releasing agents (Table 3-4). The phenolphthalein-containing stimulants (e.g., Ex-lax) are the type used most often in bulimia.[114] They function by stimulating the myenteric plexus to enhance the secretion of water and electrolytes into the bowel and inhibit the colon from resorbing water.[115] Therefore, they only affect fluid retention not calorie absorption. Laxatives have been shown to eliminate only about 12% of calories consumed.[75,114] Stress the fact that the weight fluctuations that the patient finds so upsetting are loss and retention of fluid. Although laxatives can be withdrawn "cold turkey" without medical sequela, tapering laxative usage is usually easier and more successful. A schedule is drawn up decreasing laxative use by whatever consistent amount the patient can tolerate, anywhere from 2 to 10 per week, and contracts are written accordingly. When daily laxative usage is very high, more than 50 per day, push for a decrease of at least 5 per week. Make sure electrolytes are being checked periodically. During withdrawal, it is important to stress adequate fluid, moderate exercise, and increased fiber to promote the natural function of the bowel. Decreasing or arresting purge behavior, particularly oral laxative abuse, is going to produce fluid retention, constipation, and bloating much like the initial reversal of starvation in anorexia.[102] If the patient cannot tolerate the constipation and it is sabotaging the tapering process, a mild bulking agent may be used.[114]

How well patients tolerate the small weight gain that is usually associated with initial recovery from bulimia is a good prognostic indicator. Patients will want to be put on a diet to control the discomfort and avoid weight gain. It is important to discourage this and yet be sensitive to the fact that bulimic patients often have a stockier build or a history of a chubby childhood. Bulimia may have allowed them to be a fashionable weight for the first time. Because a history of heaviness may indicate a naturally higher weight due to genetic predisposition, many bulimic patients' metabolism has slowed somewhat to allow them to maintain their lower weights. Retaining the calories they normally purge will tend to increase their weights back toward their premorbid weights.[95,116] The estimated metabolic decrease that typically results from bulimia is 10 to 15% on the average, with a range of 5 to 35%.[51] Therefore, the target energy level should be adjusted for a lowered metabolism as if the patient were more sedentary than she is.[19] Recovering bulimic patients need an average of 25 to 28 kcal/kg/day to maintain weight versus normal controls, who need an average of 30 to 32 kcal/kg/day.[60] Bulimic patients who have a history of anorexia nervosa are the exception. They may require slightly more kilocalories to maintain normal weight than the average.

Introduction of Healthy Eating Behaviors

Concomitant with the above emphasis on purging cessation, it is important to work toward healthy eating habits in the same manner. Factual nutrition and phys-

Table 3-4 Common Nonprescription Laxatives

Type	Mechanism	Mode	Speed	Actions	Kinds
Can be dangerous if taken in excess					
Stimulants	Increases stool's bulk and water content	Mouth or Rectal	6–12 hr / 15–60 min	Addictive / Excessive fluid loss	Aloe / Biscodyl / Cascara / Castor Oil / Phenolphthalein / Senna
Saline	Draws water into the bowel	Mouth or Rectal	1–6 hr / 2–15 min	Contraindicated if kidney disease	Mg salt / PO_4 salt / Tartar
Stool softeners	Penetrates and softens stool	Mouth or Rectal	12–72 hr / 2–15 min	Interferes with nutrient absorption	Sulfosuccinate / Ducosate
Generally regarded as safe					
Bulk-forming	Increases stool's volume and water content	Mouth	12–72 hr	Requires additional water	Bran / Cellulose / Gum / Psyllium
Lubricants	Makes fecal matter slippery	Mouth or Rectal	6–8 hr / 2–15 min	None	Mineral oil
Hyperosmotic	Increases water content of stool	Rectal	15–60 min	Similar to saline but no side effects	Glycerin sorbitol
CO_2-releasing	Creates gentle pressure	Rectal	5–30 min	None	Suppository

Source: Reprinted with permission. *Physician's Desk Reference for Nonprescription Drugs.* Copyright 1993. Oradell, NJ: Medical Economics Company.

ical fitness education about the "bottom-line" needs of the human body should be provided. The target calorie level will be approached over time from a level that the patient can tolerate without feeling deprived while she works on the cessation of the purging process. Remember that the term *binge* may not mean the same thing to the patient as it does to you. In Beglin and Fairburn's study, bulimic patients rated the sense of loss of control as the most important characteristic in defining a binge.[69] In this same study, bulimic patients defined a "large amount of food" as ranging from just one candy bar to more than 3000 calories in one sitting. Recognize that this means what a normal person would consider an occasional treat, a candy bar, is a cardinal sin to a bulimic patient. She may need to keep these foods "off-limits" in her mind at the beginning of treatment. In fact, usually one of the last things a bulimic patient in recovery is able to do is allow herself to eat a small amount of sweets without guilt. Because the patient is afraid of this uncontrolled eating, the thought of increasing food intake outside of bingeing is terrifying. Initially, the patient may not be able to handle more than contracting to eat an orange or a few carrots at a specific time each day without purging them. This is acceptable. If the patient can succeed at this, foods can be added gradually until she is retaining a normal number of calories. The patient needs tremendous amounts of encouragement and the allowance to fail in making these small steps toward better nutrition.

Strategies

In setting goals with this population, use a very logical approach. Some researchers suggest approaching the behavior as a problem to be solved with repetitive use of the following steps: identify problems; target the problem that the patient is most motivated to work on; list all possible solutions; choose a particular solution to attempt; and devise a procedure for implementation.[19,108] This method gives the patient a consistent, factual piece of ammunition against her impulses. Large goals such as cessation of purging and resumption of a three-meals-per-day eating pattern can be set for "sometime in the future," but subgoals need to be small—something that can be attained on a weekly basis.

Self-monitoring will help identify the pieces of the problem. Records should be kept of how much of what was eaten when and where. Thoughts and feelings both before and after as well as the circumstances surrounding the eating episode will prove informative. As treatment progresses, it may be useful to graph the patient's binge/purge cycles, weight, meal frequency, and exercise to track problems, progress, and treatment direction.

Once a problem is identified, solutions can be found and ranked for practicality. Then, the most pragmatic solution can be selected and a contract written (Exhibit 3-9).[117–121] The proper use of these techniques requires extensive training.

Exhibit 3-9 Cognitive-Behavioral Techniques

Response tapering: patient contracts over time to incrementally decrease the frequency of a purging behavior

Response delay: patient contracts over time to incrementally delay the occurrence of the purging behavior for a longer amount of time

Stimulus control: patient attempts to positively change the environment in such a way that a "trigger" for bingeing is no longer present or reduced in intensity

Distraction: patient recognizes the emotional state that produces a binge/purge cycle and diverts herself with another activity

Support networking: "cry for help" is made to a professional or an involved friend to avoid the behavior

Relaxation: patient uses learned relaxation techniques to consciously lower the anxiety level that produces a binge

Sublimation: patient replaces the binge/purge cycle with an agreed on healthier coping mechanism

Visualization: patient forms a specific mental image of handling the threat of a binge/purge cycle and then follows through on this scenario

Response-prevention: patient is presented with a "trigger" food or another binge/purge-producing situation in the presence of the therapist and prevented from handling the "test" by bingeing and/or purging

Reframing: patient is taught to "catch" a negative thought sequence as it starts and remodel it into a more positive thought sequence

---

Prognosis

Recovery from an eating disorder depends on patients' readiness to give up their preoccupation with food, weight, and body image and get on with the rest of their lives. However, even with a motivated patient, therapy is a long-term complex process that takes a great deal of patience and honesty on the parts of both the clinician and the patient. It is essential to take the time to establish rapport with the patient, understanding where she is coming from and the speed at which she is capable of going toward wellness. Open communication must be maintained between members of the therapy team to coordinate the direction of treatment and avoid manipulation during this process. Even in the best of circumstances, without comorbidity and within a supportive environment, a minimum of 16 weeks of focused short-term therapy is required. With any complicating factor, a full year of psychological and behavioral treatment is recommended.[19,27]

Follow-up studies[99,107,122–124] of anorexia nervosa report these approximate statistics: (1) essential recovery in 20 to 25% of cases; (2) persistent eating and weight difficulties in addition to continued psychological problems in 20 to 30%

of cases; (3) recurrent mood and behavior disorders (e.g., depression, bulimia, obsessive-compulsive disease) at a normal body weight in 20 to 30% of cases; and (4) chronic, intractable anorexia in 20 to 25% of cases. Chronic anorexia shortens the lifespan and can be fatal at any point in the disease process. Estimates of deaths, usually due to cardiac complications or renal failure, range from 2 to 20% of cases.[40,122] Poor prognostic indicators are comorbidity with depression or personality disorder, lower premorbid weight, concomitant purging, and continued environmental conflict.[125] A positive prognostic indicator was the anorexic patient's ability to leave home and form a partner relationship with a peer.[126]

Follow-up studies[127,128] on bulimia report these approximate statistics: (1) essential recovery in 30% of cases; (2) partial recovery or marked improvement in 45 to 50% of cases; and (3) chronic symptoms in 25% of cases. Poor prognostic indicators are increased frequency of purging, lower premorbid body weight, and presence of comorbidity (e.g., depression or personality disorder, as with anorexia).[127,129,130] Family environment was also a major factor in prognosis. Strong social support was predictive of recovery,[127] whereas continued conflict and control issues impeded progress in treatment.[131]

Concluding Remarks on Therapy Issues

Recovery is achieved in stages. From the outset, the patient, not the family or therapist, must be motivated for her to get well. If there is no motivation because the patient is too thin and her ability to reason is compromised, the first job of the therapy team is to correct this situation. Sometimes, even with the best of intentions and treatment, this fails. Allowing a patient to walk away from treatment when she is not ready to get well is very difficult, but it is the action that keeps the door open for the patient to return in the future. If there is motivation, you must resist the temptation to tell the patient everything you know to help her get better in the first few sessions. These are very intelligent, but very scared and unassertive, women. Let the patient set the pace and do the work.

You are one of the coaches. Your job is to keep the patient on track once the pace has been set. To do this, we would emphasize three characteristics you must develop to work well with these patients:

1. *Be consistent.* Keep your role defined as the nutritionist who is there to help her with her fear of food and lack of proper nutrition. If the patient brings up therapy issues during your session, be empathic but refer her back to her primary therapist. Keep a set weekly appointment time during which you work methodically and systematically on the patient's recovery.

2. *Be goal-directed.* The patient will have trouble breaking her illness down into steps toward wellness that she is able to take. Help the patient make sure her subgoals for herself are realistic, incremental, achievable, and measurable. If in doubt, set your sights lower rather than higher; consistent, progressive success is the desired end result. Record the subgoal and homework assignment for each week. Make sure you come back to them in the next session. This will send the message that you are serious about your work together and expect her to uphold her end of the bargain.

3. *Be nonjudgmental.* If the patient does not succeed in her subgoal, accept it, and concentrate immediately on examining why this happened and how the problem can be overcome. The patient has been taught that failure is not OK, but failure is part of life. You must model dealing with failure constructively for her so that she can continue to learn that it is OK and just another aspect of normal life.

Again, we encourage anyone interested in dealing with this population to become trained in psychology as well as nutrition. This population can be very emotionally draining if you have not built the defenses and acquired the arsenal of techniques necessary to work successfully with them. It can be very frustrating, but the rewards of steering a young person back toward good health and high self-esteem are well worth it.

CASE STUDIES

Case 1

Janey is in tenth grade. She is an A student, serves on Student Council, sings in chorus and the church choir, takes piano and dance lessons, and is very active in Future Leaders of America. Everything is always under control, done on time, and "by the book." But something is wrong. Janey does not "hang out" with friends after school. She is not interested in boys. She does not even come to the cafeteria at lunch-time to hear the latest gossip—and she does not eat. The latest baggy fashions hide exactly how much weight she has lost, but you know it is a lot because you can see it in her face. Her smile is brittle as if her face may crack. Her laugh is forced, and her eyes often look empty, hollow as if Janey is far away. If someone expresses concern and offers her half their sandwich, Janey will either politely decline or "pick at it" for a while and then cram it into the ledge under the table when she thinks no one is looking. Janey will always say that she is doing fine but seems driven to study or practice or "work" on something all the time. Janey has anorexia nervosa (restricting type).

Janey's self-monitoring instrument might show the following daily scenario. She had 1 measured oz of dry 100% fiber cereal for breakfast. Lunch was skipped on several days. On the days that she ate lunch, it consisted of one slice of low-fat cheese on one slice of diet bread with mustard and exactly six carrot sticks. She jogged 4 to 5 miles at a slow pace every day after school. She expressed feelings of guilt on the days that her run did not take a full hour because she would then worry whether she had burned up all her food for that day. This fear would result in skipping lunch the subsequent day. Dinner was required to be eaten with the family at Janey's house. Janey described her feelings at dinner as anxious because "everyone is watching what I eat." She reported taking one small serving of each item that her mother cooked. For example, one evening she ate one chicken leg with the skin removed, the smallest baked potato (of which she ate the skin, not the starchy inside), and one spoonful of peas (some of which she probably managed to drop on the floor on the way to her mouth). She recorded drinking several 2-liter bottles of diet caffeinated soda after school and throughout the evenings.

Janey is 162.5 cm (64 in.) tall, which is assumed to be her adult height as menarche occurred at age 12 years. Until recently, she had weighed 61.3 kg (135 lb). Over the past 5 months, her weight has dropped to 40.0 kg (88 lb), which is 73% of IBW for her small frame, 54.5 kg (120 lb). Usual recommended calorie intake is approximately 1800 kcal/day to maintain a normal weight. The weight loss depresses the BMR to approximately 1000 kcal/day. The increased energy demand of the 5-mile jog raises the EEN to 1300 to 1400 kcal/day. However, intake has been less than 500 kcal/day. In this case, the initial calorie level would be set at 750 kcal/day and increase 100 to 200 kcal/day until the expected basal calorie needs are met. The food would be given in six small feedings as Janey's stomach cannot tolerate large volumes at once. Ideally, over the course of the next 3 weeks, the kilocalorie level would be increased 300 kcal/wk to 1900 kcal/day, at which Janey should be gaining approximately 0.5 kg/wk. As she recovers, the calories needed for continued weight gain will increase to 2400 to 2500 kcal/day and may reach more than 3000 kcal/day dependent on the amount and type of exercise she is allowed. When weight stabilizes, BMR, TEA, and TEF will all normalize to some extent; maintenance calories are estimated at 1900 to 2100 kcal/day.

Case 2

Sally is a sophomore at the state university. In high school, she was the class secretary, the homecoming queen, a member of two winning varsity teams, and an A/B student. Now she feels lost in a sea of unfamiliar faces where all the other girls are prettier than she is, the athletes are better than she could ever hope to be even if all she did was practice sports, and she is a number, not the star pupil, in her academic classes. She joined a sorority and a school organization to try to fit in, but it seems to have made matters worse. She feels as if she is expected to be the perfect sorority sister and organization member yet still take care of her appearance, stay in shape, and keep her grades up. On the surface, it seems as if Sally is doing just that, but those few who know her well suspect otherwise. She has been moody; happy-go-lucky one day, then sad and withdrawn the next. Her room-mate notices that she stays up very late at night and spends a lot of time in the bathroom. Her "big-sister" thinks she parties too hard on the weekend, then runs herself ragged during the week to get her work done. When confronted, she is either defensive, admits to bouts of depression over "how does everyone else do it?" or may, with relief, admit to having bulimia nervosa.

Sally's self-monitoring instrument might show the following alternate daily scenario. Sally awoke every morning with a firm resolve to "make up for yester-day." She avoided breakfast and lunch by drinking diet soda, chewing sugarless gum, and staying around people. Each day in the beginning of the week she made it to "gym time" without any food, recording her feelings as "good." She allowed herself an "energy bar" before exercising to motivate herself to work out harder. After an hour on the stair-machine, she had a salad and a baked potato for dinner with her friends at the sorority house. Each evening, she consumed more diet soda and chewing gum while she studied until the wee hours of the morning. Each evening, however, the time at which she recorded starting to binge became progressively earlier until, on Thursday, she stayed downtown alone and ate an entire pizza for dinner before returning to the sorority house. The recorded content of the binges was very vague (i.e., part of a box of cookies, a lot of ice cream, etc.), and purging was indicated by an asterisk beside the food rather than filling out the appropriate column. Feelings in the evening were completely avoided.

Sally is 167.6 cm (66 in.), which is her adult height. Her weight fluctuates between 64 to 68 kg (140 to 155 lb) depending on the time of day in relation to her fast/binge/purge cycle. Sally bemoans these weight fluctuations as "a con-stant fight with the same 10 to 15 lb of fat" because her weight was a constant 65 kg (143 lb) in high school. She now thinks that even that is too heavy and that she should weigh the 59 kg (130 lb) that she was told was the ideal weight for her height by her sorority sisters. In reality, these weight fluctuations are fluid shifts; they also occurred (to a lesser degree) in high school; and her weight is essen-tially unchanged. A recommended weight range for Sally, given her medium frame and greater than average muscle mass, is 62 to 68.5 kg (136 to 151 lb). The notion of 59 kg (130 lb) must be discredited emphatically. Usual recommended calorie intake would be 1900 to 2100 kcal/day with her activity level. Due to the daily bulimic cycle, intake recommendations would be decreased 10% to 1700 to 1900 kcal/day. However, actual intake has fluctuated anywhere from 500 to 3000 kcal/day. In this case, an initial target calorie level may or may not be set. The general goal would be to get Sally to eat something during the day so that she is not physically starved each evening. Sally may start with a bagel for breakfast and an apple for lunch. Ideally, over the course of the next few months, the amount eaten during the day would increase, and the frequency of and the amount eaten during binges would decrease. Purging would also become less frequent. Weight should eventually stabilize around her usual weight in high school. Maintenance calorie level should stabilize at approximately 1700 to 1800 kcal/day. This value is calculated using the formula 925 kcal/day × BSA (here, BSA = 1.85) for a weight-stable patient.

REFERENCES

1. American Psychiatric Association. *Diagnostic and Statistical Manual of Mental Disorders*. 4th ed. Washington, DC: American Psychiatric Association; 1994.

2. Bruch H. Conceptual confusion in eating disorders. *J Nerv Ment Dis*. 1961;133:46–54.

3. Fukagawa N. Eating disorders: diagnosis and management. *Semin Pediatr Gastroenterol Nutr*. 1992;3:1–2.

4. Halmi K, Casper R, Eckert E, Goldberg S, Davis J. Unique features associated with age of onset of anorexia nervosa. *Psychiatry Res*. 1979;1:209–215.

5. Bruch H. Four decades of eating disorders. In: Garner DM, Garfinkel P, eds. *Handbook of Psychotherapy for Anorexia Nervosa and Bulimia*. New York, NY: The Guilford Press; 1985.

6. Halmi K, Falk J, Schwartz E. Binge-eating and vomiting: a survey of a college population. *Psychol Med*. 1981;11:697–706.

7. Drewnowski A, Yee D, Krahn D. Bulimia in college women. *Am J Psychiatry*. 1988;145:753–755.

8. Carlat D, Camargo C. Review of bulimia nervosa in males. *Am J Psychiatry*. 1991;148:831–843.

9. Fairburn C, Cooper J. Self-induced vomiting and bulimia nervosa: an undetected problem. *BMJ*. 1982;284:1153–1155.

10. Hart K, Ollendick T. Prevalence of bulimia in working and university women. *Am J Psychiatry*. 1985;142:851–854.

11. McKenna M. *College Mental Health and Eating Disorders. Anorexia and Bulimia: New Theories and Current Treatment*. 1990: 98–108.

12. Fairburn C, Welch S, Hay P. The classification of recurrent overeating: the "binge eating disorder" proposal. *Int J Eating Disord*. 1993;13:155–159.

13. Spitzer R, Stunkard A, Yanovski S, et al. Binge eating disorder should be included in DSM-IV: a reply to Fairburn et al.'s "The classification of recurrent overeating: the binge eating disorder proposal." *Int J Eating Disord*. 1993;13:161–169.

14. Strober M. Family-genetic studies of eating disorders. *J Clin Psychiatry*. 1991;52:9–12.

15. Mitchell JE, Hatsukami D, Eckert ED, Pyle RL. Characteristics of 275 patients with bulimia. *Am J Psychiatry*. 1985;142:482–485.

16. Halmi K. Comorbidity of psychiatric diagnosis in anorexia nervosa. *Arch Gen Psychiatry*. 1991;48:712–718.

17. Rutherford J, McGuffin P, Katz R, Murray R. Genetic influences on eating attitudes in a normal female twin population. *Psychol Med*. 1993;23:425–436.

18. Holland A, Sicotte N, Treasure J. Anorexia nervosa: evidence for a genetic basis. *J Psychosom Res*. 1988;32:561–571.

19. Johnson C, Connors M. *The Etiology and Treatment of Bulimia Nervosa*. New York, NY: Basic Books; 1987.

20. Kassett J, Gershon E, Maxwell M, et al. Psychiatric disorders in the first-degree relatives of probands with bulimia nervosa. *Am J Psychiatry.* 1989;146:1468–1471.

21. Leibowitz S. The role of serotonin in eating disorders. *Drugs.* 1990;39:33–48.

22. Jimerson D, Lesem M, Hegg A, Brewerton T. Serotonin in human eating disorders. *Ann NY Acad Sci.* 1990;600:532–544.

23. Jimerson D, Lesem M, Kaye W, Hegg A, Brewerton T. Eating disorders and depression: is there a serotonin connection? *Biol Psychiatry.* 1990;28:443–454.

24. Lacey JH, Smith G. Bulimia nervosa: The impact of pregnancy on mother and baby. *Br J Psychiatry.* 1987;150:777–781.

25. Brinch M, Isager TK. Anorexia nervosa and motherhood: reproduction pattern and mothering behavior of 50 women. *Acta Psychiatr Scand.* 1988;77:611–617.

26. Minuchin S, Rosman B, Baker L. *Psychosomatic Families: Anorexia Nervosa in Context*. Cambridge, Mass: Harvard University Press; 1978.

27. Garner DM, Garfinkel PE. *Handbook of Psychotherapy for Anorexia Nervosa and Bulimia*. New York, NY: The Guilford Press; 1985.

28. Schwartz R, Barrett M, Saba G. Family therapy for bulimia. In: Garner D, Garfinkel P, eds. *Handbook of Psychotherapy for Anorexia Nervosa and Bulimia*. New York, NY: The Guilford Press; 1985.

29. Stein A, Fairburn C. Children of mothers with bulimia nervosa. *BMJ.* 1989;299:777–778.

30. Abraham S, Carroll M, Najjar M, Fulwood R. *Obese and Overweight Adults in the United States*. National Center for Health Statistics, Public Health Service, U.S. Department of Health and Human Services; 1983.

31. Garner D, Garfinkel P, Schwartz D, Thompson M. Cultural expectations of thinness in women. *Psychol Rep.* 1980;47:483–491.

32. Wiseman C, Gray J, Mosimann J, Ahrens A. Cultural expectations of thinness in women: an update. *Int J Eating Disord.* 1992;11:85–89.

33. Nylander I. The feeling of being fat and dieting in a school population: epidemiological interview investigation. *Acta Socio-med Scand.* 1971;3:17–26.

34. Storz N, Greene W. Body weight, body image and perception of fad diets in adolescent girls. *JNE.* 1983;15:15–18.

35. Moore D. Body image and eating behavior in adolescent girls. *AJDC.* 1988;142:1114–1118.

36. Lucas A. Towards the understanding of anorexia nervosa as a disease entity. *Mayo Clin Proc.* 1981;56:254–264.

37. Ploog D. The importance of physiologic, metabolic, and endocrine studies for the understanding of anorexia nervosa. In: Pirke KM, Ploog D, eds. *The Psychobiology of Anorexia Nervosa*. Berlin: Springer-Verlag; 1984:1–4.

38. Williamson D. *Assessment of Eating Disorders: Obesity, Anorexia and Bulimia Nervosa*. New York, NY: Pergamon Press; 1990.

39. Bray G. Definition, measurement, and classification of the syndrome of obesity. *Int J Obes.* 1978;2:99–112.

40. Haller E. Eating disorders: a review. *West J Med.* 1992;157:658–662.

41. Kerr J, Skok R, McLauglin T. Characteristics common to females who exhibit anorexic or bulimic behavior: a review of current literature. *J Clin Psychol.* 1991;47:846–853.

42. Brownell K. The yo-yo trap. *Am Health.* 1988;3:78–84.

43. Brownell K. Metabolic effects of repeated weight loss and regain in adolescent wrestlers. *JAMA.* 1988;260:47–50.

44. Garfinkel P, Moldofsky H, Garner D. The heterogeneity of anorexia nervosa. *Arch Gen Psychiatry.* 1980;37:1036–1040.

45. Kaplan A, Woodside D. Biological aspects of anorexia nervosa and bulimia nervosa. *J Consult Clin Psychol.* 1987;55:645–653.

46. Highet R. Athletic amenorrhea. An update on aetiology, complications and management. *Sports Med.* 1989;7:82–108.

47. Brownell K, Greenwood M, Stellar E, Shrager E. The effects of repeated cycles of weight loss and regain in rats. *Physiol Behav.* 1986;38:459–464.

48. Pertschuk MJ, Crosby LO, Mullen JL. Nonlinearity of weight gain and nutrition intake in anorexia nervosa. In: Darby PL, Garfinkel PE, Garner CM, Coscina DV, eds. *Anorexia Nervosa: Recent Developments in Research.* New York, NY: Alan R. Liss; 1983:301–310.

49. Keys A, Brozek J, Henschel A, Mickelsen O, Taylor H. *The Biology of Human Starvation.* Minneapolis, Minn: University of Minnesota Press; 1950.

50. Comerci G. Medical complications of anorexia nervosa and bulimia nervosa. *Med Clin North Am.* 1990;74:1293–1309.

51. Kaplan AS. Biomedical variables in the eating disorders. *Can J Psychiatry.* 1990;35:745–753.

52. Van Binsbergen C, Hulshof K, Wedel M, Odink J, Coelingh-Bennink H. Food preferences and aversions and dietary pattern in anorexia nervosa patients. *Eur J Clin Nutr.* 1988;42:671–678.

53. Gwirtsman H, Kaye W, Curtis S, Lyter L. Energy intake and dietary macronutrient content in women with anorexia nervosa and volunteers. *J Am Diet Assoc.* 1989;89:54–57.

54. Moreiras-Varela O, Nunez C, Carbajal A, Morande G. Nutritional status and food habits assessed by dietary intake and anthropometrical parameters in anorexia nervosa. *Int J Vitam Nutr Res.* 1990;60:267–274.

55. Thibault L, Roberge A. The nutritional status of subjects with anorexia nervosa. *Int J Vitam Nutr Res.* 1987;57:447–452.

56. Bakan R, Birmingham C, Aeberhardt L, Goldner E. Dietary zinc intake of vegetarian and non-vegetarian patients with anorexia nervosa. *Int J Eating Disord.* 1993;13:229–233.

57. Gwirtsman H, Kaye W, Obarzanek K, et al. Decrease caloric intake in normal-weight patients with bulimia: comparison with female volunteers. *Am J Clin Nutr.* 1989;49:86–92.

58. Walsh BT, Kissileff HR, Cassidy SM, Dantzic S. Eating behavior of women with bulimia. *Arch Gen Psychiatry.* 1989;46:54–58.

59. Abraham SF, Beumont PJV. How patients describe bulimia or binge eating. *Psychol Med.* 1982;12:625–635.

60. Weltzin TE, Fernstrom MH, Hansen D, McConaha C, Kaye WH. Abnormal caloric requirements for weight maintenance in patients with anorexia and bulimia nervosa. *Am J Psychiatry.* 1991;148:1675–1682.

61. Johnson C. Diagnostic survey for eating disorders. Appendix to initial consultation for patients with bulimia and anorexia nervosa. In: Garner DM, Garfinkel PE, eds. *Handbook of Psychotherapy for Anorexia Nervosa and Bulimia.* New York, NY: The Guilford Press; 1985.

62. Garner D, Garfinkel P. The eating attitudes test: an index of the symptoms of anorexia nervosa. *Psychol Med.* 1979;9:273–279.

63. Garner D, Olmsteard M, Polivy J. The development and validation of a multidimensional eating disorders inventory of anorexia nervosa and bulimia. *Int J Eating Disord.* 1983;2:15–35.

64. Cooper Z, Fairburn CG. The eating disorder examination: a semi-structured interview for the assessment of the specific psychopathology of eating disorders. *Int J Eating Disord.* 1987;6:1–8.

65. Garner D, Garfinkel P. Body image in anorexia nervosa: measurement, theory and clinical implications. *Int J Psychiatry Med.* 1981;11:263–284.

66. Williamson D, Davis C, Goreczny A, Blouin D. Body image disturbances in bulimia nervosa: influences of actual body size. *J Abnorm Psychol.* 1989;98:97–99.

67. Gottesman E, Caldwell W. The body-image identification test: a quantitative projective technique to study an aspect of body image. *J Gen Psychol.* 1966;108:19–33.

68. Beumont P, Chambers T, Rouse L. The diet composition and nutritional knowledge of patients with anorexia nervosa. *J Hum Nutr.* 1981;35:265–273.

69. Beglin SJ, Fairburn CG. What is meant by the term "binge"? *Am J Psychiatry.* 1992;149:123–124.

70. Walsh B. Diagnostic criteria for the eating disorders in DSM-IV: work in progress. *Int J Eating Disord.* 1992;11:301–304.

71. Bruch H. Family background in eating disorders. In: Anthony E, Koupernik C, eds. *The Child in His Family.* New York, NY: John Wiley & Sons; 1970.

72. Lucas A. "Pigging Out." *JAMA.* 1982;247:82–93.

73. Kissileff HR, Walsh BT, Kral JG, Cassidy SM. Laboratory studies of eating behavior in women with bulimia. *Physiol Behav.* 1986;38:563–570.

74. Kaye W, Weltzin T, Hsu L, McConaha C, Bolton B. Amount of calories retained after binge eating and vomiting. *Am J Psychiatry.* 1993;150:969–971.

75. BoLinn GW, Santa Ana CA, Morawski SG, Fordtran JS. Purging and calorie absorption in bulimic patients and normal women. *Ann Intern Med.* 1983;99:14–17.

76. Grant A, DeHoog S. *Nutritional Assessment and Support.* Seattle, Wash: Northgate Station; 1985.

77. Actuaries Society, Association of Life Insurance Medical Directors of America, 1. Metropolitan Height and Weight Tables. *Stat Bull.* 1983.

78. Hamill P, Drizd T, Johnson C, et al. Physical growth: National Center for Health Statistics percentiles. *Am J Clin Nutr.* 1979;32:607–629.

79. Tanner J, Whitehouse R. Clinical longitudinal standards for height, weight, height velocity, and weight velocity, and the stages of puberty. *Arch Dis Child.* 1976;51:170–179.

80. Gibson R. *Principles of Nutrition Assessment.* New York, NY: Oxford University Press; 1990.

81. Siervogel R, Roche A, Himes J, Chumlea W, McCammon R. Subcutaneous fat distribution in males and females from 1 to 39 years of age. *Am J Clin Nutr.* 1982;36:162–171.

82. Jelliffe DB. *The Assessment of the Nutritional Status of the Community Series.* Monograph. 1966;53:240.

83. Frisancho A. New standards of weight and body composition by frame size and height for assessment of nutritional status of adults and the elderly. *Am J Clin Nutr.* 1981;40:808–819.

84. Hooker C, Hall R. Nutritional assessment of patients with anorexia and bulimia; clinical and laboratory findings. *Psychiatr Med.* 1989;7:27–37.

85. Jackson A, Pollack M. Prediction accuracy of body density low body weight and total body volume equations. *Med Sci Sports.* 1977;9:197–201.

86. Jackson A, Pollack M, Ward A. Generalized equations for predicting body density of women. *J Sci Sports.* 1980;12:175–178.

87. Siri W. Body composition from fluid spaces and density. In: Brozek J, Honschel A, eds. *Techniques for Measuring Body Composition.* Washington, DC: National Academy of Sciences; 1961:223–224.

88. Brozek J, Grande F, Anderson J, Keys A. Densitometric analysis of body composition: revision of some quantitative assumptions. *Ann NY Acad Sci.* 1963;110:113–140.

89. Lohman T. Skinfolds and body density and their relation to body fatness: a review. *Hum Biol.* 1981;2:181–225.

90. Lohman T, Roche A, Martorell R. *Anthropometric Standardization Reference Manual.* Champagne, Ill: Human Kinetics Books; 1988.

91. Devlin J, Walsh B, Kral J, et al. Metabolic abnormalities in bulimia nervosa. *Arch Gen Psychiatry.* 1990;47:144–148.

92. Krahn D, Rock C, Dechert R, Nairn K, Hasse S. Changes in resting energy expenditure and body composition in anorexia nervosa patients during refeeding. *J Am Diet Assoc.* 1993;93:434–438.

93. Apovian CM, McMahon M, Bistrian BR. Guidelines for refeeding the marasmic patient. *Crit Care Med.* 1990;18:1030–1033.

94. Casper RC, Schoeller DA, Kushner R, Hnilicka J, Gold ST. Total daily energy expenditure and activity level in anorexia nervosa. *Am J Clin Nutr.* 1991;53:1143–1150.

95. Walker J, Roberts S, Halmi K, Golberg SC. Caloric requirements for weight gain in anorexia nervosa. *Am J Clin Nutr.* 1979;32:1396–1400.

96. Crawford J, Terry M, Rourke G. Simplification of drug dosage calculation by application of the surface area principle. *Pediatrics.* 1950;5:783–790.

97. Solomon SM, Kirby DF. The refeeding syndrome: a review. *JPEN.* 1990;14:90–97.

98. Cueller RE, VanThiel DH. Gastrointestinal consequences of the eating disorders: anorexia nervosa and bulimia. *Am J Gastroenterol.* 1986;81:1113–1124.

99. Hall A, Slim E, Hawker F, Salmond C. Anorexia nervosa: long-term outcome in 50 female patients. *Br J Psychiatry.* 1984;145:407–413.

100. Beresin EV, Gordon C, Hergog DB. The process of recovering from anorexia nervosa. *J Am Acad Psychoanal.* 1989;17:103–130.

101. Havala T, Shronts E. Managing the complications associated with refeeding. *Nutr Clin Prac.* 1990;5:23–29.

102. Comeric GD. Fluid and electrolyte and drug therapy considerations in the management of eating disorders. *Semin Adolesc Med.* 1986;2:37–46.

103. Vaisman N, Rossi MF, Corey M, et al. Effect of refeeding on the energy metabolism of adolescent girls who have anorexia nervosa. *Eur J Clin Nutr.* 1991;45:527–537.

104. Apfelbaum MB, Lacatis D. Effect of calorie restriction and excessive caloric intake on energy expenditure. *Am J Clin Nutr.* 1971;24:1405–1409.

105. American Dietetic Association. *Handbook of Clinical Dietetics.* New Haven, Conn: Yale University Press; 1992.

106. Garfinkel P, Garner D. *Anorexia Nervosa: A Multidimensional Perspective.* New York, NY: Brunner/Mazel; 1982.

107. Crisp AH. Treatment and outcome in anorexia nervosa. In: Goldstein RK, ed. *Eating and Weight Disorders: Advances in Treatment and Research.* New York, NY: Springer; 1983:203–233.

108. Agras WS. *Eating Disorders: Management of Obesity, Bulimia, and Anorexia Nervosa.* New York, NY: Pergamon Press; 1987.

109. Mitchell J, Bantle J. Metabolic and endocrine investigating in women of normal weight with the bulimic syndrome. *Biol Psychol.* 1983;18:355–365.

110. Palla B, Litt I. Medical complications of eating disorders in adolescents. *Pediatrics.* 1988;81:613–623.

111. Hall RCW, Beresford TP. Medical complications of anorexia and bulimia. *Psychol Med.* 1989;7:164–192.

112. Hofland SL, Dardis PO. Bulimia nervosa: associated physical problems. *J Psychosoc Nurs.* 1992;30:23–27.

113. Murray R, Granner D, Mayes P, Rodwell V. *Harper's Biochemistry.* 22nd ed. Norwalk, Conn: Appleton & Lange; 1990.

114. Vann JR, Saylor KE. Laxative abuse: a hazardous habit for weight control. *College Health.* 1989;37:227–230.

115. *Physician's Desk Reference for Nonprescription Drugs.* Oradell, NJ: Medical Economics Co; 1993.

116. Lacey JH, Gibson E. Does laxative abuse control body weight? A comparative study of purging and vomiting bulimics. *Hum Nutr Appl Nutr.* 1985;39:36–42.

117. Beck A. *Cognitive Therapy in Clinical Practice: An Illustrative Casebook.* New York, NY: Routledge Press; 1989.

118. Freeman A, Greenwood V. *Cognitive Therapy: Applications in Psychiatric and Medical Settings.* New York, NY: Human Sciences Press; 1987.

119. Freeman A, Simon K, Buetler L, Arkowitz H. *Comprehensive Handbook of Cognitive Therapy.* New York, NY: Plenum Press; 1989.

120. Kalodner C, DeLucia J. The individual and combined effects of cognitive therapy and nutrition education as additions to a behavior modification program for weight loss. *Addict Behav.* 1991;16:255–263.

121. Stern R, Drummond L. *The Practice of Behavioral and Cognitive Psychotherapy.* Cambridge: Cambridge University Press; 1991.

122. Theander S. Outcome and prognosis in anorexia nervosa and bulimia: some results of previous investigations, compared with those of a Swedish long-term study. *J Psychiatr Res.* 1985;19:493–508.

123. Toner B, Garfinkel P, Garner D. Long term follow-up of anorexia nervosa. *Psychosom Med.* 1986;48:520–529.

124. Jarman F, Rickards W, Hudson I. Late adolescent outcome of early onset anorexia nervosa. *J Paediatr Child Health.* 1991;27:221–227.

125. Banas A, Januszkiewicz-Grabias A. An attempt to formulate prognosis for anorexia nervosa on the basis of follow-up data. *Psychiatr Pol.* 1992;26:483–489.

126. Hentze M, Engel K. Prognostic factors for long-term survival in anorexia nervosa. *Z Klin Psych Psychopathol Psychother.* 1991;39:173–181.

127. Fahy T, Russell G. Outcome and prognostic variables in bulimia nervosa. *Int J Eating Disord.* 1993;14:135–145.

128. Johnson-Sabine E, Reiss D, Dayson D. Bulimia nervosa: a 5-year follow-up study. *Psychol Med.* 1992;22:951–959.

129. Olmsted M, Kaplan A, Rockert W. Rate and prediction of relapse in bulimia nervosa. *Am J Psychiatry.* 1994;151:738–743.

130. Steiger H, Leung F, Thibaudeau J, Houle L. Prognostic utility of subcomponents of the borderline personality construct in bulimia nervosa. *Br J Clin Psychol.* 1993;32:187–197.

131. Blouin J, Carter J, Blouin A, et al. Prognostic indicators in bulimia nervosa treated with cognitive-behavioral group therapy. *Int J Eating Disord.* 1994;15:113–123.

4

❧

Food Consumption Patterns in Women

Pamela S. Haines

Each society develops particular foodways through which food is acquired and consumed. In the United States, women have traditionally assumed much of the responsibility for food acquisition activities for both themselves and the family. To understand what women of the year 2000 will be eating, it is important to consider the wide range of factors that have influenced food consumption patterns of women over time.

Food consumption patterns of U.S. women today are determined by the environment in which food is selected, personal and cultural preferences, economic conditions, level of education, and frequently, conflicting personal goals and social roles. Although it remains true that food serves as a channel through which women can uniquely define their own place within the household and through which value and meaning are conveyed and received, the social, economic, and physical environments in which food decisions are made have changed dramatically over the years, and the food consumption patterns of women reflect these changes.

FOOD CONSUMPTION DETERMINANTS IN WOMEN

A conceptual framework that includes both environmental and individual behavior perspectives to describe food consumption patterns is illustrated by the 1989 report of the ad hoc Expert Panel on Nutrition Monitoring (Figure 4-1)[1]. This theoretical model examines the relationships between determinants of food choice, food and nutrient intakes, and nutritional and health status outcomes in one general conceptual model.

Many economic, social, psychological, and cultural patterns contribute to the development, change, and maintenance of dietary intake patterns. No single discipline has been found that can adequately explain why people eat as they do.

NATIONAL FOOD SUPPLY → FOOD DISTRIBUTION → CONSUMPTION → NUTRIENT UTILIZATION → HEALTH OUTCOME

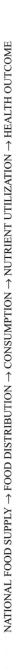

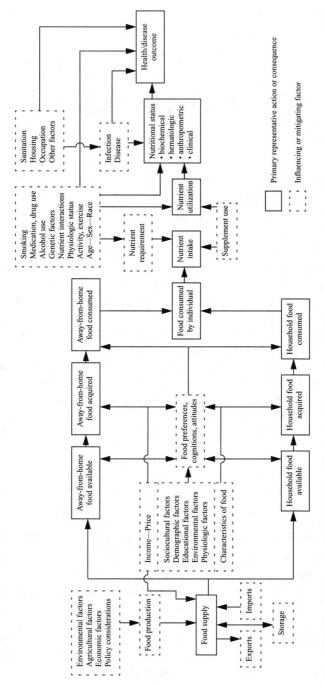

Figure 4-1 General Conceptual Model for Food Choice, Food and Nutrient Intake, and Nutritional Health Status *Source:* Reprinted from *An Update Report on Nutrition Monitoring,* US Department of Health and Human Services and US Department of Agriculture, DHHS Pub No 89-1255, September 1989.

Several chapters in this book expand on selected topics such as nutrition across the life cycle, eating disorders, pregnancy, vegetarianism—all conditions that influence the choices women make about what they eat. Some food intake determinants reviewed in this chapter include:

- food supply changes—How does the proliferation of new products and the growth of away-from-home food influence diet?
- demographic and socioeconomic—How do income and employment practices influence consumption patterns?
- access to and use of information—What is the impact of education on dietary practices? Where do consumers get information about diet, food, and health? How does the availability of information, per se, alter diet?
- perceived social roles—How do changing social roles influence food decisions of women?
- health attitudes, beliefs, and life style—How does the awareness of diet and health influence diet? How do life-style differences contribute to differences in dietary practices in women?

Impacts of a Changing Food Supply

One of the most significant demographic shifts over the past 50 years has been that the rate of population growth is declining and the population is growing older and living longer. The number of people 65 years and older is projected to more than double in the next 50 years, and an aging America will be more concerned about the availability of products to meet their special health needs. Due to differential birth rates and immigration, the ethnic mix of the U.S. population is changing, with the fastest growing ethnic groups being Hispanics and Asians.[2]

Sensitive to the marketing opportunities provided by demographic changes, the food industry has and is introducing foods targeted to particular segments of the population. Every year new food products are introduced, reflecting different packaging or applications of new food technologies to achieve some aspect of product differentiation, in terms of safety, cost, convenience, nutrition, or perishability.[3] In 1985, 5600 new food products were introduced, and in 1989, 9200 new products were on the market.[2]

The food industry has responded to the population-wide interest in improved nutrition by creating a range of products designed to address preferences for reductions in calories, sodium, cholesterol, and fat.[4] Although sales of high-intensity sweeteners and fat-substitute-containing foods have captured increasing market shares, there is still little evidence that use of such foods has an impact on the overall diet quality of women. Data from long-term studies are limited, but shorter-term studies suggest that replacement of sugars with high-intensity sweeteners results in a small net reduction in energy intake.[5] Energy reduction is lowest among nondieting consumers who select few items and is greatest among individuals actively attempting to restrict intake. Inadequate evidence is available to determine if consumption of fat-substitute-containing foods results in net dietary reductions in fat and/or energy.[6–8] To date, no study has fully examined the diet and nutritional status impacts of adoption of fat- and sweetener-substitute-containing foods in population level samples of women. Some have predicted, however, that one of the less obvious impacts of the increasing availability of designer foods is that the consumer seemingly loses the incentive to need to know anything about nutrition or the quality of diet or how much food constitutes a healthy diet.[9]

The food supply has also changed in the kinds of food opportunities away-from-home. Women of the 1990s can choose food from a wide variety of distributional channels, including diverse sit-down, fast-food, ethnic, and pizza restaurants as well as the workplace cafeteria. Despite the growth in availability of food outside the home, the healthfulness of food consumed away from home has been criticized.[10,11] Although some have suggested that the extent of away-from-home consumption is so modest that overall diet quality is not affected,[12] evidence exists that the extent of away-from-home eating is increasing. Among women surveyed as part of the 1989 to 1991 Continuing Survey of Food Intake by Individuals (CSFII), over a dietary assessment period of 3 days, 69% of all women aged 20 years and older consumed something away from home at least once. Over a 3-day period, 85% of all teenagers, 75% of women in their 40s, 59% of women in their 60s, and 44% of women in their 70s consumed some kind of food away from home. The food energy contribution of food away from home averaged 23%, ranging from a high of 31% among teenage girls aged 12 to 19 years and decreasing to 25% for women in their 30s and 17% for women in their 60s to a low of 11% among women aged 70 and older.[13]

The nutritional impacts of away-from-home eating are not straightforward.[12,14,15] Among women surveyed as part of the 1987–1988 Nationwide Food Consumption Survey (NFCS), mean daily energy intakes across women classified into patterns of eating ranged from a low of 1393 calories among women in a pattern with 25 to 30% cafeteria food to a high of 1682 calories among women with 25 to 30% consumed as a guest, a difference approaching about 20% of the mean adult female intake. Women in many away-from-home eating patterns had energy intakes similar to intakes of women in patterns without a significant amount of away-from-home food. There were significant differences, however, in fat and micronutrient densities between women consuming predominantly food at home versus those in restaurant and fast-food patterns. Mean caloric intake was about 1475 kcal among women classified in restaurant and fast-food patterns versus 1523 kcal in home-food based women. However, presence in the restaurant, cafeteria, or fast-food eating patterns was associated with an increased percentage of energy contributed by fat and reduced percentages of the recommended dietary allowance (RDA) consumed for calcium, dietary fiber, vitamins A and C, and folacin.[16]

Demographic and Socioeconomic Influences

Traditional consumer demand theory used by economists has consistently confirmed relationships between income, prices, and food consumption patterns. Income-, own-, and cross-price elasticities have been estimated for commodity categories to describe these economic phenomena. Household sociodemographic characteristics are important determinants of both food expenditures and nutrient intake.[17] Axelson[18] found that income-food expenditure or income-food use relationships are more likely to show positive associations than are income-nutrient intake studies, which frequently show conflicting or no association. The United States has experienced a significant increase in per capita income over the past 30 years, and this increase in available resources has had a significant impact on food consumption patterns.

As per capita or household income increases, people often eat more food and/ or substitute preferred items. Away-from-home consumption increases with increasing income level. Although expenditures on food are positively associated with increasing income, above an income threshold at which adequate quantities of food can be purchased, the nutritional quality of diets is not consistently related to income level. At higher income levels, additional income is often associated with purchase of additional discretionary food and greater expenditures for improved "quality" of food, in which quality might be defined in terms of added convenience, packaging, macronutrient modification, or special production methods such as organically grown or hormone-free. For some, such purchases improve the nutrient density of the diet; for others, discretionary purchases contribute disproportionate quantities of fat, sugars, and sodium.

As an example of one representative income and diet study, Thompson et al[19] examined food sources of fat and dietary fiber in women surveyed as part of the 1985 to 1986 U.S. Department of Agriculture (USDA) CSFII by income level. Lower-income women (less than 130% of poverty) consumed fewer daily servings of total vegetables, fewer raw vegetables, less juice, less solid fruit, less total grains, less whole-grain bread, and less higher-fiber cereal than did women in higher-income categories. Mean dietary fiber was also lower in women in households with incomes less than 185% of poverty. Food sources of fat also differed across income levels. Total and saturated fat intakes were less in lower-income women as was the percent of energy from fat. Other studies have observed either contrasting or no association between dietary intakes and income. In a probability sample of adults in the Twin Cities area of Minnesota, Kushi et al[20] concluded that women with higher incomes had superior diet quality, with lower Keys dietary scores and higher polyunsaturated fatty acid intakes.

Most studies have not used regression analyses to identify the independent effect of income on dietary outcomes, and this has contributed to different estimates of the effect of income. Murphy et al[21] used multivariate methods in a sample of women from the 1987–88 NFCS and found no association between income and either the percentage of energy from fat or the number of low intake nutrients (defined as less than 67% of the RDA) for women aged 19 and older when income was defined as above or below 100% of the federal poverty level. In a second study using regression analysis to examine the relationship of income to diet in a national sample of women from the 1989 Diet and Health Knowledge Survey (DHKS) and the 1989 CSFII, income was unrelated to absolute intakes of dietary lipids, fiber, calcium, cholesterol, or vitamin E or C. However, income in excess of 450% of the federal poverty level was associated with a higher percentage of energy from fat (+2.0%), lower percentage energy from carbohydrate (–2.8%), and greater daily servings of fruit and vegetables but fewer grains and legumes.[22]

Another good example of how demographic trends have influenced eating patterns can be seen by examining the impact of the working woman. One of the fastest growing life-style profiles is that of the working woman with family. The labor force participation rate for women increased from 34.8% in 1960 to 56.6% in 1988.[2] From 1960 to 1988, the percentage of working mothers with children younger than six years increased from 19% to 57%, and the percentage is expected to rise to 66% by 1995.[23] This increase has been attributed to several changing economic, social, and demographic factors including a greater demand for female labor, a rise in female wages, lower birth rates, and shifting cultural and economic norms making it acceptable and/or necessary for women to work.[24]

Two primary pathways through which female employment may influence food choices have been suggested.[25,26] Higher household income generated with employment should result in increased expenditure (consumption) for all normal (in the economic sense) foods, with increases proportional to the size of income elasticity for each commodity. Second, if time is considered as a resource that is to be allocated (spent), then consumption of time-intensive foods should be reduced among working women, and consumption of time-saving foods should increase. Food-related activities are some of the most time-consuming of all household tasks, and several studies have determined that employed women decrease meal preparation time through increased use of convenience foods.[27,28] Also, in another time-related effect, female employment outside the home has been positively related to increased food consumption away from home.[25,29,30]

Using data from the 1984 Family Food Expenditure Survey of Canada and a 2-week household food diary, Horton and Campbell[25] concluded that in households where the female head of household is employed outside the home full time, household availability of calories, fat, carbohydrate, calcium, iron, thiamin, and niacin is lower than in households where the woman works part time or is not engaged in market employment. However, these nutrient results reflect household availability rather than consumption and cannot be tied to the actual dietary consumption patterns of women. In 1985 CSFII data, 19-to-50-year-old women employed full time had lower mean intakes of milk, cereals, and pastas but higher intakes of total fats and oils, salad dressings and beverages.[31] However, the only differences observed by employment status of the 27 nutrients and dietary components evaluated were that employed women consumed more fat but less vitamin A and C and carotenes than did women who worked part time or those not employed outside the household.

Access To and Use of Information

The level of formal education has frequently been a strong predictor of food-related behaviors and attitudes.[18] If one accepts the conceptual framework in which food consumption is not only an end in itself but becomes an input into creation of other desired outcomes such as good health, then level of education can be thought of as a variable in determining how efficiently time and resources are used to produce a healthy diet, which, in turn, contributes to production of improved overall levels of health.[26] A woman with higher educational attainment should have both greater knowledge of what she should eat and how to best purchase and prepare it. Given comparable time and income to work with, the better educated woman should be able to use resources more efficiently to produce the desired level of diet quality and health. Clearly, many other factors motivate behavior, but in multivariate examinations of education and diet, educational level has consistently been independently associated with greater awareness of diet and health relationships and consumption of healthier diets.[22,32–35]

A recent survey of how Americans are making food choices examined sources of information about diet and health.[36] Women reported that they got information about food and nutrition from magazines (40%), newspaper articles (17%), television (18%), books (18%), and physician (16%). Only 6% of all women reported obtaining food and nutrition information from food labels. However, when asked "how likely are you to change you eating habits as a result of what you read in magazines, the newspaper," etc., based on only those who had used specific sources, less than 10% of all respondents said that it was very likely that they would change their eating habits based on what they read in magazines or the newspaper or saw on television. By contrast, 68% responded that they would be likely to change on the advice of a physician or dietitian. This suggests that when assessing the impact of education on diet, assessment of not only information availability but also information credibility is needed if the goal is to determine the potential for behavior change.

Assessment of exposure to relevant food and nutrition education is difficult. Consumers obtain information about food and diet in many places other than formal schooling. Existing studies that use years of formal schooling actually capture a constellation of variables including exposure to relevant health information during formal schooling, sensitization to diet, health-relevant information from informal sources, literacy level, motivation to search out information, and other unmeasured factors that characterize individuals who are able to achieve higher levels of formal education.

Perceived Social Roles

Social roles also condition the eating patterns of women. Fifty years ago, Lewin[37] tried to combine the analytic approaches of cultural anthropology and psychology to investigate why people eat what they eat. He described the gatekeeper role in the now classic "channel theory" stemming from examination of "how food comes to the table and why." Today, as more women are in the work force, husbands participate in more meal planning and preparation tasks and have more involvement in nutrition decisions and family health goals.[38,39] However, the woman still retains a major portion of the food and nutrition roles, including ensuring that the family is provided with regular and balanced meals and nutrition, avoiding conflicts over food, and establishing shared nutrition goals and patterns of eating with her partner.[39,40]

Several authors have attempted to identify role expectations and determine how conflicting role expectations may influence food behaviors. For example, Roland and Harris[41] explored behaviors arising from internal conflicts between the role of the working woman and "the good mother." Kirk and Gillespie[40] conducted focus groups to identify role expectations of "young family life cycle" working mothers. Five roles, labeled "nutritionist," "economist," "manager-organizer," "meaning-creator," and "family diplomat" were identified. Family meals reflect both the perceived expectations of the spouse as well as "family diplomat" foods (e.g., foods that cater to children's preferences to reduce disharmony). Because women would prepare and consume a different mix of foods if they were not balancing multiple roles, this suggests that some level of role confluence may be needed if women are to be expected to successfully consume a healthy personal diet and also meet family needs and expectations.

From an empirical standpoint, no data exist to measure role perceptions related to food in nationally representative samples of data. Characterization of this set of profiles would fill one gap in our understanding of the independent factors that influence food consumption decisions of women.

Health Attitudes, Beliefs, and Life-Style Patterns

As illustrated earlier in Figure 4-1, a host of life-style factors influence food behaviors. Limited empirical evidence identifies life-style factors as determinants of dietary practices, and information is less available and standardized in national data sets than for other dietary determinants.

Health Attitudes and Beliefs

Analysis of survey data from the 1989 CSFII and 1989 DHKS has provided the most recent opportunity to enhance our understanding of the factors that both determine health attitudes and beliefs about food and nutrition and the extent to which knowledge and attitudes independently predict dietary intake differences.

In results drawn from a sample of meal planner/preparers, individuals who expressed personal importance of following the U.S. Dietary Guidelines consumed approximately 5 g less total fat than did those who did not report such personal importance.[22] Such women also consumed a greater percentage of energy from carbohydrates, more fruits and grains, and less dietary cholesterol and sodium. However, no differences were observed in percentage of calories from fat or number of servings of vegetables consumed daily.

Awareness of diet and health associations has also been useful in explaining dietary differences in both food and nutrients.[22] Results are not always, however, in the expected direction. In multivariate analyses of data from the 1989 DHKS, greater awareness of diet and disease was associated with more adequate intakes of dietary fiber, calcium, vitamin C, and servings of fruits and vegetables. However, "aware" consumers also consumed more calories, fat, and saturated fat.

Although much more is known about nutrition knowledge and attitudes in small nonrepresentative samples of individuals, more information is needed at the population level. Characterization of a range of attitudes toward diet and dietary change, coupled with information related to current and past diet, is needed.

Relative Weight and Weight Management Strategies

A preoccupation with body weight and body image is related to a significant prevalence of short-term and chronic dieting among American women. In the National Health and Nutrition Examination Survey (NHANES) III, 35% of women aged 20 to 74 years were classified as overweight.[42] The prevalence of overweight in women increases with age and differs by ethnicity. Despite the fact that the prevalence of obesity is higher in older women, the incidence of overweight is highest in 35- to 44-year-old women and declines with age.[43] More African-American women than white women are overweight. A heightened sensitivity to relative weight has contributed to widespread prevalence of dieting and other weight management strategies.

In recent estimates obtained from the Behavioral Risk Factor Surveillance System (BRFSS), it has been estimated that 44% of teenage women and 38% of adult women were attempting to lose weight at any given time, whereas another 26% and 28%, respectively, were attempting to maintain weight.[44-46] The prevalence of dieting has markedly increased since the 1950s and 1960s when approximately 14% of women reported that they were currently dieting.[47] In 1988, approximately 27% of dieting women were chronic dieters or had been dieting continuously for more than 1 year.[43]

How dieting behavior affects food choices and dietary patterns among women can be illustrated by how women choose to lose weight. The most common methods were eating fewer calories (84%) and increasing physical activity (60 to 63%) in a national survey.[46,48] By self-report, hypocaloric diets seem to be the weight loss regime of choice among younger women,[49,50] but other forms of weight reduction range from skipping meals (44% of teenage women reported this strategy in 1990) to much smaller numbers of women who report using diet pills or vomiting.

Supplement Use

In data obtained from the CSFII 1989–91, 44% of all women aged 20 and older reported using some kind of dietary supplement.[13] Mean use of multivitamins with iron or some other mineral was 31%, whereas use of calcium supplements averaged 13% (ranging from a low of 7% in women aged 20 to 39 but increasing to 19% among women aged 60 and older).

How supplements are defined contributes to some of the differences in usage rates. In the 1987 National Health Interview Survey (NHIS) 27% of all surveyed women reported use of some kind of daily supplement, ranging from use of multiple-type vitamins to supplements of single nutrients (such as calcium or vitamins A, C, and/or E).[51] White women aged 55 to 74 years reported the highest daily supplement use (39%), compared to black and Hispanic women (17 and 21%, respectively). Among all women, multivitamins were most commonly used (20%) followed by calcium (10%) and vitamin C (8%). In NHANES II data,[52] a modest age-related supplement use rate was found. Thirty-eight percent of women aged 18 to 50 used supplements compared to 44% of women 51 to 74 years.

Bender et al[53] report that individuals with more self-reported health problems are likely to use dietary supplements but that supplement use is greatest among those who perceive their own health to be excellent and lowest among those who perceive their health to be poor. Thus, it is frequently observed that women who regularly use dietary supplements such as multivitamins and minerals have nutrient intake profiles that, exclusive of the contribution of the nutritional supplement, exceed intakes of other women.

Smoking and Alcohol Use

Several studies have suggested that the diets of women smokers differ from diets of nonsmokers. Such dietary differences may exacerbate the health impacts of cigarette smoking. Analysis of data from the CSFII 1985, NHANES II, and other community-based samples conclude that women smokers consume fewer fruits and vegetables than do nonsmokers but tend to consume more beverages including coffee, soft drinks, and alcohol. Nutrient intakes and nutrient densities of female smokers are consistently lower for vitamin C, carotenes, and dietary fiber. For example, in 1985 CSFII women, smokers consumed 64 mg/day vitamin C daily versus intakes of 88 mg/day among never-smokers. Dietary fiber intakes ranged from 10.2 to 11.9 g/day. CSFII never-smokers consumed 1% of energy from alcohol; quitters and current smokers consumed 3%.[54] In contrast to other studies that have studied only men or included men and women, none of the above studies found a difference in energy intake between female smokers and nonsmokers. Also, there were no differences in intakes of fat or dietary cholesterol in either the analysis of NHANES II or 1985 CSFII data, although differences in dietary lipids were observed in the community-based samples.[54-57]

Alcohol use is another health behavior that varies widely across women. Estimates reported in *Health, United States, 1992*[58] indicate that in 1990, 51% of women were currently using some form of alcohol. Rates were higher among younger women than older (59% among 25- to 44-year-olds, 47% among 45- to 64-year-olds, and 31% among women aged 65 and older). Rates of alcohol use among white women exceeded rates among black women (e.g., 65 versus 38% among women younger than 45, and 44 versus 25% among women 45 years and older). In 1990, 29% of all women reported that they consumed no alcohol; 46% reported that they consumed up to three drinks per week. An additional 21% were classified as moderate drinkers (e.g., 4 to 13 drinks per week), and 3% were classified as heavy drinkers, drinking two or more drinks a day, or 14 per week.

A growing number of researchers are suggesting that health behaviors tend to cluster.[59,60] Smoking and alcohol use are two such interdependent health and life-style factors. It is clear that many of the dietary patterns of women smokers are less healthful than those of nonsmokers. It is more difficult to characterize alcohol use, so fewer studies have examined dietary patterns by level of usual alcohol use in national-level data sets. It is well recognized, however, that alcohol use dilutes the apparent fat density of diets (e.g., diets of drinkers are lower in percentage of energy from fat because of the energy contributed by alcohol), making such diets appear to be more healthy than they actually are.

DIETARY PATTERNS IN WOMEN

Although much of the population work describing the development of food consumption patterns has been gender-neutral, it is possible to describe several factors that have had a significant impact on dietary trends in women over the past 20 years.

Food consumption patterns in women are diverse and have changed over time. Although there are quantitative and some qualitative differences between the diets of men and women, there are larger qualitative differences across groups of women. One of the most important determinants of diet in women is age. From existing analyses, it is impossible to determine whether the observed differences in diet associated with age result from a pure effect of age, a cohort effect (e.g., women born at the same time whose behaviors are influenced by the same social and political conditions), a stage of life-cycle effect, a time effect, or some combination of these. Although there are also very clear differences in the diets of women from differing ethnic and cultural backgrounds, the discussion that follows examines dietary differences across the life cycle as these differences are common to women from all cultures.

Examination of trends in food consumption can be accomplished by using one or more of the three levels of data currently collected to assess the American diet.[61] Availability of information at the level of the U.S. food supply, at the household food use level, and at the individual food intake level provides a range of ways to examine consumption. Food supply data have been collected since the turn of the century. Per capita trends estimated from these food disappearance data do not, however, reflect actual food consumption by individuals but rather the per person availability of food that is sold from wholesale and retail outlets. Household-level food use information has been collected by the federal government for more than 50 years and reflects food brought into the household over a 7-day period. However, household food use data cannot identify how food was distributed among household members. Since 1965, the federal government has sponsored collection of dietary intake data from individual household members. The predecessors of the National Nutrition Monitoring System (NNMS), the 1965 to 1966 USDA NFCS, and the NHANES I-1971–74 provided the first of a series of nationally representative individual-level estimates of food consumption. Although women are not the sole focus of the NNMS, data are available that allow examination of dietary trends in women over time.

Table 4-1 illustrates food supply trends between 1970 and 1990 and reflects the shifts in availability of food for human consumption. Food supply data suggest an increase in total meats, poultry, and fish; total fat; grains and cereals; fruits; and vegetables. Declines in red meat are offset by increases in poultry (71%) and fish and shellfish (25%). Total food supply fat increased between 1970 and 1990, but large increases in vegetable fats were countered, in small part, by declines in ani-

Table 4-1 Food Supply Trends, 1970 to 1990

	Pounds Available per Capita[a]		
	1970	*1980*	*1990–1991*
Total meats, poultry, fish	177	179	185
Red meats	132[b]	126	112
Poultry	34	41	58
Fish, shellfish	12	12	15
Total fat	53	57	63
Vegetable fat	39	45	53
Animal fat	14	12	10
Refined sugar	102	84	65
Corn sweeteners	19	39	73
Low-calorie sweeteners	6	8	22
Grains and cereals	135	146	183
Fruit	96	103	112
Vegetables[c]	82	87	104
Potatoes	59	49	44

[a]Per capita food consumption is calculated by dividing the total amount of food disappearance by the U.S. total population.
[b]For example, 132 lbs. of red meats per man, woman, and child in the United States was available for consumption in 1970.
[c]Limited to 17 commercial market items but does not include potatoes.
Source: Reprinted from *Health, United States 1992,* National Health Statistics, DHHS Pub No 93-1232, 1993.

mal fat. Although use of refined sugar declined by about one-third, use of corn sweeteners and other low-calorie high-intensity sweeteners increased dramatically (284% and 267%, respectively). The per capita food supply of cereals and grains increased approximately 35% between 1970 and 1990. Fruit and vegetable availability also increased, although about 25% fewer potatoes were distributed in 1990 than in 1970.

Although food supply level data provide a useful way to examine the big picture of food consumption trends, they do not provide a good picture of what any one group of individuals is actually eating. Even per capita consumption figures mask differences between consumption practices of individuals who use selected foods and those who do not when food is grouped into categories for which many persons consume no food.[62] Tables 4-2 to 4-5 and Figures 4-2 to 4-4 reflect actual consumption behaviors by women surveyed as part of the NFCS 1977–78 and the CSFII 1989–91. Data reflect the percentage of women consuming any food in a given food group over a 3-day period to better reflect usual consumption of foods as well as nutrients. From the perspective of the nutrition educator, persons often first decide whether to consume a particular kind of food at all and then decide

Table 4-2 Women's Dietary Trends: Percentage of Women Consuming Selected Dairy Products, 1977–78 NFCS and 1989–91 CSFII, Weighted Data

Foods	All Ages	12–18 Yr	19–29 Yr	30–49 Yr	50–59 Yr	60–69 Yr	70+ Yr
Low-fat dairy	57	54[a]	50	53	70	59	67
		(+27)[b]	(+21)	(+24)	(+38)	(+17)	(+36)
Whole-fat dairy	35	52	40	32	21	31	32
		(–30)	(–24)	(–23)	(–34)	(–26)	(–30)
Low-fat cheeses	12	5	13	10	12	17	18
		(NC)[c]	(+4)	(NC)	(NC)	(+1)	(NC)
Regular cheeses	47	47	53	50	46	39	32
		(+7)	(+7)	(+6)	(+4)	(+2)	(–1)

[a]Numbers without parentheses indicate the percentage of women consuming any food from each group over a 3-day period, 1989–91 CSFII.
[b]Numbers in parentheses indicate the percentage increase or decrease observed between 1977 and 1991 (e.g., the percentage of women consuming low-fat dairy products increased from 27% in 1977 to 1978 to 54% in 1989 to 1991, an increase of 27% of all women).
[c]NC, no change.

how much of that food they will consume. A two-step method of describing food consumption gives different information than does per capita intake and is useful from the nutrition education standpoint.

Food Group Consumption Trends in Women

Tables 4-2 to 4-5 provide trend data estimated from the two-step approach, using weighted samples of women surveyed in the NFCS 1977–78 and the CSFII 1989–91. Across adult women, consumption patterns vary widely by age, and results are stratified to reflect differences across the life cycle. Tables reflect the proportion of the age-specific population who consumed any food from a given food group during the 3 days of dietary intake collected in 1989 to 1991. Numbers in parentheses indicate the increase or decrease in the proportion of the population consuming a given type of food since 1977 to 1978.

The second stage of the two-step analysis, grams consumed per user, are not reported here as there was less change in portion sizes over time than there was in the proportion of women consuming food from a food group. A few of the grams-per-user results do echo common health messages as suggested in *Dietary Guidelines for Americans*.[63] For example, there were declines in grams consumed of all kinds of beef and pork among users between 1977 and 1991. Among persons reporting use of milk products, average grams consumed declined, but consumption declined much more among women using whole-milk products.[33]

Table 4-3 Women's Dietary Trends: Percentage of Women Consuming Meat, Fish, Poultry, and Eggs (1977–78 NFCS and 1989–91 CSFII, Weighted Data)

Foods	All Ages	12–18 Yr	19–29 Yr	30–49 Yr	50–59 Yr	60–69 Yr	70+ Yr
Low-fat beef/ pork	45	45[a] (+6)[b]	44 (+11)	47 (+13)	49 (+16)	47 (+19)	39 (+12)
Medium-fat beef/ pork	50	57 (–8)	49 (–16)	54 (–13)	49 (–18)	44 (–16)	41 (–15)
High-fat beef/ pork	11	15 (–32)	14 (–30)	10 (–36)	9 (–32)	7 (–32)	6 (–31)
Low-fat poultry	40	33 (+15)	37 (+17)	39 (+18)	45 (+19)	52 (+31)	42 (+21)
Medium-fat poultry	25	28 (–7)	27 (–5)	25 (–8)	21 (–12)	16 (–18)	26 (–8)
Low-fat lunchmeat	18	18 (+11)	20 (+12)	17 (+9)	21 (+14)	14 (+7)	14 (+8)
Medium-fat lunchmeat	8	17 (–5)	6 (–5)	7 (–2)	10 (+3)	8 (+2)	5 (–2)
High-fat lunchmeat	30	33 (–16)	28 (–17)	32 (–12)	28 (–11)	27 (–9)	32 (NC)[c]
Low-fat fish	25	13 (–4)	21 (NC)	30 (+8)	27 (+6)	30 (+11)	23 (+10)
Medium-fat fish	12	9 (–9)	12 (–4)	12 (–5)	13 (–6)	15 (–3)	16 (+1)
Egg products	36	32 (–11)	35 (–17)	37 (–17)	38 (–20)	33 (–26)	37 (–5)

[a]Numbers without parentheses indicate the percentage of women consuming any food from each group over a 3-day period, 1989–91 CSFII.
[b]Numbers in parentheses indicate the percentage increase or decrease observed between 1977 and 1991.
[c]NC, no change.

The food grouping system on which results are based was developed using major food groupings traditionally used by USDA to describe food consumption. However, to further describe high- and low-fat and fiber foods, fat and dietary fiber composition were used to develop more finely defined food groups. Nutrient thresholds were first established to ensure that there would be a meaningful difference in absolute quantity of nutrient across food groups. The second threshold criteria were designed to distinguish between consumer behaviors, such as the skinning of poultry or fat trimming on meats. See Popkin et al[33] for more detail on the creation of the food grouping system. Table 4-6 contains examples of foods within food groups.

Table 4-4 Women's Dietary Trends: Percentage of Women Consuming Breads and Grains,[a] (1977–78 NFCS and 1989–91 CSFII, Weighted Data)

Foods	All Ages	12–18 Yr	19–29 Yr	30–49 Yr	50–59 Yr	60–69 Yr	70+ Yr
Lower-fat white breads	53	64 (–13)	54[b] (–13)[c]	53 (–17)	44 (–24)	50 (–18)	51 (–20)
Lower-fat whole-grain breads	51	27 (NC)[d]	49 (+12)	51 (+15)	63 (+19)	63 (+20)	57 (+16)
Higher-fat white breads	57	54 (–10)	55 (NC)	57 (NC)	63 (+12)	58 (+8)	55 (+9)
Higher-fat whole-grain breads	18	18 (+7)	17 (+6)	21 (+12)	20 (+11)	14 (+5)	13 (+5)
Pasta/rice/cooked cereals	42	37 (–3)	42 (+5)	42 (+4)	43 (+7)	42 (+4)	50 (+5)
Lower-fiber ready-to-eat cereals	24	39 (+2)	23 (+4)	17 (+3)	25 (+9)	22 (–3)	29 (NC)
Higher-fiber ready-to-eat cereals	23	16 (–5)	20 (+3)	21 (+5)	28 (+6)	27 (+5)	34 (+5)

[a]See Table 4-6 for definition of breads and grains.
[b]Numbers without parentheses indicate the percentage of women consuming any food from each group over a 3-day period, 1989–91 CSFII.
[c]Numbers in parentheses indicate the percentage increase or decrease observed between 1977 and 1991.
[d]NC, no change.

Dairy Product Consumption

In 1989 to 1991, 57% of all women reported consumption of low-fat dairy products, but only 35% reported consuming whole-fat dairy products (see Table 4-2). The proportion of all women consuming low-fat and skim milk products increased with age, and numbers consuming whole-milk products (milk, yogurts) declined with increasing age. Women older than the age of 50 were more likely to use lower-fat dairy products, whereas those 30 and younger were more likely to use whole-fat dairy products. Similar age-related associations were observed for consumption of low-fat and regular cheeses.

Over time, use of whole-milk dairy products declined substantially, with 23 to 34% fewer women consuming these products in 1989 to 1991 versus 1977. Increases in the age group-specific proportions of lower-fat dairy product consumers ranged from 17 to 38% in the same period. Since 1965, the substitution of lower-fat milk products has been substantial, as in 1965 nearly 60% of all consumers reported consumption of whole-milk products, but only 7% reported consuming low-fat or skim milk products.

Table 4-5 Women's Dietary Trends: Percentage of Women Consuming Desserts, Snacks,[a] Fats, and Oils (1977–78 NFCS and 1989–91 CSFII, Weighted Data)

Foods	All Ages	12–18 Yr	19–29 Yr	30–49 Yr	50–59 Yr	60–69 Yr	70+ Yr
Low-fat desserts	18	21[b] (−6)[c]	11 (−4)	17 (−2)	18 (−6)	21 (−4)	30 (+2)
High-fat desserts	61	62 (−12)	56 (−2)	60 (+1)	65 (+4)	62 (+2)	68 (+7)
Low-fat salty snacks	7	7 (+2)	9 (+5)	7 (+3)	8 (+5)	8 (+6)	2 (NC)[d]
High-fat salty snacks	50	57 (+4)	48 (+5)	52 (+11)	46 (+6)	50 (+13)	42 (+5)
Sugar and jellies	61	54 (−19)	56 (−14)	60 (−13)	65 (−6)	66 (−9)	73 (−4)
Candy	18	20 (−2)	19 (+7)	17 (+7)	18 (+8)	17 (+8)	14 (+7)
Butter	18	18 (−14)	17 (−14)	24 (−9)	21 (−13)	22 (−8)	21 (−7)
Margarine	50	39 (−2)	45 (+3)	49 (+5)	57 (+9)	57 (+4)	65 (+8)
Low-fat salad dressing	9	1 (NC)	5 (+3)	10 (+7)	14 (+10)	9 (+6)	13 (+11)
Regular salad dressing	56	53 (+1)	51 (−8)	59 (−5)	63 (+3)	57 (+7)	50 (+7)

[a]See Table 4-6 for definition of low-fat/high-fat salty snacks and desserts.
[b]Numbers without parentheses indicate the percentage of women consuming any food from each group over a 3-day period, 1989–91 CSFII.
[c]Numbers in parentheses indicate the percentage increase or decrease observed between 1977 and 1991.
[d]NC, no change.

Numbers of women reporting cheese consumption have changed very little between 1977 and 1989 to 1991. However, consumption percentages do not reflect use of cheeses in mixed or ethnic dishes, so reported rates underestimate current consumption and underestimate temporal trends. However, the percentage of women reporting cheese consumption in 1989 to 1991 is still nearly twice the rate observed in 1965.

In many broad commodity categories, consumption of foods with visible fat has declined. This was not observed for cheese, in which the fat content is less visible and, until more recently, the fat content has not been well recognized. In part due to changes in the use of mixed dishes and ethnic foods and in part in response to other health messages related to calcium, consumption of this signifi-

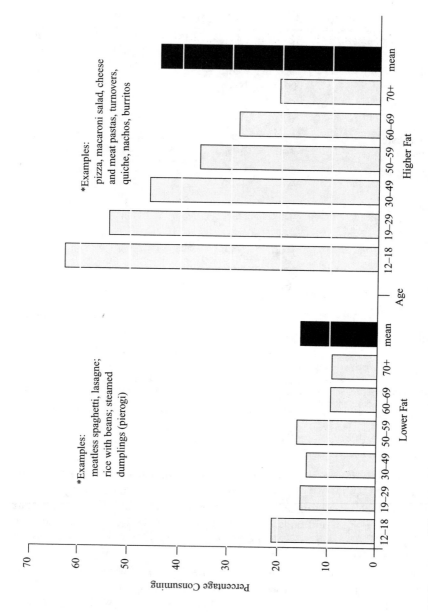

Figure 4-2 Percentage of Women Consuming Grain-Based Dishes* (1989–91 CSFII, by age group, 3 days, weighted data)

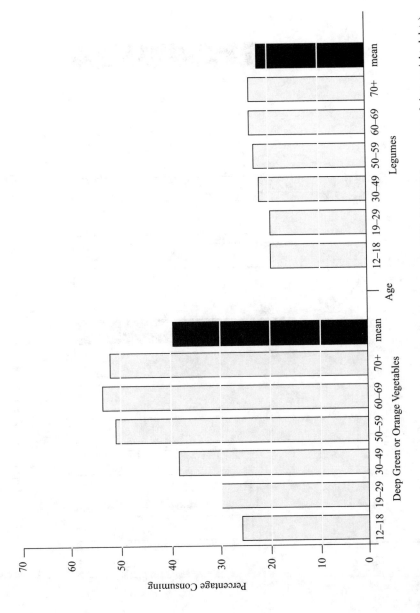

Figure 4-3 Percentage of Women Consuming Green and Orange Vegetables and Legumes (1989–91 CSFII, by age group, 3 days, weighted data)

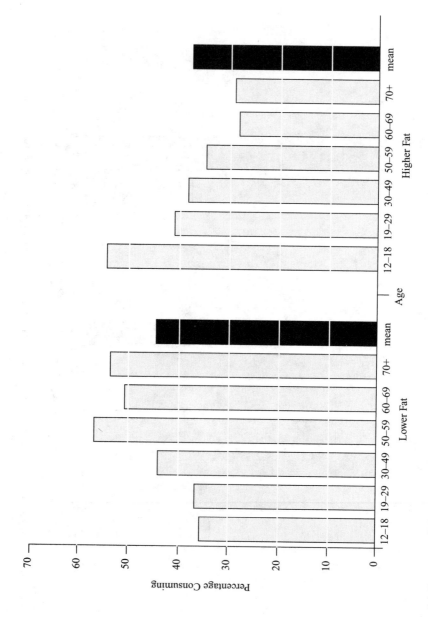

Figure 4-4 Percentage of Women Consuming Potatoes (1989–91 CSFII, by age group, 3 days, weighted data)

Table 4-6 Representative Foods, UNC Food Grouping System

Food Group	Representative Foods
Low-fat milk and milk products	2% Milk, skim milk
High-fat milk and milk products	Whole milk
Low-fat cheeses	Cottage cheese
High-fat cheeses	American, cheddar
Low-fat beef and pork	Ham, beef roast (lean only)
Medium-fat beef and pork	Lean ground beef, lean beef roast
High-fat beef and pork	Regular ground beef, beef pot roast
Low-fat poultry	Skinned chicken breast, turkey
High-fat poultry	Chicken or turkey salad, chicken or turkey pot pie, fried chicken
Low-fat fish	Tuna (canned), water packed
High-fat fish	Fried perch, fish (cooking method not specified)
Low-fat luncheon meats	Lean sliced ham, turkey ham, low-fat hot dogs
High-fat luncheon meats	Pork sausage, bologna, beef hot dogs
Low-fat salad dressings	Low-calorie French and Italian dressings
High-fat salad dressings	Mayonnaise, Italian and French dressings
Low-fat desserts	Gelatin dessert, angel food cake
High-fat desserts	Ice cream, apple pie, butter or sugar cookies, cakes
Low-fat salty snacks	Pretzels
High-fat salty snacks	Saltines, potato chips
Eggs and egg dishes	Fried egg, boiled egg, omelet
Legumes	Pinto beans, pork and beans
Low-fat, low-fiber breads	White bread
Low-fat, high-fiber breads	Wheat or whole-grain bread, bagels
High-fat, low-fiber breads	Rolls (white, soft)
High-fat, high-fiber breads	Cornbread, bran muffin
Pasta, rice, and cooked cereals	Oatmeal, rice, pasta salad
Low-fiber ready-to-eat cereals	Cornflakes, wheat flakes, Cheerios
High-fiber ready-to-eat cereals	Shredded wheat, bran cereal, raisin bran
Low-fat, grain-based mixed dishes	Meatless pasta dishes
High-fat, grain-based mixed dishes	Macaroni and cheese, pizza, burritos
Citrus fruits and juices	Orange juice
Other fruits	Banana, apple, strawberries, cantaloupe
Noncitrus fruit juices	Apple juice, cranberry juice
Fruit drinks	Cranberry cocktail, cranberry-apple juice drink, fruit-flavored drink
Low-fat potatoes	Baked potato, mashed potato
High-fat potatoes	Home fries, potato salad, French fries
Green and orange vegetables	Carrots, broccoli, spinach
Low-fiber other vegetables	Lettuce, tomatoes, onions, celery, green beans
High-fiber other vegetables	Green peas, corn
Coffee	Coffee (ground and instant)
Tea	Tea, hot, iced
Regular soft drinks	Soft drink (cola)
Diet soft drinks	Soft drink (sugar-free)

cant source of fat and saturated fat has increased over time in women of all ages. Until recently, lower-fat cheese alternatives have been used sparingly, presumably in part because of undesirable organoleptic qualities.

Meat, Poultry, and Fish Consumption

Beef and pork are commonly consumed foods among women, but significant shifts in the kinds of meat consumed have occurred over time. Consumption of lower-fat beef, pork, poultry, and fish increased between 1977 and 1989 to 1991 (see Table 4-3). These food groups included lean and/or trimmed beef and pork, broiled or skinned poultry, and broiled or baked fish and tuna canned in water. Declines in the numbers of women consuming medium-fat beef and pork (which included regular hamburger, leaner roasts and chops) continued, whereas more than 30% fewer women in each age group consumed any beef or pork that was classified as high fat (untrimmed roasts, chops, steaks) in 1989 to 1991 as compared with 1977. Differences in consumption of poultry products varied considerably by age. Women younger than 30 were nearly as likely to consume a poultry that was fried or with skin (medium-fat poultry) as they were to consume the lower-fat poultry alternatives (e.g., broiled or skinned). However, women older than 30 were much more likely to select lower-fat poultry. Egg consumption patterns were nearly identical across the age categories of women. Rates of consumption declined for women of all ages. But declines were much steeper among older women up to 70 years of age.

Several authors have correctly suggested that part of the observed decline in meat product consumption can be explained by the increased use of food mixtures and frozen convenience meals. Figure 4-2 illustrates the age-specific use of low- and higher-fat grain-based food entrees, which include many of the ethnic Italian, Mexican, and Chinese foods that rely less on meat but more on grains and vegetables. Examples include spaghetti and meat sauce, stir-fry, pizza, burritos, and pasta salads. As can be seen in Figure 4-2, use of mixed dish foods is consistently greatest at younger ages. Between 1977 and 1989 to 1991, rates of consumption of higher-fat grain-based mixed dishes increased most among younger women, ranging from 27% more consumers among 12- to 18-year-olds (e.g., 63% versus 36%) to 9% more consumers among 70+-year-olds (20% versus 11%) in 1989 to 1991 versus 1977.

Popkin et al[33] reported an increase from 28 to 47% of women aged 19 to 50 years consuming higher-fat grain-based entrees between 1977 and 1985, with concurrent increases from 76 to 104 g consumed per user per day. Per capita consumption increased from 20 to 48 g/day. In data also from the 1985 CSFII, the percentage of meat, poultry, and fish products consumed as mixtures increased from 35 to 49% of all meats consumed between 1977 and 1985. The proportion of all grain products consumed by women as grain-based mixtures increased from 27% in 1977 to 35% in 1985.[64]

Grains and Cereal Consumption

Consumption of other grain-based products has also shifted over time in women. For example, although white breads are still consumed by large proportions of women, fewer women consumed lower-fat white bread products in 1989 to 1991 when compared with 1977 (e.g., 53% in 1989 to 1991 in contrast to 72% in 1977). Consumption of whole-grain breads, crackers, rolls, etc., increased between 1977 and 1989 to 1991 for all but teenage women. As seen in Table 4-4, consumption of whole-grain products (breads, bagels) increased with increasing age among women younger than 70 years of age. Consumption of higher-fat white breads was comparable across the age spectrum, with approximately 57% of all women reporting consumption of some kind of rolls, biscuits, cornbread, or other sweet breads such as pancakes, croissants, etc. Although lower-fiber ready-to-eat (RTE) cereals were more likely to be consumed by teenage girls (39%) in 1989 to 1991, higher-fiber RTE cereal consumption was lowest among teenagers and increased with age. Among women aged 30 and older, slightly more reported consuming a higher- versus lower-fiber RTE cereal. In data not shown from the 1987 NFCS, the ratio of high to lower dietary fiber RTE cereal consumers was greater in 1987 than in 1989 to 1991. It is likely that the relative increase in RTE higher-fiber cereal consumption observed in 1987 reflects, in part, the transient increase in advertising for high-fiber cereals that occurred with use of the first health claims on RTE cereal boxes.

Overall, increases observed in the numbers of women consuming whole-grain products were offset by smaller numbers consuming traditional white bread products. Other smaller increases in rice, pasta, and higher-fat breads and grains were also observed in 1989 to 1991, but the consumption of these kinds of grain-based products cannot totally explain the sizable increase in food supply disappearance data for grain products. It is likely that part of the food supply increase can be accounted for by increases in mixed dishes as well as salty snack food consumption.

Fruit and Vegetable Consumption

In contrast to the marked consumption changes observed in women's diets in dairy and meat products, there were fewer real trends in consumption of fruits and vegetables between 1977 and 1989 to 1991. Differences in fruit and vegetable consumption were observed, however, across the different age categories of women in the 1989–91 survey. A slightly larger proportion of women older than the age of 60 consumed citrus fruit or juice than did younger women (e.g., 58% of women aged 70 and older versus 41% of teenagers aged 12 to 18). Similarly, women older than the age of 50 were more likely to report consumption of other kinds of noncitrus fruit than were younger women (e.g., 77% of women aged 70 and older, 65% of women aged 60 to 69, versus 46% of women younger than 30). By contrast, younger women were slightly more likely to consume noncitrus fruit juices and fruit drinks than were older women.

In 1989 to 1991, twice as many women aged 50 and older consumed a deep green or orange vegetable than did the youngest women in the sample (e.g., more than 50% versus 26%) (see Figure 4-3). Between 1977 and 1989 to 1991, the numbers of youngest women consuming deep green and orange vegetables declined slightly, whereas approximately 10% more women aged 50 to 70 reported consumption, increasing the age-related consumption differential. Other shifts in vegetable consumption over time occurred in the areas of higher-fiber vegetables such as corn and lima beans and legumes and soy products. Consumption declined over time in these food groups, with the steepest declines observed among younger women. Approximately 22% of all women reported consumption of legumes and 42% reported consumption of a higher-fiber vegetable in 1989 to 1991. In the only exception to this trend, slightly more women aged 60 and older consumed legumes in 1989 to 1991 than in 1977.

Potato consumption reflects another generational trend (see Figure 4-4). In 1977, consumption was fairly constant across the age spectrum as about 55% of all women consumed lower-fat potatoes. Between 1977 and 1989 to 1991, consumption of lower-fat varieties of potatoes (boiled, baked, etc.) declined from 1977 levels across all age categories (45% of all women reported consuming any lower-fat potatoes in 1989 to 1991), but the declines were greatest at younger ages. In 1989 to 1991, consumption ranged from approximately 50+% among women older than 50 years to 36% among women younger than 30. By contrast, women younger than 20 years of age were most likely (55%) to report consumption of high-fat potatoes (most generally French fries). Consumption declined with increasing age, with those least likely to consume fast foods and those women in the age categories demonstrating the greatest fat avoidance (the 60- and 70-year-olds), only half as likely to consume higher-fat potato products (28%). (It should be noted that the existing analysis does not identify if butter or margarine is added to a naturally lower-fat product such as potato. So, whereas the fat content of prepared and processed foods such as French fries or potato salad is obvious, the ultimate fat contribution of fats and dressings added to foods such as baked potatoes is less clear.)

Fats and Oils Consumption

Older women were more likely to add margarine to food than were younger women in 1989 to 1991 (see Table 4-5). Approximately 18% of all women used butter and 50% of all women reported use of added margarine. Women younger than 30 were slightly less likely to report butter or margarine consumption than were older women, a difference that increased between 1977 and 1989 to 1991. From existing analyses of trend data, it is unclear if results reflect a greater predisposition to use added fat or simply that the food choices of younger and older women differ. Younger women are more likely to consume prepared and mixed dishes that already include fat, whereas older women consume more foods in which the fat is traditionally added at the table at the time of consumption. Differences in use of regular salad dressings were not great across the age range of women, although use of low-fat dressings was greater among women older than 30.

Several studies have found that salad dressing contributes a significant and growing proportion of fat to the diets of women.[19,65,66] As secular trends have resulted in consumption of more fresh salads, consumption of salad dressing among women has increased as well. It will be interesting to see if food supply increases in no-fat versions of salad dressing will ultimately result in a "fat correction factor" as increasing numbers of women select low- or no-fat versions of salad dressing in place of regular versions.

Snacks and Desserts Consumption

Despite the growing indications of health-consciousness among women, women still consume a significant amount of intake from snacks and desserts. The rates of consumption of desserts remained rather stable between 1977 and 1991, although some declines were observed in teenage women (see Table 4-5). Also, across the broad categories of sweets and salty snack foods, there were fewer differences across women of different ages than for some of the other food categories. For example, between 56% and 68% of women in any age category consumed high-fat desserts during the 3 days of dietary data collection. Desserts included not only the grain-based cakes and cookies but also pies and frozen dairy desserts such as ice cream. Consumption of lower-fat desserts (items such as angel food cake or sherbets) was lowest among women ages 19 to 29 and higher among teenagers and women aged 60 and older. More than 61% of all women reported using some kind of sugar or jelly-type product over the 3 days of dietary intake surveyed. Fewer younger women (54% among teenagers) reported sugar consumption than did older women (73% among 70+-year-olds). By contrast, consumption of candy declined slightly with age. Similarly, teenage women were more likely to consume higher-fat salty snack foods than were older women (e.g., 57% among the 12- to 18-year-olds versus 42% among the 70-year-olds).

In general, between 1977 and 1989 to 1991, the proportion of women reporting consumption of desserts declined among teenagers, but remained fairly constant or increased slightly for all other women. The proportion reporting salty snacks increased over time but was more than countered by declines in the number of women reporting consumption of added sugars. Interestingly, rates of dessert consumption are positively correlated with education level in women. That is, more highly educated women are more likely to consume desserts, and among those who consume desserts, better educated women consume more (unpublished observations). Such results suggest the multiple factors that influence food choices and argue for a broad understanding of overall food and nutrient intake patterns to characterize the overall quality of diet.

Diet Quality in Women

Although food group consumption trends provide a good picture of changes occurring in consumption in women of all ages, as suggested earlier, food use data alone are not adequate to define the quality of diet. Several standards have been used to assess diet quality in populations. Nutrient-based measures include evaluation of absolute nutrient intakes and intakes relative to standards such as the RDA as well as evaluation of nutrient densities for foods and macronutrients. Dietary diversity can be measured relative to food pyramid recommendations or other servings-per-day recommendations, such as consumption of five or more servings of fruits and vegetables or six or more servings of grains per day as suggested in the dietary guidelines. A few aggregate measures of diet quality have been used in population surveys.

So, relative to accepted standards, what is the quality of diet in women? Are food consumption trends suggestive of healthier diets?

Nutrient Intakes

Table 4-7 provides some of the most recent nationally representative nutrient intake data describing diets of women aged 12 years and older. Mean caloric intake for women aged 20 and older was 1556 kilocalories/day, and daily caloric intake decreased with increasing age. Mean total fat intake was 60.2 g/day, with 33.9% of energy consumed as fat among women aged 20 and older. Dietary fiber averaged 12.3 g/day while mean dietary cholesterol was 231 mg/day. Dietary fiber increased with increasing age, but dietary cholesterol declined with age.

When nutrient intakes of women are evaluated in relative terms (Table 4-8), women aged 20 and older reported consuming a mean of 74% of the recommended energy allowance (REA). Age group-specific means relative to the RDA indicate that despite relatively low caloric intakes, in 1989 to 1991, all age group average intakes for women exceeded 100% of the RDA for protein, vitamins A and C, and folate (as well as thiamin, riboflavin, niacin, vitamin B_{12}, and phosphorus in data not shown). Among women aged 12 and older, age group-specific relative intakes of vitamin E, calcium, and zinc were consistently less than 100%

Table 4-7 Mean Nutrient Intakes, Women Aged 12 Years and Older (1 Day, 1989 to 1991, CSFII)

Age (Yr)	Kilo-calories (g)	Total Fat (g)	Saturated Fat (g)	% Energy from Fat	% Energy from Saturated Fat	Dietary Fiber (g)	Cholesterol (mg)
12–19	1748	67.4	25.2	33.7	12.6	11.6	223
20–29	1655	63.5	22.5	34.0	11.9	11.6	250
30–39	1658	65.5	22.9	34.6	12.1	12.0	249
40–49	1520	60.3	20.6	34.7	12.0	11.5	238
50–59	1482	57.1	19.3	33.7	11.4	12.5	221
60–69	1498	56.9	19.3	33.3	11.4	14.0	222
70–79	1366	50.1	16.7	31.9	10.7	13.2	180
80+	1390	52.0	17.8	32.2	11.2	13.7	191
20 and older	1556	60.2	20.8	33.9	11.7	12.3	231

Source: Reprinted from *Continuing Survey of Food Intakes by Individuals, 1989–1991,* US Department of Agriculture, 1994.

of the RDA. When compared with similar analyses of women's diets in 1977 and 1985, more current intakes were somewhat lower for food energy. The percentage of the mean RDA for vitamin C continued to increase from 128% in 1977 to 133% in 1985 to 147% in 1991. Calcium as a percentage of the RDA dipped slightly below levels observed in 1985, but population mean relative intakes of iron, folacin, and zinc increased over time. The mean iron intake as a percentage of the RDA increased from 61% in 1985 to 93% in 1991 in women older than 20 years.[13,67] Mean zinc as a percentage of the RDA increased from 60% in 1985 to 75% in 1991. Vitamin E as a percentage of the RDA declined slightly from 1985 levels of 97% to 87% in 1989 to 1991.

In USDA data not shown,[13] when nutrient densities (e.g., nutrient intakes per 1000 kilocalories) are examined, the nutrient density of dietary fiber increases with age, as do the densities of vitamins A and C, carotenes, and folate, as well as densities of potassium, magnesium, iron, and zinc. However, neither calcium, phosphorus, nor sodium densities vary much by age.

Macronutrient density measures, such as the percentage of energy from fat, have become common yardsticks of the American diet. Healthy People 2000,[68] national health promotion and disease prevention objectives, recommends a reduction of dietary fat intake to an average of 30% of calories or less and average saturated fat intake to less than 10% of calories among people aged 2 years and older. Although such measures do not necessarily reflect the quality of the entire diet (see Patterson et al[69]), comparisons of the percentage of food energy consumed as fat have provided one means of tracking population dietary quality. Peterkin[67] summarizes changes in women's diets between 1977 and 1985 and

Table 4-8 Nutrient Intakes as a Percentage of 1989 Recommended Energy Allowance (REA) and Recommended Dietary Allowance (RDA): Women Aged 12 Years and Older (Mean per Day, 1 Day, 1989 to 1991, CSFII)

Age (Yr)	% REA	Protein	Vitamin A	Vitamin E	Vitamin C	Folate	Calcium	Iron	Zinc
12–19	79	146	97	78	161	134	66	79	77
20–29	74	134	101	84	145	118	68	80	75
30–39	75	131	101	88	134	116	83	80	75
40–49	69	125	105	82	128	109	72	75	73
50–59	77	127	121	86	151	123	77	113	76
60–69	79	127	142	97	171	136	77	127	80
70–79	72	112	132	81	175	131	70	115	68
80+	73	108	150	91	167	133	78	119	69
20 and older	74	127	114	87	147	120	75	93	75

Source: Reprinted from *Continuing Survey of Food Intakes by Individuals, 1989–1991,* US Department of Agriculture, 1994.

reports that the percentage of energy from fat declined from 41 to 37% during that time. The most recent data (see Tables 4-7 and 4-9) indicate that the mean percentage of energy from fat among adult women has dropped to 34%, a level still above the year 2000 objective, but a level much closer than 15 years ago. Table 4-9 illustrates that growing numbers of women of all ages are meeting the total fat guidelines. Older women are more likely to have diets that meet the guidelines. Thirty-one percent of women aged 60 and older have total fat intakes that are 30% of energy or less, as compared with 18% of teenage women.

Fruit, Vegetable, and Grains Servings

Healthy People 2000,[68] recommends an increase in the amount of complex carbohydrate-containing foods consumed. The objective of five or more daily servings of vegetables (including legumes) and fruits and six or more daily servings of grain products is double the baseline measure of 2.5 servings of vegetables and fruits and three servings of grains consumed daily by women (CSFII 1985). Several additional national data sets provide estimates that show trends in consumption of the numbers of servings of fruits, vegetables, and grains.

In NHANES II (1976-1980)[70] 25% of white women and 19% of black women consumed three or more servings of vegetables daily. 32% and 24%, respectively, consumed two or more servings of fruit daily; Only 9% of white women and 5% of black women consumed five or more servings of fruits and vegetables daily.

Table 4-9 Percentage of Women by Category of Percentage Energy from Fat: Women Aged 12 Years and Older (3 Days, 1989 to 1991, CSFII)

	% Energy from Fat		
	<30	>30 but <40	>40
Age (yr)	% Individuals		
12–19	17.9	61.1	21.0
20–29	25.9	55.6	18.5
30–39	21.7	54.9	23.5
40–49	20.2	50.9	28.9
50–59	25.8	54.7	19.4
60–69	30.6	50.1	19.3
70+	32.1	54.4	13.6
Women 20 and older	25.2	53.6	21.1

Source: Reprinted from *Continuing Survey of Food Intakes by Individuals, 1989–1991,* US Department of Agriculture, 1994.

Among primary meal planner/preparers surveyed as part of both the CSFII 1989 and the DHKS, 50% of women consumed fewer than one serving of fruit daily and fewer than 1.5 servings of vegetables daily. Approximately 15% of the sample consumed the recommended five or more daily servings of fruits and vegetables, 25% consumed between three and five servings daily, and the remaining 60% consumed fewer than three total servings daily. Only about 10% of female primary planner/preparers consumed six or more servings of grains daily, 50% consumed 3.7 or fewer servings per day, and approximately 15% of 1989 DHKS women consumed two or fewer servings of grains daily.[22]

Most recently in 1991, the 5 a Day for Better Health program sponsored by the National Cancer Institute and the Produce for Better Health Foundation conducted a nationally representative baseline survey of fruit and vegetable consumption patterns of adults aged 18 and older. The estimated daily fruit and vegetable consumption of adult women was 3.7 servings per day. When asked the number of servings of fruits and vegetables one should eat each day, 58% of all women responded that two or fewer servings per day was sufficient; 24% thought four or more servings should be consumed daily. When results of the baseline survey were summarized, authors concluded that women, people older than age 65, and those with more education and/or income consumed more fruits and vegetables compared with other groups in each category.[71]

When comparing estimates of fruit, vegetable, and grain consumption, some methodological issues may bias estimates. First, not all studies that estimate fruit, vegetable, and grain servings per day include estimates of food included in mixed dishes. Several researchers[69,70,72] have demonstrated the importance of separating components of mixed dishes, salads, and soups to appropriately count servings of fruits, vegetable, and grain. Second, differences in the definition of a serving size may result in differences in estimates across different studies.

Regardless of the method used to count servings of fruits, grains, and vegetables in the diet, it is clear that large proportions of American women fail to consume adequate numbers and varieties of fruits, vegetables, and grains on a daily basis. Consumption patterns of younger women lag behind those of older women, despite the greater caloric intakes of younger women. Some dietary transitions are clear. Many women have heard the dietary fat and dietary cholesterol messages and have made food changes, which are reflected in lower total intakes of fat and dietary cholesterol. Across all persons, the percentage of food energy from fat has declined steadily since the mid-1970s. This decline results from food supply as well as conscious food behavior changes. Dairy, meat, and egg consumption changes are consistent with nutrient quality differences observed over time in the diets of women. It is clear that the dietary messages regarding reducing selected sources of dietary fat and cholesterol have been heard.

It is also clear that the messages related to increasing consumption of selected fruits, vegetables, and grains are not as familiar and have not yet been adopted by the numbers of individuals that have been able to change dietary patterns related to fat. The national promotion by the 5 a Day for Better Health program has had an impact on awareness, as has the introduction of the Food Guide Pyramid.[73] However, it is unlikely that increasing awareness, without concurrent food supply and behavior-oriented interventions, will accomplish the desired population increase in complex carbohydrate-containing foods.

To improve the quality of women's diets with respect to fruits, vegetables, and grains, it is perhaps relevant to examine what we have learned about adopting and maintaining changes in dietary fat intakes.[74,75] Experience with the Women's Health Trial indicates that women who were successful in decreasing and maintaining reductions in dietary fat were initially successful in reducing visible fats and oils. Examples include use of diet salad dressings and margarines. However, decreasing fat from grain products was more difficult. Women were initially successful by substituting specially manufactured foods to achieve the dietary fat goals. When women were required to significantly modify the dietary pattern by avoiding core foods such as beef and pork or replacing high-fat foods such as desserts or mixed dishes, success in achieving and maintaining change was more limited. The limited availability of reduced-fat grain products is a food supply difference that may shift during the later part of the 1990s as additional fat-modified grain products arrive on grocers' shelves. Palatable food supply introductions could improve the probability that women will continue to increase consumption of complex carbohydrate grain-based products. However, the prevalent concern of many women for weight management, coupled with the long-standing impression that many grain products are "fattening" may make increasing grain consumption more difficult than reducing sources of visible fats.

Increasing fruit and vegetable consumption presents another challenge. The problem is not that women eat too much or the wrong kind but rather that they consume too little. If prior experience in dietary modification is a guide, this guideline will require significant social marketing to suggest acceptable strategies for changing basic patterns of eating. Modifications in the perceptions of palatability, the convenience of fruits and vegetables as stand-alone foods that can be consumed as snacks or fast foods, as well as the ease of preparation for at-home consumption, will be needed to significantly increase population-level consumption levels.

Indices of Overall Diet Quality

The diversity of food consumption practices suggests that an overall index reflecting consensus food and nutrient recommendations would be useful in evaluating the overall quality of the diet of American women. Several such indices have been or are being developed. The diet quality index (DQI) provides the first published example of the usefulness of an aggregate index measuring overall diet quality.[69] This particular index scales eight distinct diet and health dietary recommendations into a single index designed to reflect a risk gradient for major diet-related chronic diseases. Possible index scores range from 0 to 16 and reflect the percentage of energy consumed as total and saturated fats, dietary cholesterol and sodium intakes, numbers of servings of fruits, vegetables, and grains, and the percentage of the RDA consumed for protein and calcium. A person achieving the desired dietary intake level in each of the eight recommendation areas would receive a score of 0. Deviations of approximately 30% from each of the desired dietary levels are scored as 1 point, while greater deviations are scored with 2 points.

Gender-specific data related to diet quality are not published.[69] However, subsequent analysis of data from women interviewed as part of the 1989 CSFII and 1989 DHKS suggests that the overall mean DQI score was slightly better for women than men (8.15 versus 8.70). Ten percent of women had scores of 5 or lower, 25% had scores of 6 or lower, while 25% had scores that exceeded 10, and 10% had scores that exceeded 11.[22] To illustrate possible scenarios that might result in this range of scores, the woman with a DQI score of 5 might meet three of the eight recommendations and be within about 30% of meeting the remaining five recommendations. In a likely scenario, the woman with a DQI score of 5 would

- Meet the following recommendations:
  1. less than 300 mg of dietary cholesterol per day = 0 points
  2. sodium intake less than or equal to 2400 mg = 0 points
  3. protein intakes not more than 100% of the RDA = 0 points

- Be within approximately 30% of the goal for the following recommendations:
  1. calcium intakes between 67 and 99% RDA rather than greater than 100 = 1 point
  2. Three to four fruit and vegetable servings per day rather than five or more = 1 point
  3. 30 to 40% of energy from fat rather than less than 30% = 1 point
  4. 10 to 13% of energy from saturated fat rather than less than 10% = 1 point
  5. Four to five servings of grains per day rather than six or more = 1 point.

The woman with a DQI score of 8 could have a score of 1 for each of the guideline's categories, whereas those with scores in excess of 8 must have one or more categories in which the diet is judged to be greatly above or below the recommended intake levels and is scored as a 2. For example, intakes of greater than 40% of energy as fat, zero to two servings of fruit and vegetables daily, or zero to three servings of grain products daily would each be scored as 2 points.

With a population mean DQI score in excess of 8 and only 25% of a sample of female primary meal planner/preparers with scores of 6 or less, a considerable amount of improvement in the diets of American women is possible. Trend estimates are unavailable at this time to track changes in overall diet quality scores, but it seems clear that a simple index can provide a useful yardstick by which to measure improvements in the American diet and will be a useful addition to the NNMS. The extent to which a dietary quality measurement such as the DQI is useful in predicting morbidity and/or mortality remains to be seen. However, as a descriptive tool, it provides a useful means of monitoring intakes of either the overall population or subgroups of interest.

OPPORTUNITIES FOR CHANGE

In an era of increasing interest in the health of women, it is natural to examine the opportunities available to improve the diets of women. Opportunities can be generally divided into environmental opportunities versus interventions that are targeted to individuals or groups of women to influence individual patterns of behavior.

Environmental-level channels offer some of the most promising avenues for continuing dietary change. Changes in the food supply have made a significant contribution to the population-level reduction in the percentage of energy from fat to current levels. As palatable substitutes become available at reasonable prices, the personal cost of making dietary change is reduced, and meaningful food changes are more likely. Food supply changes must, however, be accompanied by consistent guidance regarding what kinds and amounts of food are needed to constitute a healthy diet. At one time, nutritionists were concerned that widespread fortification would lead to the "nutrification" of the food supply, or viewing foods only in terms of a select range of nutrients provided. The increased use of fat and sweetener substitutes again has the potential to blur the "quality" of potential food choices by narrowing the evaluation of the quality of a given food to its contribution of fat or sweetener. If a potato chip no longer contains fat, is it a good food choice? Food supply change is probably necessary to facilitate continued healthful dietary change, but alone it will not be sufficient to help the average woman design a healthful diet given the range of natural and engineered foods available.

This suggests that the second opportunity for change must include intervention efforts that help the average consumer make food choices from among increasing options. Consumers still need to recognize that a healthy diet can be described in terms of what it contains, as well as what it limits. Adoption of educational approaches based on the food guide pyramid and based on nutrition labeling is an area in which to begin. But just as food supply changes will not be sufficient to facilitate healthful diets across the broad population, traditional nutrition education, without meaningful behavior change strategies, will not be sufficient to achieve our dietary goals either. We must learn more about the behavioral barriers that exist regarding adoption of dietary patterns that are more dense in complex carbohydrate-containing foods. Whether barriers relate to eating out, feeling deprived, time pressures, hectic life style making planning difficult, presence or lack of friend or family support, economic or other reasons, we need to identify cost-effective ways of matching change strategies to the individuals who need them. The strategies must relate to the use of food—the basic commodity of the diet, rather than some proximal nutrient-based goal. The necessity of incorporation of a behavioral component cannot be emphasized enough. The challenge of educating the nutrition educators of tomorrow is providing a sense of the "big picture" and a vision of all the possibilities available to those who work with the public, as well as the skills to tailor a behaviorally oriented change program for a single individual or a community. No longer are skills in nutrition science sufficient. The nutrition practitioner of tomorrow must posses skills in political science, health communications, creative partnershiping, and financing. No longer acting as the sole educator, the new nutritionist must serve in the capacity of the visionary and leader as well as manager of people and resources.

Some institutional avenues exist through which to increase the promotion of healthier diets for women, but in general adult health promotion efforts receive only a very small portion of the health dollar. A broader institutional infrastructure is needed to support nutrition in health promotion, as well as in treatment of disease. Without such community capacity, access to nutrition information will be limited to women with the education, motivation, or economic means to pay for such services.

Although widespread structural change is needed in how we as a nation finance health promotion, several opportunities do exist in both the public and private sector. The Supplemental Food Program for Women, Infants, and Children (WIC) is a public source of individualized nutrition education for low-income pregnant, postpartum, and breastfeeding women. Despite heavy caseloads and the limited age and economic range of the female population served, health promotion including both education and behavior change to achieve normal diets for adult women should be incorporated into WIC education programs. Among older women, the Nutrition Program for Older Americans, administered by the Administration on Aging of the DHHS, could serve as a vehicle to foster better dietary choices. Currently, nutrition education is mandated only semiannually, and program staff rarely includes professional nutrition staff at the local level. Reauthorized in 1992, new provisions of the Older American Act encourage provision of services related to health promotion, so new opportunities exist for nutrition professionals to reach older women through this venue.

Fewer avenues currently exist with which to reach women between the ages of childbearing and retirement. Inclusion of nutrition counseling as a reimbursable service as part of national health care reform or as part of private health insurance policies would provide a significant avenue for reliable nutrition information. Reliable health promotion information available through the worksite is increasingly an option. A recent survey by the Office of Disease Prevention and Health Promotion of the U.S. Public Health Service suggests that the numbers of worksites with 50 or more employees that offered some kind of nutrition programming increased from 16 to 31% between 1985 and 1992.[76] The National Cancer Institute of the NIH currently sponsors the evaluation of a range of nutrition-related worksite cancer prevention programs. Worksite or other organizational-level channels provide access to groups of women not reached before with nutrition and health information.

Health communications is a broad area currently encompassing multiple kinds of media. Coordinated programs using social marketing techniques carefully designed to accomplish explicit behavioral goals are needed to reach the mass of women living in differing environments with different life styles and purchasing patterns. In particular, the potential exists for electronic media to provide an opportunity to educate in a cost-effective way. Perhaps the nutritionist of the future should consider running a computer bulletin board/clearinghouse as a source of information, sharing, and social support for food and nutrition-related information. CD-ROM or its future version of electronic media provides access to pictures, sound, and motion, as well as more traditional text. Interactive computing services provide another opportunity for creative sharing and problem solving for diverse groups. Even in traditional worksite settings, desktop publishing has made the creation of exciting written materials within the reach of even the most limited health department budget.

Improving the diet of the American woman will not happen in a vacuum. Social and economic changes influence the resources available and the roles each woman adopts in day-to-day activities. By anticipating and working within our changing environment and looking to both public and private organizations to coordinate the series of efforts needed to reach women diverse in age, race, education, income, and life-style philosophy, all women can have better access to a safe and healthy diet.

References

1. U.S. Department of Health and Human Services and U.S. Department of Agriculture. *An Update Report on Nutrition Monitoring.* September 1989. DHHS Pub No. (PHS) 89-1255.

2. Senauer B, Asp E, Kinsey J. *Food Trends and the Changing Consumer.* St. Paul, Minn: Eagan Press; 1991.

3. National Research Council. *Designing Foods: Animal Products Options in the Marketplace.* Washington, DC: National Academy Press; 1988.

4. Smith RE. Food demands of the emerging consumer: the role of modern food technology in meeting the challenge. *Am J Clin Nutr.* 1993;58:307s–312s.

5. Rolls B. Effects of intense sweeteners on hunger, food intake, and body weight: a review. *Am J Clin Nutr.* 1991;53:872–878.

6. Stern JS, Hermann-Zaidins MG. Fat replacements: a new strategy for dietary change. *J Am Diet Assoc.* 1992;92:91–93.

7. Mela DL. Nutritional implications of fat substitutes. *J Am Diet Assoc.* 1992;92:472–476.

8. Beaton GH, Tarasuk V, Anderson GH. Estimate of possible impact of non-calorie fat and carbohydrate substitutes on macro-nutrient intake in the human. *Appetite.* 1992;19:87–103.

9. Gussow J, Akabas S. Are we really fixing up the food supply? *J Am Diet Assoc.* 1993;93:1300–1304.

10. Hurley J, Schmidt S. Chinese food: a wok on the wild side. *Nutr Action Newsletter.* September 1993.

11. Hurley J, Schmidt S. Mexican food: oile. *Nutr Action Newsletter.* July/August, 1994.

12. Reis CP, Kline K, Weaver SO. Impact of commercial eating on nutrient adequacy. *J Am Diet Assoc.* 1987;87:463–468.

13. U.S. Department of Agriculture, Agriculture Research Service. *Food and Nutrient Intakes by Individuals in the United States, 1 Day, 1989–91. Continuing Survey of Food Intake by Individuals, 1989–91.* NFS Report No. 91-2.

14. Enns CW, Guenther PM. Women's food and nutrient intakes away from home, 1985. *Family Econ Rev.* 1988;1:9–12.

15. Haines P, Hungerford D, Popkin B, Guilkey D. Eating patterns and energy and nutrient intakes of US women. *J Am Diet Assoc.* 1992;92:698–704, 707.

16. Haines P. *Executive Summary. Dietary Status and Eating Patterns.* January 1993. Final Technical Report for USDA Cooperative Agreement no. 58-3198-9-069.

17. Davis CG. Linkages between socioeconomic characteristics, food expenditure patterns, and nutritional status of low income households. *Am J Agric Econ.* 1982;64:1017–1025.

18. Axelson ML. The impact of culture on food-related behavior. *Annu Rev Nutr.* 1986;6:345–363.

19. Thompson FE, Sowers MF, Frongillo EA, Parpia BJ. Sources of fiber and fat in diets of US women aged 19 to 50: implications for nutrition education and policy. *Am J Public Health.* 1992;82:695–702.

20. Kushi LH, Folsom AR, Jacobs DR, Luepker RV, Elmer PJ, Blackburn H. Educational attainment and nutrient consumption patterns: the Minnesota Heart Survey. *J Am Diet Assoc.* 1988;88: 1230–1236.

21. Murphy SP, Rose D, Hudes M, Viteri FE. Demographic and economic factors associated with dietary quality for adults in the 1987–88 Nationwide Food Consumption Survey. *J Am Diet Assoc.* 1992;92:1352–1357.

22. Haines P. *Executive Summary. Knowledge and Attitudes Related to Dietary Choices among US Men and Women. The 1989 Diet and Health Knowledge Survey and the 1989 Continuing Survey of Food Intakes by Individuals.* June 1994. Final Technical Report for USDA Cooperative Agreement no. 58-3198-0-052.

23. U.S. Bureau of the Census. *Statistical Abstract of the United States.* Washington, DC; 1990.

24. Johnson RK, Crouter AC, Smiciklas-Wright H. Effects of maternal employment on family food consumption patterns and children's diets. *J Nutr Educ.* 1993;25:130–133.

25. Horton S, Campbell C. Wife's employment, food expenditures, and apparent nutrient intake: evidence from Canada. *Am J Agric Econ.* 1991;73:784–794.

26. Popkin BM, Haines PS. Factors affecting food selection: the role of economics. *J Am Diet Assoc.* 1981;79:419–425.

27. Redman B. The impact of women's time allocation on expenditure for meals away from home and prepared foods. *Am J Agric Econ.* 1980;62:234–237.

28. Capps O, Tedford JR, Havlick J. Household demand for convenience and nonconvenience foods. *Am J Agric Econ.* 1985;67:862–869.

29. McCracken VA, Brandt JA. Household consumption of food away-from-home: total expenditure by type of food facility. *Am J Agric Econ.* 1987;69:274–284.

30. Kinsey J. Working wives and the marginal propensity to consume food away from home. *Am J Agric Econ.* 1983;65:10–19.

31. Tippett KS, Cristofar S. Dietary intakes by employment status. *Fam Econ Rev.* 1988;1:11–13.

32. Popkin B, Guilkey D, Haines P. Food consumption changes of adult women between 1977 and 1985. *Am J Agric Econ.* 1989;71:949–959.

33. Popkin B, Haines P, Reidy K. Food consumption trends of US women: patterns and determinants between 1977 and 1985. *Am J Clin Nutr.* 1989;49:1307–1319.

34. Shea S, Stein AD, Bach CE, et al. Independent associations of educational attainment and ethnicity with behavioral risk factors for cardiovascular disease. *Am J Epidemiol.* 1991;13:567–582.

35. Cotugna N, Subar AF, Heimendinger J, Kahle L. Nutrition and cancer prevention knowledge, beliefs, attitudes and practices: the 1987 National Health Interview Survey. *J Am Diet Assoc.* 1992;92:963–968.

36. American Dietetic Association and the International Food Information Council. *How Are Americans Making Food Choices?* Chicago,Ill: American Dietetic Association, 1994.

37. Lewin K. Forces behind food habits and methods of change. In: National Research Council, ed. *The Problem of Changing Food Habits.* Washington, DC: National Academy Press; 1943.

38. Schafer RB, Schaefer E. Relationship between gender and food roles in the family. *J Nutr Educ.* 1989;21:119–126.

39. Devine CM, Olsen CM. Women's perceptions about the way social roles promote or constrain personal nutrition care. *Women Health.* 1992;19:79–95.

40. Kirk MC, Gillespie AH. Factors affecting food choices of working mothers with young families. *J Nutr Educ.* 1990;22:161–168.

41. Roland A, Harris B. *Career and Motherhood—Struggles for a new identity.* New York: Human Sciences Press; 1979.

42. Kuczmarski RJ, Flegal KM, Campbell SM, Johnson CL. Increasing prevalence of overweight among U.S. adults: the National Health and Nutrition Examination Surveys, 1960–1991. *JAMA.* 1994;272:205–211.

43. Williamson DF. Epidemiologic analysis of weight gain in US adults. *Am J Clin Nutr.* 1991;7:285–286.

44. Serdula MK, Colins ME, Williamson DF, Anda RF, Pamuk E, Byers TE. Weight control practices of U.S. adolescents and adults. *Ann Intern Med.* 1993;119:667–671.

45. Williamson DF, Serdula MK, Anda RF, Levy A, Byers T. Weight loss attempts in adults: goals, duration, and rate of weight loss. *Am J Public Health.* 1992;82:1251–1257.

46. NIH Technology Assessment Conference Statement. Methods for voluntary weight loss and control. *Nutr Rev.* 1992;50:340–345.

47. Dwyer JT, Mayer J. Potential dieters: who are they? *J Am Diet Assoc.* 1970;56:510–514.

48. Horm F, Anderson K. Who in America is trying to lose weight? *Ann Intern Med.* 1993;119:672–676.

49. Kirkley BG, Burge JC. Dietary restriction in young women: issues and concerns. *Ann Behav Med.* 1989;11:66–72.

50. Arrington R, Bonner J, Still KR. Weight reduction methods of college women. *J Am Diet Assoc.* 1985;85:483–484.

51. Subar AF, Block G. Use of vitamin and mineral supplements: demographics and amounts of nutrients consumed. *Am J Epidemiol.* 1990;132:1091–1101.

52. Koplan JP, Annest JL, Layde PM, Rubin GL. Nutrient intake and supplementation in the United States (NHANES II). *Am J Public Health.* 1986;76:287–289.

53. Bender MM, Levy AS, Schucker RE, Yetley EA. Trends in prevalence and magnitude of vitamin and mineral supplement usage and correlation with health status. *J Am Diet Assoc.* 1992;92:1096–1101.

54. Larkin FA, Basiotis PP, Riddick HA, Sykes KE, Pao EM. Dietary patterns of women smokers and non-smokers. *J Am Diet Assoc.* 1990;90:230–237.

55. Subar AF, Harlan LC, Mattson ME. Food and nutrient intake differences between smokers and non-smokers in the US. *Am J Public Health.* 1990;80:1323–1329.

56. Strickland D, Graves K, Lando H. Smoking status and dietary fats. *Prev Med.* 1992;21:228–236.

57. McPhillips JB, Eaton CB, Gans KM, et al. Dietary differences in smokers and nonsmokers from two southeastern New England communities. *J Am Diet Assoc.* 1994;94:287–292.

58. National Center for Health Statistics. *Health, United States 1992.* Hyattsville, MD: Public Health Services; 1993. DHHS Publication no. (PHS) 93–1232.

59. Bradstock K, Forman MR, Binkin NJ, et al. Alcohol use and health behavior lifestyles among women: the Behavioral Risk Factor Surveys. *Addict Behav.* 1988;13:61–71.

60. Patterson RE, Haines PS, Popkin BM. Health lifestyles chosen by US adults. *Prev Med.* 1994;23:453–460.

61. U.S. Department of Health and Human Services and U.S. Department of Agriculture. *Nutrition Monitoring in the United States. A Report from the Joint Nutrition Monitoring Evaluation Committee.* Washington, DC: Public Health Service; July 1986. DHHS Pub no. (PHS) 86-1255.

62. Haines P, Guilkey D, Popkin B. Modeling food consumption decisions as a two-step process. *Am J Agric Econ.* 1988;70:543–552.

63. U.S. Department of Agriculture and U.S. Department of Health and Home Services. *Dietary Guidelines for Americans.* 1990. Home and Garden Bulletin no. 232.

64. U.S. Department of Agriculture. *1990 Agricultural Chartbook.* 1990. Agricultural Handbook no. 689.

65. Krebs-Smith SM, Cronin FJ, Haytowitz DB, Cook DA. Food sources of energy, macronutrients, cholesterol, and fiber in diets of women. *J Am Diet Assoc.* 1992;92:168–174.

66. Popkin B, Haines P, Patterson R. Dietary changes in older Americans, 1977–1987. *Am J Clin Nutr.* 1992;55:823–830.

67. Peterkin B. Women's diets: 1977 and 1985. *J Nutr Educ.* 1986;18:251–257.

68. U.S. Department of Health and Human Services. *Healthy People 2000 National Health Promotion and Disease Prevention Objectives.* 1991. DHHS Publication no. (PHS) 91-50212.

69. Patterson RE, Haines PS, Popkin BM. Diet quality index: capturing a multidimensional behavior. *J Am Diet Assoc.* 1994;94:57–64.

70. Patterson BM, Block G, Rosenberger WF, Pee D, Kahle LL. Fruit and vegetables in the American diet: data from the NHANES II Survey. *Am J Public Health.* 1990;80:1443–1449.

71. Subar AS, Heimendinger J, Krebs-Smith SM, Patterson BH, Kessler R, Pivonka E. *5 a Day for Better Health: A Baseline Study of Americans Fruit and Vegetable Consumption.* Rockville, Md: National Institutes of Health, National Cancer Institute, Division of Cancer Prevention and Control; 1991.

72. Krebs-Smith SM, Cronin FJ, Haytowitz DB, Cook DA. Contributions of food groups to intakes of energy, nutrients, cholesterol, and fiber in women's diets: effect on method of classifying food mixtures. *J Am Diet Assoc.* 1990;90:1541–1546.

73. U.S. Department of Agriculture. *The Food Guide Pyramid.* 1992. Home and Garden Bulletin no. 252.

74. Burrows ER, Henry HJ, Bowen DJ, Henderson MM. Nutritional applications of a clinical low fat dietary intervention to public health change. *J Nutr Educ.* 1993;25:167–175.

75. Kristal AR, White E, Shattuck AL, et al. Long-term maintenance of a low-fat diet: durability of fat-related dietary habits in the Women's Health Trial. *J Am Diet Assoc.* 1992;92:553–559.

76. Interagency Board for Nutrition Monitoring and Related Research. *Nutrition Monitoring in the United States. Chartbook I: Selected Findings from the National Nutrition Monitoring and Related Research Program.* Hyattsville, Md: Public Health Service; 1993. DHHS Publication no. (PHS) 93-1255-2.

5

 है।

Diet, the Menstrual Cycle, and Sex Steroid Hormones

Christy C. Tangney

This chapter includes a review of (1) the phases of the menstrual cycle including a brief description of the interrelationships among the sex steroid hormones; (2) the effect of the menstrual cycle on food intake and nutrient use; (3) the role of dietary composition on serum sex steroids and menstrual function; (4) diet, nutritional supplements, and premenstrual syndrome; and (5) under- and overnutrition and fertility.

MENSTRUAL CYCLE

Phases

Menstruation marks the beginning of a new cycle with the first day of menses being day 1. The other three phases are (1) the follicular (or postmenstrual) phase, during which follicular development occurs; (2) the periovulatory period, when final maturation of the oocyte and its release into the reproductive tract occurs; and (3) the luteal (or premenstrual) phase, when the corpus luteum secretes hormones to facilitate and prepare for implantation.

During the active reproductive years, the median interval between menstrual periods is 28 days.[1] However, the length of the menstrual cycle can be highly variable.[2] Much of the variability is due to differences in follicular phase length, as the luteal phase is usually about 12 to 15 days long.[3]

One method of describing menstrual cycles is by documenting the time of ovulation. If the day of the gonadotrophin surge or ovulation can be determined—specifically, follicle-stimulating hormone (FSH) and luteinizing hormone (LH)—clinicians will label this day 0 (Figure 5-1). With this method, follicular-phase days are those that occur as negative numbers as they occur before the rise (days −12 to 0). Conversely, luteal-phase days are positive numbers as they occur after

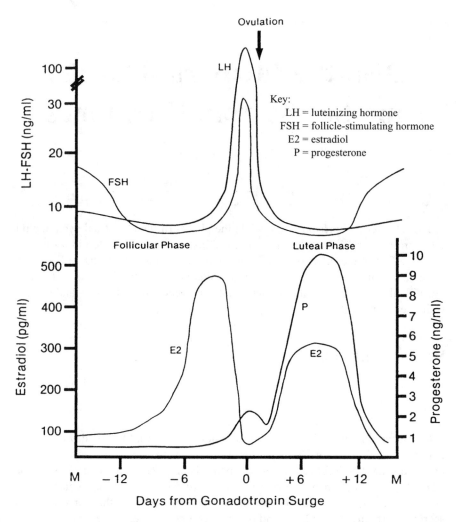

Figure 5-1 Hormone Profiles during the Menstrual Cycle (day 0 = day of gonadotrophin surge, days –12 to 0 = follicular phase, days +1 to +12 = luteal phase) *Source:* Reprinted from *The Menstrual Cycle: Physiology, Reproductive Disorders, and Infertility* by M Ferin, R Jewelewicz and M Warren (p 6) with permission of Oxford University Press, © 1993.

the surge (days +1 to 12). Commercial kits to pinpoint ovulation by measuring gonadotrophins are available to the public.

Another method to approximate ovulation and the luteal phase is by daily monitoring of the basal body temperature (BBT).[3–5] A marked rise in BBT occurs about 2 days after the LH peak; the temperature remains elevated for the entire luteal phase and falls close to menses (Figure 5-2). BBT rises because progesterone acts on the thermoregulatory center in the anterior hypothalamus to increase temperature.[3] When progesterone levels drop, BBT declines accordingly. If pregnancy occurs, the BBT will stay elevated. For accurate assessment, patient cooperation in charting BBT is essential. The coverline method[6] is another method to estimate ovulation by using daily BBTs.

The most accurate method of determining menstrual phase is by measuring blood levels of estradiol-17β (E_2), progesterone (P), and if possible FSH and LH (see Figure 5-1). During the menstrual cycle, E_2 exhibits a bimodal pattern. The first peak, which occurs a day before the LH surge, marks the late follicular phase. After ovulation, a drop in E_2 secretion is followed by a second rise corresponding to the formation of the corpus luteum. The rise and fall of serum P (or sodium pregnanediol-glucuronide, the major urinary progestin metabolite) parallel the activity of the corpus luteum and, thus, may be used to confirm ovulation and proper functioning of the corpus luteum. Thus, P is elevated only during the luteal phase. FSH also exhibits two peaks, the first of which initiates follicular development and the second occurs at ovulation. LH peaks at ovulation, too.

When no clinical or biochemical measures are available to discern the menstrual phase, two surrogate approaches may be used. If menstrual histories are available, cycle length may be defined as the number of days between the onset of two consecutive menstrual periods. Because luteal-phase length is relatively constant,[3] the 14 days before menses onset are identified as the luteal phase. The remaining days, starting on the first day of menstruation, represent the follicular phase.[7,8] Alternatively, one may "standardize" the cycle data to 28 days. With this approach, the luteal 14-day period is still maintained, but the days during the follicular phase are forced into a standard 14-day numbering sequence. This method is often used when menstrual histories are incomplete with regard to cycle length.

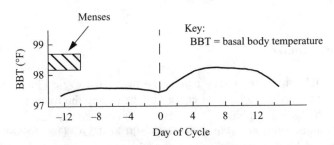

Figure 5-2 Basal Body Temperatures during the Menstrual Cycle (day 0 = day of gonadotrophin surge, days −12 to 0 = follicular phase, days +1 to +12 = luteal phase) *Source:* Reprinted from *Reproductive Endocrinology: Physiology, Pathophysiology and Clinical Management* by SSC Yen and RB Javve (p 852) with permission of WB Saunders, © 1977.

Because the accuracy of these surrogate methods vary, comparisons among studies that used different methods are difficult.

Sex Steroid Hormones

Sex hormones belong to three major classes, which are all synthesized from cholesterol. These classes are distinguished by the number of carbon atoms present in the structure. The three classes are:

1. C21 series, the progestins
2. C19 series, the androgens
3. C18 series, the estrogens

The pathway for converting cholesterol to pregnenolone is identical in adrenal, ovary, and testis. Thus, pregnenolone is a key precursor of all steroid hormones[9] (Figure 5-3).

The progestins and estrogens are the predominant sex hormones in women. P is the most abundant progestin. It is secreted by the follicle and corpus luteum during the periovulatory and luteal phases. Estrogens are a family of hormones (Figure 5-3). E_2 is the predominant estrogen in premenopausal women. E_1 is the major source of estrogens in postmenopausal women. Estriol (E_3) is the least potent and least abundant estrogen in premenstrual women; it is derived from E_1 and is produced by the placenta during pregnancy. Estrone sulfate is a major metabolite of estrogen present in blood (45 to 50% of the estrogen in blood) and has a concentration ten times higher than E_1 or E_2.[10]

PATTERNS OF FOOD INTAKE ACROSS THE MENSTRUAL CYCLE

Total Energy Intake

Energy intake appears to vary across the menstrual cycle (Table 5-1). Most investigators report an increase in energy intake during the luteal phase as compared with the follicular phase.[7,8,11–18] This premenstrual increase in energy consumption ranges from an additional 87 to 500 kcal/day. The variability in the increase could be due to methodologic problems. In these studies, food consumption was assessed by many days of self-reported food records or weighed food intakes. However, the phase of the cycle was set at one time point—either during the 3 or 10 days before menstruation (for luteal phase) or during the 3 or

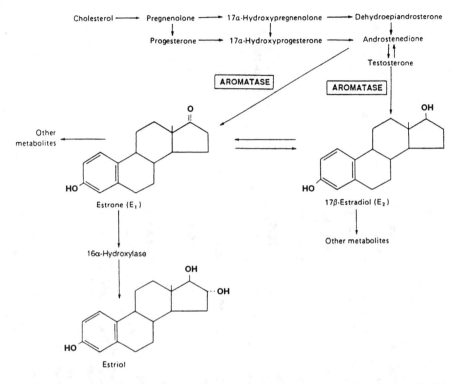

Figure 5-3 Synthesis of Sex Steroid Hormones *Source:* Reprinted from *Review of Medical Physiology,* ed 16 (p 401) by WF Ganong with permission of Appleton & Lange, © 1993.

10 days after menstruation (for the follicular phase).[14] Thus, the exact phase of the cycle was estimated and not definitively determined by blood analyses or other methods.

The Beltsville One-year Dietary Intake Study[19] provided a unique opportunity to examine the relationship between dietary patterns and menstrual cyclicity, because 29 participants recorded their food intakes for 365 days. Unfortunately, the 14 premenopausal women only provided menstrual history information during four 1-week balance periods.[8] Therefore, information was available only for those periods instead of the whole year. As shown previously, energy intakes were significantly greater (about 90 kcal) during the luteal phase as compared with the follicular phase.

More recently, Barr et al[17] studied energy intakes across six cycles in women with or without ovulatory disturbances. Again, women with normal cycles consumed an average of 300 more calories during the luteal phase. However, women who did not ovulate consumed about the same number of calories during the dif-

Table 5-1 Energy Intakes throughout the Menstrual Cycle[a]

Study	Subjects (n)	Premenstrual/Luteal (L)	Menses (M)	Postmenstrual/Follicular (F)	Ovulation (O)	Energy Difference (kcal)
Dalvit, 1981[11]	8	1789 ± 74		1286 ± 57		503
Manocha et al, 1986[13]	11	1620 ± 83		1300 ± 87		320
Gallant et al, 1987[14]	10	1933 ± 109		1498 ± 120		435
Lissner et al, 1988[7]	23	2335		2248		87[b] 100–150[c]
Gong et al, 1989[15]	7	2040 ± 156	1887 ± 230	1833 ± 146	1766 ± 252	214 (L–F)[d] 283 (L–O)[d]
Lyons et al, 1989[16]	18	2198 ± 86	2155 ± 100	2012 ± 69	1874 ± 81	324 (L–O)[d]
Tarasuk and Beaton, 1991[8]	14	1912		1822		90[b] 106[c]
Fong and Kretsch, 1993[23]	9	2501 ± 180	2453 ± 196		2243 ± 285	NS
Barr et al, 1995[17]	29	2225 ± 120		1922 ± 105		303

[a]Values are mean caloric intake ± SEM. All are statistically significant unless NS (no significant differences) is listed.
[b]Significant difference between premenstrual and postmenstrual phases, for Tarasuk and Beaton, 14-day comparisons, while for Lissner et al, 10-day comparisons.
[c]Significant peak-to-trough differences obtained with curve-fitting analyses.
[d]Significant differences located between phases using multiple comparison tests.

ferent phases. Most previous studies did not document ovulation. Thus, the variability in energy intakes observed could be due to the inclusion of women with anovulatory cycles.

Energy intakes have been plotted by hormone fluctuations to see if the two parameters could be related. Lissner et al[7] plotted group energy intakes as a function of a standardized 28-day cycle and then compared these plots with graphs of serum P and E_2 levels.[18] The pattern for both hormones reflected that of energy intakes. Two periodic effects were observed: one peak during the luteal phase and a second smaller peak during the follicular phase (Figure 5-4). The two peaks, approximately 2 weeks apart, reflected an increment of 200 kcal. Stated another way, two declines in caloric intake are observed—one during menstruation and

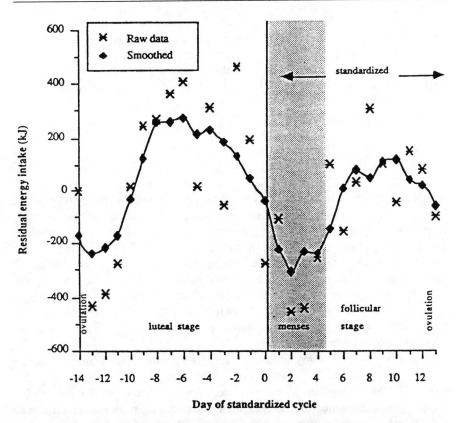

Figure 5-4 Cyclic Pattern of Energy Intakes Plotted across a Standardized Menstrual Cycle (day 0 = 0 menstruation, day 1 to 12 = follicular phase, day −14 to −1 = luteal phase) *Source:* Adapted with permission from *American Journal of Clinical Nutrition* (1988;48:956–962), Copyright © 1988, American Society for Clinical Nutrition.

another around ovulation. Others have confirmed a fall in energy intake at ovulation.[15,16] With similar curve-fitting techniques, Tarasuk and Beaton[8] estimated peak-to-trough differences of approximately 106 kcal.

Overall, energy intakes vary by the menstrual phase when the menstrual cycle is ovulatory. One very controlled metabolic study failed to find changes in energy intake across the menstrual cycle.[20–23] However, ovulation was not confirmed by BBT, and a very small sample size was used. Thus, discrepancies in the literature could be due to (1) failure to document ovulation, (2) small sample sizes, (3) imprecise methods used to measure food intake, or (4) whether subjects were free-living or in a metabolic ward. Although the metabolic unit provides considerable study control, a limitation is that such an environment may be stressful and have a negative effect on food selection.

In support of the observed decline in energy intake during ovulation, a similar inverse relationship between E_2 levels and food intake has been documented in rhesus monkeys. The highest food intake was observed during the luteal or postovulatory phase and lowest during the time of expected ovulation.[21,22] One common interpretation of these findings is that estrogen has an inhibitory effect on appetite. However, plots of energy intake and hormones from Lissner et al[7] suggest that E_2 levels across the cycle parallel and, therefore, positively relate to energy intake patterns.

Variability in Dietary Components

Identifying which macronutrients or dietary components might be responsible for the changes in energy intake has been less consistent and far from compelling. Only one study[12] found that carbohydrate was the source of increased energy intake observed during the luteal phase (Table 5-2). Fong and Kretsch[23] found that consumption of sugar-containing soft drinks was greater during the luteal phase, but the impact on total carbohydrate consumption was not significant. The trend for greater carbohydrate consumption in the luteal phase has been observed in another small sample.[16] Therefore, anecdotal reports of increased carbohydrate consumption in the luteal phase have not been confirmed by research conducted to date.

Similarly, only two of five groups[8,14] observed greater fat consumption during luteal or premenstrual days (Table 5-3). Furthermore, the Beltsville group[8] found that cyclic patterns of absolute fat intake, fat density, and protein intake were superimposable on those for energy intake. Estimating peak (luteal) to trough (follicular) differences were 8.9 g for fat and 2.9 g for protein intake (absolute intakes). Abraham et al[20] also found significant increases in both fat and protein intakes during the luteal phase. However, no paired analyses were performed. Only one study[16] found differences in protein intakes during the menstrual cycle

Table 5-2 Carbohydrate Intakes throughout the Menstrual Cycle[a]

Study	Premenstrual/ Luteal (L)	Menses (M)	Postmenstrual/ Follicular (F)	Ovulation (O)	Significance
Dalvit-McPhillips, 1983[12]	257 ± 13		133 ± 7		Yes
Gallant et al, 1987[14]	211 ± 18		172 ± 15		No
Gong et al, 1989[15]	62 ± 16[b]	54 ± 10	50 ± 9	56 ± 21	No
Lyons et al, 1989[16]	263 ± 13	263 ± 14	252 ± 11	235 ± 14	O < L
Tarasuk and Beaton, 1991[8]	220		213		No
	116 g/1000 kcal		118 g/1000 kcal		No
Fong and Kretsch, 1993[23]	297 ± 33	303 ± 20	278 ± 17	267 ± 27	No

[a]Carbohydrate intake is expressed in grams. Values are mean intake ± SEM.
[b]These authors report sucrose intakes, not total carbohydrates.

Table 5-3 Fat Intakes throughout the Menstrual Cycle[a]

Study	Premenstrual/ Luteal (L)	Menses (M)	Postmenstrual/ Follicular (F)	Ovulation (O)	Significance
Dalvit-McPhillips, 1983[12]	62 ± 4		62 ± 4		No
Gallant et al, 1987[14]	81 ± 6		61 ± 7		Yes
Lyons et al, 1989[16]	88 ± 4	87 ± 5	80 ± 3	78 ± 3	No
Tarasuk and Beaton, 1991[8]	80		73		Yes
	41.3 g/1000 kcal		39.5 g/1000 kcal		Yes
Fong and Kretsch, 1993[23]	116 ± 11	111 ± 14	110 ± 14	103 ± 18	No

[a]Fat intake is expressed in grams. Values are mean intake ± SEM.

(Table 5-4). The inconsistent results among the various studies are probably attributable to the insufficient number of days sampled to provide accurate estimates of macronutrients. Intakes of other nutrients (vitamin E, selenium, carotenes, and cholesterol) were found to be consistent across the menstrual cycle.[24]

In summary, most studies suggest that voluntary food intake or energy intake varies across the menstrual cycle. The peak intake occurs during the luteal phase and ranges in magnitude from 80 to 500 kcal. This variability in intake across the menstrual cycle exceeds that reported for weekend-weekday differences.[16,25] If nutritionists acknowledge the need to include at least 1 weekend day when planning food intake studies, recognition of the variability that menstrual cyclicity may contribute should also be made. Because of this source of intraindividual variation in food energy consumption, nutrition researchers may collect dietary intake data during each menstrual phase or for the entire cycle.

Because of the recognized variation in energy intakes attributable to menstrual cyclicity, Eck and coworkers[26] examined food intakes of 28 women to determine whether a 7-day block might serve as an accurate substitute for the entire menstrual cycle. On the basis of food records kept for two cycles, these authors found that the sequence of days 5 through 11 (follicular phase) reflected the best estimate of actual intake, predicting more than 85% of the variance for the entire cycle. On the basis of the previously discussed patterns in energy intake, it is not unexpected that this block would underestimate cycle mean intakes by an average of 65 kcal. Unfortunately, selection of the 7-day blocks were not based on established clinical or biochemical markers of menstrual timing. Each research group must wrestle with the ideal number of days needed to accurately sample intakes of food energy and other nutrients during that phase or the entire cycle. The number of days will depend on the dietary components or nutrients to be quantified as well as the sample of women selected for study.

NUTRIENT USE DURING THE MENSTRUAL CYCLE

Energy Expenditure

Since the 1920s, estimates of energy expenditure in eumenorrheic women have been determined.[27,28] More recent studies confirmed that basal metabolic rate (BMR) does vary significantly during the menstrual cycle (Table 5-5). Specifically, BMR rises 7 to 10 days before menses, drops at menses, remains at its lowest level 1 week before ovulation, and then gradually rises again. The average difference from zenith to nadir ranged from 142 to 359 kcal/day or during the luteal phase, an 11 to 14% increase in BMR has been reported.[29,30] As seen with energy consumption across the menstrual cycle, BMR only increases when ovulation occurs.[30] Subjects on oral contraceptives that suppress ovulation, experi-

Table 5-4 Protein Intakes throughout the Menstrual Cycle[a]

Study	Premenstrual/ Luteal (L)	Menses (M)	Postmenstrual/ Follicular (F)	Ovulation (O)	Significance
Dalvit-McPhillips, 1983[12]	50 ± 2		49 ± 3		No
Gallant et al, 1987[14]	76 ± 7		52 ± 3		Yes
Lyons et al, 1989[16]	73 ± 2	69 ± 4	68 ± 3	63 ± 4	O < L
	67		66		No
Tarasuk and Beaton, 1991[8]	36.6 g/1000 kcal		36.8 g/1000 kcal		No
Fong and Kretsch, 1993[23]	81 ± 8	77 ± 8	76 ± 7	75 ± 8	No

[a]Protein intake is expressed in grams. Values are mean intake ± SEM.

Table 5-5 Patterns in Energy Expenditure across the Menstrual Cycle

Study	Phase in Which Expenditures Were High	Phase in Which Expenditures Were Low	Diet	Significance
Solomon et al, 1982[29]	Luteal	Menses and follicular	Defined formula diets adjusted to maintain body weights	Cyclic patterns BMR varied significantly (359 kcal) with menstrual cycle phase
Webb, 1986[30]	Luteal	Preovulatory or late follicular	Mixed diets presented with caloric value to match energy expenditures	142-kcal difference significant for both direct and indirect calorimetry
Bisdee et al, 1989[32]	Late luteal: sleep metabolic rate	Late follicular: sleep metabolic rate	Meals in metabolic setting matching energy expenditures and prior records	Only sleep metabolic rate varied by about 6.1%

ence no change in energy expenditures across the menstrual cycle. However, when pills were discontinued, a 14% increase in expenditure occurred during the 2 weeks after ovulation.

Change in BMR may be mediated in part by P, which is known to increase body heat production.[31] The secretion pattern for P coincides with the observed timing of BMR changes: that is, there is a luteal rise in P, followed by a postmenstrual fall. Solomon and coworkers[29] contend that the chronology suggests that P, not E_2, is the more dominant effector in BMR changes. Although Webb[30] found no significant correlation between energy expenditures and urinary pregnanediol levels, Bisdee et al[32] did observe a significant correlation between BBT and the log urinary pregnanediol excretion for the same periods when the data for all subjects were combined. The etiology of these changes in energy metabolism across the menstrual cycle remains uncertain, but the observation that changes in BMR do exist in menstruating women is strongly supported by all these studies.

Nitrogen

Nitrogen balance studies have shown cyclic changes in nitrogen utilization in young women for sequential menstrual cycles.[29,33] Urinary nitrogen excretion exhibited a significant biphasic pattern across the menstrual cycle in every subject: rising immediately after menses to a nadir at ovulation, rising sharply during the early luteal phase, and falling again just before or with the onset of menstruation. The increase in urinary nitrogen excretion during the early luteal or postovulatory phase has been confirmed recently.[23]

There is a striking relationship between increased nitrogen excretion during the luteal phase and increments in energy intake and expenditure for many of the studies reviewed.[7,29] However, muscle-protein breakdown is probably not the origin of the increased urinary nitrogen levels because no differences were seen in plasma branched-chain amino acids or urinary 3-methylhistidine excretion between follicular and luteal phases.[34] Also, whole-body protein turnover, when measured randomly across the menstrual cycle, did not exhibit any detectable menstrual cycle effects.[35] Despite the stability of these parameters, a rise in urinary nitrogen excretion during the luteal phase has been observed. Therefore, the mechanisms underlying changes in nitrogen excretion remain ill-defined. If nitrogen excretion reflects nitrogen use, these findings suggest that protein allowance varies with menstrual timing. The pattern observed may reflect the rhythmic gain and loss of soft-tissue nitrogen by women. Further study is required.

Iron Nutriture

Physiologic changes such as fluctuations in fluid volume, blood loss, and loss of iron in menstrual blood may affect test results for iron status.[36] However, little information exists regarding the magnitude of such influences within a single menstrual cycle.[37] Kim and coworkers[38] examined the data from 1712 eumenorrheic women, 18 to 44 years of age, in the Second National Health and Nutrition Examination Survey (NHANES II). Adjusted mean values of hemoglobin (3 g/L difference), transferrin saturation (3.6% difference), and serum ferritin (6.8 µg/L difference) were lowest for those women whose samples were drawn during menses and highest for those drawn during the luteal or late luteal phase. Estimated prevalence of impaired iron status based on the ferritin model[39] was highest for women sampled during the menstrual phase and lowest during the luteal phase and in the late luteal phase. Similar differences in prevalence estimates were also observed with the mean corpuscular volume.[36] These data imply a woman is more likely to be diagnosed as iron-deficient if the blood sample is obtained during menstruation than at other phases. Failure to control for menstrual phase when bloods are sampled can add to measurement error and confound interpretation of data in premenstrual women.

ROLE OF DIET ON SEX STEROID HORMONES

Diet composition, both from a qualitative and quantitative perspective (i.e., vegan diets or low-fat dietary patterns), has been suggested to affect menstrual cyclicity and reproductive performance. It is surprising how often diet is mentioned as the probable cause of oligomenorrhea or amenorrhea, when, in fact, so little effort has been made to carefully document dietary patterns of subjects. Very few studies actually used diet as a treatment variable. Furthermore, dietary descriptions are often incomplete, and dietary descriptors, such as "vegetarian" diets, are confounded by other dietary constituents, such as fat or dietary fiber. In other words, menstrual cycles could be affected not only by a vegetarian diet but also by diets that vary in fat, fiber, or other nutrients.

Vegetarian Diets

The effects of vegetarian versus Western diets on sex hormones have been investigated. When nine premenopausal, vegetarian, black women were placed on a meat-containing diet, the follicular phase was significantly increased (mean of 4.2 days).[40] Concomitantly, FSH increased and E_2 decreased significantly. Others[41] have shown that E_2 is significantly decreased when subjects change to a vegetarian diet. Conversely, when 16 omnivorous, white women were placed on a meatless diet for 2 months, they experienced shorter follicular phases (mean, 3.8 days) during the second cycle.[42] These women also had a decreased frequency of LH peaks and increased LH concentrations after two injections of LH releasing hormone. These changes in hormones observed are similar to changes seen in women with irregular menstrual cycles. Because both the episodic release of FSH and LH[43] and a specific ratio of FSH to LH[44] are critical for follicular development, it appears that diet explains some of the dysfunction observed in menstrual cycles, such as periodicity, anovulatory cycles, and amenorrhea. Which diet component is responsible for changes in menstrual activity is not discernible from these studies because all macronutrients were changed along with the presence or absence of meat.

Cross-sectional studies[45,46] have also compared estrogen levels in small numbers of premenopausal women consuming vegetarian or omnivorous diets. Vegetarian women excreted more fecal estrogens, less urinary estrogens, and had 15 to 20% lower plasma estrogen (E_1, E_2, and E_3) levels than nonvegetarian women. Thus, dietary patterns were related to the sex hormone milieu that affects follicular development and maturation. Regrettably, few details about the dietary composition, the participants, or subject compliance to the diet were provided. Again, if calories, fat, cholesterol, and fiber intakes were all different between groups, these differences could confound the results.

Further evidence of a relationship between diet and menstrual function is a higher rate of abnormal cycles observed in women consuming vegetarian diets. The prevalence of menstrual irregularities (three to ten menses per year) was 26.5% in vegetarians (lacto- or lacto-ovo, $n = 34$) versus 4.9% in nonvegetarians (omnivores, $n = 41$).[47] As expected, nonvegetarian women reported consuming more protein and cholesterol and less carbohydrate, polyunsaturated fats, magnesium, vitamin B_6, and dietary fiber. Thus, any of these dietary variables could be related to menstrual function. Using logistic regression analyses, the nutrients positively associated with menstrual regularity were protein/kJ and cholesterol/kJ ratios. Irregularities were associated with increasing dietary fiber/kJ and increasing magnesium/kJ ratios. Therefore, no relationship between fat intake and menstrual function was observed. However, both groups of women consumed about the same amount of fat regardless of meat consumption. The association between fiber and menstrual irregularity has been observed by others.[48,49] Wheat bran, in particular, lowers serum estrone and E_2.[49]

Low-Fat versus High-Fat Diets

Because some of the vegetarian studies could be confounded by differences in fat content, a few controlled studies have addressed the impact of either meatless diets (both high or low fat) versus meat-containing diets (both high or low fat) on sex steroids and menstrual function. Using a random crossover design, Hagerty et al[50] compared the effects of low-fat (25% calories) and high-fat (46% calories) lacto-ovovegetarian diets on plasma and urinary hormone levels of six women in a metabolic unit. Diets were isocaloric, and similar in proportions of protein, fiber, polyunsaturated:saturated fat ratio (P:S), and cholesterol. Three menstrual phases were identified by daily BBTs and hormone determinations (including LH, prolactin, P, and the estrogens). Dietary fat produced no significant differences in plasma or urinary hormone levels during the three phases. Thus, in lacto-ovovegetarians short-term changes in the amount of fat consumed did not have an effect on sex hormones.

Collaborators from USDA and the National Cancer Institute (NCI)[51–53] examined the effect of high- and low-fat meat-containing diets on hormones, lipids, and menstrual function in 31 premenopausal women. Again, a randomized, cross-over design was used. First, women were placed on the high-fat diets (40% kcal as fat) for four cycles, then they switched to the low-fat (20%) diets for four cycles. The diets had a P:S ratio of 0.3 or 1.0. All meals were prepared at the Beltsville Human Nutrition Research Center. Menstrual cycle and menses length data were recorded by subjects, excluding the data of the first cycle to rule out a carryover effect. Low-fat diets produced three main effects: (1) a significant increase in cycle length (average 1.3 days), (2) a significant increase in the duration of menses (0.5 days), and (3) a significant increase in follicular phase (average of 0.9 days). Similarly, McIntosh and coworkers[54] found that a change in menstrual cycle length of 1 day generally reflects a change in follicular length of 0.77 days. Therefore, in omnivorous women changing to a low-fat diet had an effect on menstrual cycle length. It increased as the result of an increase in the menstrual and follicular phases.

Other hormone changes were also observed. Regardless of dietary treatment, insulin and growth hormone concentration were significantly higher during the luteal phase as compared with the follicular phase.[53] These investigators propose that elevated luteal insulin and growth hormone concentration may partially explain the increased caloric requirements reported by others[29–31] during this period. This speculation is intriguing but must await further confirmation. Other hormonal changes seen on low-fat diets include significantly lower cortisol and dehydroepiandrosterone (DHEA). Because cortisol and DHEA are derived from the same precursor, pregnenolone, low-fat diets either may decrease pregnenolone levels or depress its conversion to these steroids. How dietary-influenced changes in cortisol and DHEA alter menstrual function is not apparent. Manipulation of the P:S ratio had no observable influence on any hormones quantified. Thus, the amount of dietary fat affects menstrual cycle length as well as other hormones that may affect caloric needs.

Total dietary fat may affect endogenous estrogens. Woods and coworkers[55] examined the effect of diet on serum estrogen levels in 17 premenopausal women in a metabolic unit. After a 4-week control dietary period designed to simulate the "Western" meat-containing diet (40% calories as fat, 400 mg cholesterol, 12 g dietary fiber, and a P:S ratio = 0.5), women were placed for an 8- to 10-week period (two cycles) on a diet with 25% calories from fat, 200 mg cholesterol, 40 g dietary fiber, and P:S ratio = 1.0. Both diets were isocaloric and contained meat products. Serum samples were obtained only during the early follicular phase after two cycles on the dietary regimen. Estrone sulfate levels decreased by approximately 50% on the low-fat, high-fiber diet. This dramatic reduction in estrone sulfate levels reflects either a reduced production of E_1 and E_2 or a shift in the metabolism of E_1 and E_2 away from sulfation toward other estrogen metabolites. Such a reduction in circulating estrogens may modify follicular development or oocyte maturation. Another possible mechanism is that the low-fat, high-fiber diet disrupts the enterohepatic circulation of estrone sulfate, which like other estrogen conjugates is excreted into the bile. With impaired enterohepatic circulation, there would be increased fecal excretion and thus lower blood concentrations.[56] Increased fecal estrogens have been reported previously in vegetarian women.[45] No significant changes were seen in any other hormone analyzed (E_1, E_2, free E_2, androstenedione, sex hormone binding globulin [SHBG], testosterone, and free testosterone). Other hormonal changes may have been detected had samples been drawn during other phases.

DIET AND PREMENSTRUAL SYNDROME

Prevalence and Definition

Five to ten percent of women experience severe premenstrual symptoms that often require medical treatment.[57] This figure represents about 3 to 7 million American women.[58] However, the definition of *premenstrual syndrome* (PMS) remains ambiguous. The term *PMS* was first used by Frank in 1931 to describe a constellation of emotional, physical, and behavioral symptoms that occur during the luteal or premenstrual phase and disappear soon after the onset of menses.[59] In 1985, an advisory committee charged to revise the Diagnostic and Statistical Manual of Mental Disorders, third edition (DSM-III), proposed the addition of a new category termed *late luteal phase dysphoric disorder* (LLPDD), as a "diagnostic category needing further study."[60] LLPDD refers to a subset of PMS in which the dominant symptoms are related to mood disturbances. In DSM-IV,[61] the term *LLPDD* was considered too cumbersome and misleading because the symptoms are not related to endocrine changes occurring during the late luteal phase but instead seem to be triggered by them. Thus, the term *premenstrual dysphoric disorder* (PMDD) has been recommended to replace LLPDD. PMDD is categorized under "Mood Disorders, Depression, Not Otherwise Specified" in the main text of DSM-IV. PMDD itself, however, remains in the appendix of DSM-IV to foster further research. The terms *PMS, PMDD,* and *LLPDD* now are used interchangeably in the literature. In this chapter, *PMS* will be used.

Several lines of evidence link PMS to cyclic hormonal changes in the menstrual cycle. First, PMS improves or resolves when ovarian secretions are diminished. Second, PMS does not appear before puberty, when the reproductive axis is inactive. Third, PMS is not present after menopause (although hormonal replacement therapy may be associated with a reappearance of symptoms). If hysterectomy does not include an oophorectomy, PMS may persist.[3]

Symptoms

Many symptoms are reported by patients with PMS, which range from depressed mood to appetite changes and insomnia (Exhibit 5-1). Symptoms of PMS are classified by the time in which they appear during the luteal phase.[3] Four patterns are most common (Figure 5-5). In most women, the symptoms either begin in the late luteal phase (pattern A) or right after ovulation (pattern B) and then terminate rapidly at menses.

Diagnosis of PMS requires the presence of five or more symptoms in the luteal phase which are absent in the menstrual and follicular phases (Exhibit 5-1). In the differential diagnosis, it is important to rule out patients with somatic or psychiatric disorders that do not show fluctuations related to the menstrual cycle. No standardized assessment form is used by practitioners, although several validated questionnaires can be used. Some examples include the Calendar of Premenstrual Experiences (COPE),[62] the Moos' Menstrual Distress Questionnaire,[63] the Menstrual Symptom Questionnaire,[64] and the Premenstrual Assessment Form.[65] Presently, there is only one way in which researchers can identify women with "true" PMS: women are given self-rating, self-report, or visual analog scales to complete for a minimum of two cycles.[66,67] Scientific criteria (internal and external validity, reliability assessments) are then applied to the ratings to identify those who have PMS.[68]

Hygienic Strategies

In a survey of 502 American physicians, 60% said they recommended dietary changes in addition to nutritional supplements for the management of PMS.[69] However, there is no consensus about what constitutes an effective nutritional program for PMS patients or whether such nutritional recommendations have any scientific basis or are safe. Safety is of particular concern with nutritional supplements. Dietary advice has included limiting consumption of refined sugar, salt, red meat, animal fats, alcohol, caffeine, tobacco, and dairy products along with recommendations to increase consumption of fish, poultry, whole grains, legumes, complex carbohydrates, green leafy vegetables, cereals, and *cis*-linolenic acid-containing foods.

Exhibit 5-1   Diagnostic Criteria for Premenstrual Syndrome

In most menstrual cycles during the past year, five (or more) of the following symptoms were present for most of the time during the last week of the luteal phase, began to remit within a few days after the onset of the follicular phase, and were absent in the week post-menses with at least one of the symptoms being 1, 2, 3, or 4:

1. Markedly depressed mood, feelings of hopelessness, or self-deprecating thoughts
2. Marked anxiety, tension, feelings of being "keyed up" or "on edge"
3. Marked affective lability (e.g., feeling suddenly sad or tearful or increased sensitivity to rejection)
4. Persistent and marked anger or irritability or increased interpersonal conflicts
5. Decreased interest in usual activities (e.g., work, school, friends, hobbies)
6. Subjective sense of difficulty in concentrating
7. Lethargy, easy fatigability, or marked lack of energy
8. Marked change in appetite, overeating, or specific food cravings
9. Hypersomnia or insomnia
10. Subjective sense of being overwhelmed or out of control
11. Other physical symptoms, such as breast tenderness or swelling, headaches, joint or muscle pain, a sensation of bloating, weight gain

Note: In menstruating women, the luteal phase corresponds to the period between ovulation and the onset of menses and the follicular phase begins with menses. In nonmenstruating women (e.g., those who have had a hysterectomy), the timing of luteal and follicular phases may require measurement of circulating reproductive hormones.

The disturbance markedly interferes with work and school or with usual social activities and relationships with others (e.g., avoidance of social activities or decreased productivity and efficiency at home and at work).

The disturbance is not merely an exacerbation of the symptoms of another disorder, such as major depressive disorder, panic disorder, dysthymic disorder, or a personality disorder (although it may be superimposed on any of these conditions).

The preceding criteria must be confirmed by prospective daily ratings during at least two symptomatic cycles. (The diagnosis may be made provisionally before this confirmation.)

Source: Reprinted from *Diagnostic and Statistical Manual of Mental Disorders,* ed 4 (pp 717–718) with permission of American Psychiatric Association, © 1994.

Diets

Most of the research concerning the diet/PMS relationship has been largely survey and cross-sectional studies instead of controlled intervention trials. A dietary survey of 39 patients with PMS and 14 control women suggested that PMS patients consumed fivefold more dairy products and threefold more refined sugar than those patients not affected by symptoms of anxiety, irritability, and nervous tension.[70] In another study, a low-fat, high-carbohydrate diet significantly reduced

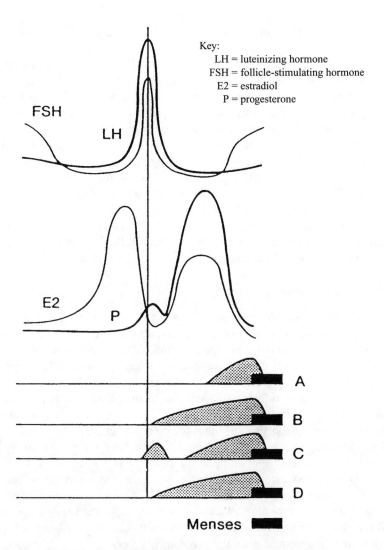

Figure 5-5 Variability in Onset of PMS Symptoms. Most patients experience patterns A or B. Shaded area represents time of symptoms. *Source:* Reprinted from *The Menstrual Cycle: Physiology, Reproductive Disorders, and Infertility* by M Ferin, R Jewelewicz and M Warren (p 201) with permission of Oxford University Press, © 1993.

breast swelling and tenderness in 21 women with long histories of severe premenstrual breast symptomatology.[71] Survey studies have also found an association between severe premenstrual symptoms and consumption of foods and beverages high in sugar content.[72] Some investigators have proposed that premenstrual lethargy, fatigue, irritability, and cravings are due to altered glucose tolerance during the luteal phase,[64] but others[73,74] have found no evidence of impaired glucose metabolism during this phase. Wurtman and coworkers[75] measured food intake in a small number of PMS and control women at an inpatient facility for 48 hours during both follicular and late luteal phases. Consumption of a carbohydrate-rich, protein-poor evening meal was found to improve moods of women with PMS, which was attributed to an increased uptake of tryptophan, a precursor of serotonin in the brain.[76] Decreased blood serotonin levels[77] and decreased platelet uptake of serotonin[78] have been observed during the luteal phase of PMS patients. Other surveys suggest an improvement of breast symptoms[79] or mood and physical changes[80,81] in patients who abstain from methylxanthine-containing foods. However, retrospective case-control studies and surveys have not certified any potential causal factors. Studies that report on the use of dietary treatments in women with carefully diagnosed PMS are uncontrolled[82,83] or combine dietary changes with other treatment components.[84]

Nutritional Supplements

Many nutritional supplements have been evaluated as potential treatment for PMS (Table 5-6). Because mood and behavior are influenced by biogenic amines and pyridoxal phosphate (which contain vitamin B_6) is an essential coenzyme for the synthesis of several of these compounds, many researchers have proposed that vitamin B_6 supplementation may alleviate some PMS symptoms. Four studies[84,86–89] found pyridoxine was superior to the placebo in improvement of symptoms. However, in one of these studies,[84] 63% of the experimental group and 40% of the placebo group improved, even though the study was double-blinded. A strong placebo effect has been previously reported in 70% of patients.[87] Another problem with these studies is the lack of a standard diagnosis of PMS. Overall, most studies have found no significant symptomatic improvement with vitamin B_6 supplementation.[87,88,90–92] Although it is widely believed that large doses of water-soluble vitamins are safe, this is not the case for vitamin B_6. Doses that averaged 120 mg/day for 6 months to 5 years caused neurologic disorders that disappeared after the supplements were stopped.[93] Sensitivity to vitamin B_6 varies from woman to woman. Other scientists believe that doses greater than 300 mg/day are risky.[94,95] Very large doses (2 g/day or more) cause ataxia or sensory neuropathy (burning or shooting pains in the extremities, numbness, clumsiness, and unstable gait).[96] Toxicity is thus dose- and time-dependent (i.e., larger doses [7 to 10 grams] cause symptoms in a shorter period [after 2 months]). To date, vitamin B_6 supplementation has provided no benefit beyond a placebo effect to PMS sufferers, and because of toxicity, use is questioned.

Another supplement, called Optivite, that is high in vitamin B_6 as well as other vitamins and minerals (See Table 5-6 for contents) has been tested. In a double-

Table 5-6 "Nutritional" Therapies for Premenstrual Syndrome

Study	Treatment; Design[a]	Measures	Methods	Findings
Abraham and Hargrove, 1980[85]	Pyridoxine; DBCO	MSQ[b]; daily weight records	25 Women: 500 mg pyridoxine or placebo daily for 3 months; MSQ and daily weighing recording	Pyridoxine superior in 22, as shown by MSQ score
Barr, 1984[86]	Pyridoxine; DBCO	Daily symptom records	48 Women: 200 mg pyridoxine or placebo daily from cycle day 10 to day 3 of menses for 2 months	Pyridoxine superior to placebo
Harrison et al, 1984[90]	Pyridoxine; SBCO	Physician's CGI[c]; PAF[d]; daily self-rating scale	Placebo for 1 cycle; nonresponders (n = 20) given 50–150 mg pyridoxine + 1.5–6.0 g L-tryptophan daily for 3 cycles	No difference between treatments
Hagen et al, 1985[88]	Pyridoxine; DBCO	Global VAS[e]; self-rating of symptoms; plasma magnesium	34 Subjects received 100 mg pyridoxine or placebo daily for 2 months; completed VAS at end of 2-month period	Treatments equivalent; order effect observed
Williams et al, 1985[87]	Pyridoxine; RDBT	Investigator's assessment; daily record of tablets taken and symptom severity	50–200 mg pyridoxine (n = 204) or placebo (n = 230) for 3 cycles	No difference between treatments, but some superiority with active treatment
Kendall and Schnurr, 1987[89]	Pyridoxine; RDBT	Daily symptom records; PAF; MDQ[f]	55 Women: 150 mg pyridoxine or placebo daily for 2 months; daily MDQ	Pyridoxine superior to placebo for autonomic and behavioral symptoms only
Malmgren et al, 1987[91]	Pyridoxine; case-control	Platelet serotonin uptake	300 mg pyridoxine or placebo daily, from cycle day 15 to day 1 of menses for 2 months	No difference between treatments
Berman et al, 1990[92]	Pyridoxine; case-control	MSQ[b]	12 Women: 250 mg pyridoxine daily for 1 month; no placebo	No significant differences between pretreatment and posttreatment scores
Chakmakjian et al, 1985[97]	Optivite[g]; DBCO	Menstrual Symptom Questionnaire (MSQ)	31 Subjects; 6 Optivite/day or placebo for 3 months; MSQ completed in weeks 2–4 of all cycles	16 preferred Optivite, 7 preferred placebo; MSQ lower for PMT-A[b] and PMT-C[b] on Optivite
Stewart, 1987[98]	Optivite; RDBT	Self-rating of symptoms	3 Months of Optivite or placebo; 119 on high dose; 104 on low dose	Optivite superior to placebo only with high dose
London et al, 1991[99]	Optivite; RDBT	Modified MSQ[b]	44 Subjects; 6 or 12 Optivite/day or placebo for 3 months; MSQ during midfollicular and late luteal phase of each cycle	All three interventions (including placebo) resulted in lower MSQ scores; 12 tablets superior to 6 tablets for weight gain and bloating symptoms only

Table 5-6 "Nutritional" Therapies for Premenstrual Syndrome (continued)

Study	Treatment; Design[a]	Measures	Methods	Findings
Thys-Jacobs et al, 1989[101]	Calcium; DBCO	Daily symptom scores; retrospective global assessments	33 Women: 1000 mg calcium carbonate or placebo daily for 3 months, fourth month symptom scoring	Calcium superior to placebo
Penland and Johnson, 1993[102]	Calcium; DBCO	MDQ[f]	10 Women: 587 mg or 1336 mg Ca daily for 4 39-day dietary periods	Higher calcium intake significantly improved mood and behavior symptoms and water retention
London et al, 1987[103]	Alpha-tocopherol; RDBT	Questionnaire based on Steiner et al[104] and Abraham[64]	400 IU (n = 22) or placebo (n = 19) for 3 months; symptoms during luteal and follicular phases for all cycles	Active treatment superior to placebo in 3 of 4 Abraham categories and Steiner symptoms, but not at $p < .05$
Callender et al, 1988[107]	Evening primrose oil (Efamol) + vitamin E supplement; DBCO	Daily symptom scores; BDI[h]	10 Women; 3000 mg Efamol + Efavit[i] or placebo from day 7 through day 1 of menses for 2 months with washout in between	Subjective improvement in 70% of active treatment; 30% of placebo cycles; no differences in BDI scores
Stephenson et al, 1988[109]	Evening primrose oil + vitamin E; RDBT	MDQ[f]	70 Women: 2-month symptom rating; 8 capsules/day; active or placebo for 3 months; MDQs completed 3 days/week	No differences between treatments
Khoo et al, 1990[108]	Evening primrose oil (Efamol); DBCO	4-Point rating scale of symptoms	38 Women met authors' criteria for PMS based on 1-month symptom rating; Efamol or placebo given for 3 months	No significant differences between treatments

[a]Designs: DBCO = double-blind crossover trial; RDBT = randomized double-blind trial; SBCO = single-blind placebo run-in; nonresponders to active treatment.
[b]MSQ = Menstrual Symptom Questionnaire; PMT-A and PMT-C = premenstrual tension syndrome subtypes A and C identified by the MSQ (Abraham[64]).
[c]CGI = Clinical Global Impression Scale.
[d]PAF = Premenstrual Assessment Form (Endicott et al[65]).
[e]VAS = Visual Analog Scale.
[f]MDQ = Menstrual Distress Questionnaire (Moos[63]).
[g]Optivite (6 capsules) provides 12,500 IU of vitamin A palmitate, 100 IU of vitamin E (as d-α-tocopherol), 100 IU cholecalciferol, 200 μg folic acid, 25 mg thiamin HCl 25 mg riboflavin, 25 mg niacinamide, 300 mg pyridoxine HCl, 62.5 μg vitamin B₁₂, 25 mg pantothenic acid, 312.5 mg choline bitartrate, 1500 mg vitamin C, 250 mg magnesium, 75 μg iodine, 15 mg iron, 0.5 mg copper, 25 mg zinc, 10 mg manganese, 47.5 mg potassium, 100 μg selenium, and 100 μg chromium. Other ingredients include calcium, citrus bioflavonoid, betaine acid HCl, pancreatin, inositol, para-amino benzoic acid, rutin, and biotin.
[h]BDI = Beck Depression Inventory.
[i]Efavit = 750 mg ascorbic acid, 30 mg zinc sulfate, and 150 mg each niacin and vitamin B₆.

blind, placebo-controlled trial, Chakmakjian and colleagues[97] found no clear indication of superiority with the preparation at six tablets daily, whereas Stewart's group[98] reported that Optivite was most efficacious at the high dose (eight tablets per day), although not at the low dose (four tablets per day). More recently, London et al[99] reported significant improvement in PMS symptoms with both a 6-tablet and 12-tablet group. Again, the placebo group also improved. The data were not analyzed to determine the extent of benefit beyond the placebo effect. Because of symptomatic improvements seen with Optivite, some researchers have suggested that symptoms occur because of marginal vitamin and mineral status. However, no evidence of deficiencies (magnesium, zinc, retinol, vitamin E, thiamin, or vitamin B_6) was observed in women with PMS.[100] More double-blind, placebo-controlled, crossover studies are needed to determine the efficacy and safety of Optivite in larger groups of women.

Several studies suggest that calcium intakes may improve PMS symptoms. In a double-blind crossover trial, 33 women given 1000 mg calcium carbonate daily for 3 months reported an improvement in symptoms.[101] In another study, nine of ten women reported significant improvement in mood and concentration, pain during menstruation, and reduced water retention with a diet containing 1300 mg calcium daily.[102] With growing numbers of women taking calcium supplements to prevent osteoporosis, the additional benefit on PMS symptoms needs further exploration.

Because of its antioxidant role, vitamin E had been investigated for a variety of diseases and conditions including PMS. In a randomized double-blind trial, women took 400 IU of vitamin E or placebo for three menstrual cycles.[103] Two questionnaires were used to assess symptoms.[64,104] Although clinical benefit was reported (i.e., some women reported improvement in a few symptoms), none of these differences were statistically significant. It has been hypothesized that vitamin E at some undetermined dose may have an effect on symptoms through regulation of prostaglandin synthesis.[105] This hypothesis needs substantiation. Further study is also needed to determine if vitamin E has any benefit beyond a placebo effect.

Another nutritional supplement examined was evening primrose oil (Efamol), which contains γ-linolenic acid (a derivative of *cis*-linoleic acid and a critical precursor of prostaglandin E_1 [PGE_1]). Levels of *cis*-linoleic acid have been reported to be increased in women with PMS as compared with control women but with lower metabolites, suggesting a low conversion rate of *cis*-linoleic acid to γ-linolenic acid.[106] Use of Efamol was proposed to overcome this defect. The weight of the three double-blind crossover studies,[107–109] however, suggests that Efamol at the doses provided is not efficacious.

Exercise

Exercise is often recommended as a treatment for PMS, but there is no published study that demonstrates its efficacy as the sole intervention. Timonen and

Procope[110] surveyed more than 700 female college students and reported that premenstrual complaints were less frequent among those who participated in sports. Prior and Vigna[111] compared the effects of exercise on premenstrual symptoms in sedentary women and runners. Increased exercise was associated with improvements in fluid and breast-related symptoms, based on daily symptom reports, as well as premenstrual dysphoria up to 6 months after initiation of an exercise program. No changes in control subjects were observed. In the strongest study design, Lemon[112] evaluated the effect of aerobic training in 32 women with prospectively confirmed PMS. Women were randomly assigned to either a high-intensity aerobic training group or a low-intensity control group. Although the high-intensity group reported greater reductions, both groups exhibited significantly fewer symptoms as compared with baseline. Further controlled studies are needed to clarify whether exercise can alleviate or mitigate physiologic or psychological symptoms of PMS.

DIET AND FERTILITY

Undernutrition

In most species, inadequate nutrition is usually accompanied by a decrease in reproductive function. Amenorrhea is a common observation in populations of women during wartime or famine. Some of the endocrine changes observed in anorexia nervosa mimic those observed in nonanorectic women who experience great weight loss. Normally, low circulating steroids result in enhanced gonadotrophin secretion. In these women, however, low serum and urinary gonadotrophin levels or altered secretion patterns (LH, in particular) are observed. Although several mechanisms are proposed for this inappropriate response, most include some form of hypothalamic dysfunction with respect to gonadotropin-releasing hormone (GnRH) release.[113] Other steroid levels are altered in anorectic women; these include elevations in serum testosterone concentrations and decreased urinary excretion of 17-ketosteroids (i.e., androsterone, epiandrosterone, etc.), possibly reflecting reduced clearance of serum androgens.[114,115] In recovering anorectic patients, weight gain usually is accompanied by a normalization of gonadotrophin and sex steroid concentrations[113] and a return to ovulatory cycles. Thus, chronic energy deprivation in anorexia results in endocrine and reproductive anomalies, which are usually restored with weight gain. In less severe anorexia, administration of GnRH will often return women to normal cycling.

The impact of short-term weight loss on the sex steroid patterns of young women of average weight has been examined. In a very small study, Kurzer and

Calloway[116] manipulated energy intakes in six healthy young women (aged 19 to 29 years) of average body composition and weight during two menstrual cycles. During the first cycle, energy intakes approximated 40 kcal/kg body weight, while for the second cycle, energy intake was reduced by 41%. Weight loss ranged from 3.2 to 6.7 kg. The two leanest women (20% body fat as compared with an average 30% for the remaining four women) became anovulatory and amenorrheic; these women lost more fat and more absolute weight than the other four women. Normal menses did not resume for these two women until 2 to 3 months later, after normal eating patterns resumed. The low-energy diet did not alter E_2, P, LH, or FSH levels across the menstrual cycle, although lower androgens were observed. SHBG levels rose during the low-energy diet and were inversely associated with body weight and adiposity. The increase in SHBG concentrations has also been observed in obese women after weight loss.[117] Thus, short-term energy deprivation in normal-weight women can affect menstrual cyclicity, but body composition of women and the rate and composition of weight loss appears to determine who may become amenorrheic. These findings need to be replicated in a larger group of women and followed once a restoration of original weight has occurred.

For more than a decade, Pirke's group[118–121] in West Germany has also studied menstrual function in healthy women following weight loss diets, albeit in a less controlled fashion. Most of their reports appear to be observational in design, with few details with respect to dietary composition or body composition. With a 2-week *starvation* period, three of five normal-weight women manifested a prepubertal LH pattern; weight losses varied between 5 and 7 kg.[118] In another study,[119] nine women on low-calorie diets (800 to 1000 kcal/day) for 6 weeks lost between 6 and 8 kg; the three who became anovulatory had extremely low E_2 levels (similar to postmenopausal levels) by the second week of dieting, with no alteration in LH secretion. These data suggest that energy deprivation (although we have no data as to the composition of such diets followed) may interfere with follicular development and ovarian estrogen production before hypothalamic stimulation of gonadotrophin release was impaired. To test this hypothesis, a follow-up study[120] in which women were studied during control and "diet" (800 kcal/day, avoiding all meat and fish) periods was conducted. Follicular growth was assessed by serial ultrasonographic examinations in addition to hormonal determinations. No follicular maturation was noted in 7 of 13 normal weight healthy women during the diet phase; the frequency and amount of LH secreted was also reduced during this period. Therefore, it seems that in severe energy deprivation, amenorrhea and a prepubertal pattern of LH secretion occur concomitantly. Even if LH patterns are not altered, inadequate follicular maturation may occur with certain weight loss regimens.

Over the past 30 years, the concept that body composition may modify menstrual cyclicity has been questioned. In recovering anorectics, normal adult LH levels occur only in women who are at more than 80% of ideal body weight (IBW).[121] Similarly, Frisch[122] reported that patients with anorexia nervosa did not menstruate before they reached at least 87% of IBW. In "average weight" women who previously have had normal menstrual function, however, the identification of a lower limit for body weight is not yet possible from existing data. How weight loss regimens and specifically what physical or dietary attributes predict aberrations in menstrual function need to be investigated.

Amenorrhea or anovulation may be considered an energy conservation mechanism. The !Kung bushwomen of the Kalahari Desert, for example, exhibit a seasonal suppression of ovulation; while carrying children, they walk a maximum of 30 miles in search of food.[123] The large metabolic demands cannot be met by caloric intake, so anovulation may be one adaptation.[124] That same mechanism may also be responsible for some instances of athletic amenorrhea, although there are probably many etiologic factors.

Overnutrition

At the other end of the continuum, obesity has also been related to menstrual function. Specifically, the number of anovulatory women increases with body weight.[125] In a recent case-control study of 597 white infertile women and 1695 primiparous white controls, Grodstein and colleagues[126] observed a similar relationship. Obese women (body mass index of 27 or greater) had a significantly higher risk of ovulatory infertility (relative risk = 3.3, 95% confidence interval: 2.2 to 4.4). Aberrations in ovulatory function and, ultimately, fertility in obese women and, in particular, for those who gain weight rapidly, have been reported by others as well.[127,128]

The increased incidence of anovulatory cycles in obese women suggests abnormal hormone release. Low levels of SHBG,[129] increased ovarian and adrenal androgen production,[116,129–131] and enhanced peripheral aromatization of androgens to estrogens[132] have been associated with body fat or obesity. Increased circulating E_1 levels may result in an inappropriate feedback to the hypothalamic-pituitary unit and increased LH secretion and hyperandrogenism. Hyperinsulinism consequent to insulin resistance in obesity may act as a further inducer of enhanced LH secretion and thereby contribute to the anomalies in follicular maturation. Also, increased levels of testosterone have been shown to inhibit follicular maturation.[133] Eumenorrheic obese women have lower total testosterone levels than amenorrheic obese women.[133] Finally, obese anovulatory women who have lost weight and subsequently began to ovulate experience an accompanying fall in plasma androgens with weight loss.[128] The level of obesity that causes anovulatory cycles is unknown. However, it is clear that diet and body weight affect menstrual function and merit further attention by nutritionists.

SUMMARY

It is clear that diet affects the menstrual cycle and that this is associated with changes in the concentration of key regulatory steroid hormones. Although it is well established that extremes in nutrient intake (i.e., undernutrition or overnutrition) are associated with a reduction in fertility, the mechanisms that account for this remain unclear. In women whose normal diet is typical of the average American diet, energy intake varies across the cycle, however, it is not clear what nutrients contribute to the increase observed in energy intake during the luteal phase versus the follicular phase. Furthermore, dietary fat intake appears to affect sex steroid hormone levels. This may provide a mechanistic basis for the observations that low-fat diets (when compared with high-fat diets) increase cycle length, increase duration of menses, and increase the duration of the follicular phase. Much remains to be learned about the biological mechanisms that account for the effects that diet has on reproductive biology. It is important to emphasize that learning about how diet affects the menstrual cycle may provide additional insights into the role that sex steroid hormones play in affecting risk of chronic disease.

References

1. Treolar AE, Boyton RE, Benn BG, Brown BW. Variation of human menstrual cycle through reproductive life. *Int J Fertil.* 1967;12:77–86.

2. Chiazze L, Brayer FT, Mascisco JJ, Parker MP, Duffy BJ. The length and variability of the human menstrual cycle. *JAMA.* 1968;203:377–380.

3. Ferin M, Jewelewicz R, Warren M. *The Menstrual Cycle: Physiology, Reproductive Disorders, and Infertility.* New York, NY: Oxford University Press; 1993.

4. Yen SSC, Jaffe RB. *Reproductive Endocrinology: Physiology, Pathophysiology and Clinical Management.* Philadelphia, Pa: WB Saunders; 1991.

5. Vollman RF. *The Menstrual Cycle.* Philadelphia, Pa: WB Saunders; 1977.

6. Hilgers TW, Bailey AJ. Natural family planning. II. Basal body temperature and estimated time of ovulation. *Obstet Gynecol.* 1980;55:333–339.

7. Lissner L, Stevens J, Levitsky DA, Rasmussen KM, Strupp BJ. Variation in energy intake during the menstrual cycle: implications for food-intake research. *Am J Clin Nutr.* 1988;48:956–962.

8. Tarasuk V, Beaton GH. Menstrual-cycle patterns in energy and macronutrient intake. *Am J Clin Nutr.* 1991;53:442–447.

9. Murray RK, Granner DK, Mayes PA, Rodwell VW. *Harper's Biochemistry.* 23rd Ed. Norwalk, Conn: Appleton & Lange; 1993.

10. Ruder HJ, Loreaux DL, Lipsett MB. Estrone sulfate: production rate and metabolism in man. *J Clin Invest.* 1972;51:1020–1033.

11. Dalvit SP. The effect of menstrual cycle on patterns of food intake. *Am J Clin Nutr.* 1981;34:1811–1815.

12. Dalvit-McPhillips SP. The effect of menstrual cycle on nutrient intake. *Physiol Behav.* 1983;31:209–212.

13. Manocha S, Choudhuri G, Tandon BN. A study of dietary intake in pre- and post-menstrual period. *Hum Nutr Appl Nutr.* 1986;40A:213–216.

14. Gallant MP, Bowering J, Short SH, Turkki PR. Pyridoxine and magnesium status of women with premenstrual syndrome. *Nutr Res.* 1987;7:243–252.

15. Gong EJ, Garrel D, Calloway DH. Menstrual cycle and voluntary food intake. *Am J Clin Nutr.* 1989;49:252–258.

16. Lyons PM, Truswell AS, Mira M, Vizzard J, Abraham SF. Reduction of food intake in the ovulatory phase of the menstrual cycle. *Am J Clin Nutr.* 1989;49:1164–1168.

17. Barr SI, Janelle KC, Prior JC. Energy intakes are higher during the luteal phase of ovulatory menstrual cycles. *Am J Clin Nutr.* 1995;61:39–43.

18. Bermant G, Davidson G. *Biological Basis of Sexual Behavior.* New York, NY: Harper & Row; 1974.

19. Mertz W, Kelsay JL. Rationale and design of the Beltsville One-year Dietary Intake Study. *Am J Clin Nutr.* 1984;40:1323–1326.

20. Abraham SF, Beaumont PJV, Argall WJ, Heywood P. Nutrient intake and the menstrual cycle. *Aust NZ J Med.* 1981;11:210–211.

21. Rosenblatt H, Dyrenfurth I, Ferin M, Vande Wiele RL. Food intake and the menstrual cycle in rhesus monkeys. *Physiol Behav.* 1980;24:447–449.

22. Kemnitz JW, Gibber JR, Eisele SG, Lindsay KA. Relationship of reproductive condition to food intake and sucrose consumption of female rhesus monkeys. In: Taub DM, King FA, eds. *Current Perspectives in Primate Social Dynamics.* New York, NY: Van Nostrand Reinhold; 1986:274–286.

23. Fong AKH, Kretsch MJ. Changes in dietary intake, urinary nitrogen, and urinary volume across the menstrual cycle. *Am J Clin Nutr.* 1993;57:43–46.

24. Tangney CC, Brownie C, Wu S-M. Impact of menstrual periodicity on serum lipid levels and estimates of dietary intake. *J Am Coll Nutr.* 1991;10:107–113.

25. Beaton GH, Milner J, Corey P, et al. Sources of variance in 24-hour dietary recall data:implications for nutrition study design and interpretation. *Am J Clin Nutr.* 1979;32:2546–2559.

26. Eck LH, Debon M, Klesges RC, Peacher-Ryan H. Gathering dietary intake during the menstrual cycle. *J Am Diet Assoc.* 1993;93(10):A-95.

27. Wakeman G. Basal metabolism and the menstrual cycle. *J Biol Chem.* 1923;56:555–567.

28. Blunt K, Dye M. Basal metabolism of normal women. *J Biol Chem.* 1921;67:69–87.

29. Solomon SJ, Kurzer MS, Calloway DH. Menstrual cycle and basal metabolic rate in women. *Am J Clin Nutr.* 1982;36:611–616.

30. Webb P. 24-hour energy expenditure and the menstrual cycle. *Am J Clin Nutr.* 1986;44:614–619.

31. Barton M, Weisner BP. Thermogenic effect of progesterone. *Lancet.* 1945;2:671–672.

32. Bisdee JT, James WPT, Shaw MA. Changes in energy expenditure during the menstrual cycle. *Br J Nutr.* 1989;61:187–199.

33. Calloway DH, Kurzer MS. Menstrual cycle and protein requirements of women. *J Nutr.* 1982;112:356–366.

34. Hrboticky N, Leiter LA, Anderson GH. Menstrual effects on the metabolism of tryptophan loads. *Am J Clin Nutr.* 1989;50:46–52.

35. Garrel DR, Welsch C, Arnaud MJ, Touriaire J. Relationship of the menstrual cycle and thyroid hormones to whole-body protein turnover in women. *Hum Nutr Clin Nutr.* 1985;29C:29–37.

36. Hallberg L, Hogdahl AM, Nilsson L, Rybo G. Menstrual blood loss—a population study. *Acta Obstet Gynecol Scand.* 1966;45:320–351.

37. Vellar OD. Changes in hemoglobin concentration and hematocrit during the menstrual cycle. I. A cross-sectional study. *Acta Obstet Gynecol Scand.* 1974;53:243–246.

38. Kim I, Yetley EA, Calvo MS. Variations in iron-status measures during the menstrual cycle. *Am J Clin Nutr.* 1993;58:705–709.

39. Pilch SM, Senti FR, eds. *Assessment of the Iron Nutritional Status of the US Population Based on Data Collected in the Second National Health and Nutrition Examination Survey 1976–1980.* Bethesda, Md: Federation of American Societies for Experimental Biology; 1984.

40. Hill PB, Garbaczewski L, Daynes G, Gaire KS. Gonadotrophin release and meat consumption in vegetarian women. *Am J Clin Nutr.* 1986;43:37–41.

41. Bennett FC, Ingram DM. Diet and female sex hormone concentrations: an intervention study for the type of fat consumed. *Am J Clin Nutr.* 1990;52:808–812.

42. Hill PB, Garbaczewski L, Haley N, Wynder E. Diet and follicular development. *Am J Clin Nutr.* 1984;39:771–777.

43. Schoemaker J, Simons AHM, Burger CW, Delemerre HA, Van Kessel H. Induction of ovulation with LH/FSH releasing hormone (LHRH). In: Roland R, Van Hall EV, Hillier SG, McNally KI, Schoemaker J, eds. *Follicular Maturation and Ovulation.* Amsterdam: Excerpta Medica; 1983:373–388.

44. DiZerega GS, Hodgen GD. Folliculogenesis in the primate ovarian cycle. *Endocr Rev.* 1981;2:27–49.

45. Goldin BR, Adlercreutz H, Gorbach SL, et al. Estrogen excretion patterns and plasma levels in vegetarian and omnivorous women. *N Engl J Med.* 1982;307:1542–1547.

46. Shultz TD, Leklem JE. Nutrient intake and hormonal status of premenopausal vegetarian Seventh-day Adventists and premenopausal nonvegetarians. *Nutr Cancer.* 1983;4:247–259.

47. Pedersen AB, Bartholomew MJ, Dolence LA, Aljadir LP, Netteburg KL, Lloyd T. Menstrual differences due to vegetarian and nonvegetarian diets. *Am J Clin Nutr.* 1991;53:879–885.

48. Wyshak G, Snow RC. Fiber consumption and menstrual regularity in young women. *J Women's Health.* 1993;2:295–299.

49. Rose DP, Goldman M, Connolly JM, Strong LE. High-fiber diet reduces serum estrogen concentrations in premenopausal women. *Am J Clin Nutr.* 1991;54:520–525.

50. Hagerty MA, Howie BJ, Tan S, Schultz TD. Effect of low- and high-fat intakes on the hormonal milieu of premenopausal women. *Am J Clin Nutr.* 1988;47:653–659.

51. Jones DY, Judd JT, Taylor PR, Campbell WS, Nair PP. Influence of dietary fat on menstrual cycle and menses length. *Hum Nutr Clin Nutr.* 1987;47C:341–345.

52. Reichman ME, Judd JT, Taylor PR, Nair PP, Jones DY, Campbell WS. Effect of dietary fat on length of the follicular phase of the menstrual cycle in a controlled diet setting. *J Clin Endocrinol Metab.* 1992;74:1171–1175.

53. Bhatena SJ, Berlin E, Judd J, et al. Hormones regulating lipid and carbohydrate metabolism; modulation by dietary lipids. *Am J Clin Nutr.* 1989;49:752.

54. McIntosh FEA, Matthews CD, Crobker JM, Broom TJ, Cox LW. Predicting the luteinizing hormone surge: relationship between the duration of the follicular and luteal phases and the length of the menstrual cycle. *Fertil Steril.* 1980;34:125–130.

55. Woods MN, Gorbach SL, Loncope C, Goldin BR, Dwyer JT, Morrill-LaBrode A. Low-fat, high-fiber diet and serum estrone sulfate in premenopausal women. *Am J Clin Nutr.* 1989;49:1179–1183.

56. Aldercreutz H, Martin F, Jarvenpod P, Fotsis T. Steroid absorption and enterohepatic recycling. *Contraception.* 1979;20:201–223.

57. Johnson SR. The epidemiology and social impact of premenstrual symptoms. *Clin Obstet Gynecol.* 1987;30:367–376.

58. US Bureau of Census. *Statistical Abstracts of the United States.* 111th ed. Washington, DC: US Government Printing Office; 1991.

59. Rapkin AJ. Premenstrual syndrome. *Clin Obstet Gynecol.* 1992;35:585–586.

60. Spitzer RL, Severino SK, Williams JBW, et al. Late luteal dysphoric disorder and DSM-IIIR. *Am J Psychiatry.* 1989;146:892–897.

61. *Diagnostic and Statistical Manual of Mental Disorders (DSM-IV).* 4th ed., Washington, DC: American Psychiatric Association; 1994.

62. Mortola JF, Girton L, Yen SSC. Diagnosis of premenstrual syndrome by a simple prospective and reliable instrument: the calendar of premenstrual experiences (COPE). *Obstet Gynecol.* 1990;76:302–307.

63. Moos RH. The development of the menstrual distress questionnaire. *Psychosom Med.* 1968;30:853–867.

64. Abraham GE. Premenstrual tension. *Curr Probl Obstet Gynecol.* 1980;3:103–124.

65. Endicott J, Nee J, Cohen J, et al. Premenstrual changes: patterns and correlates of daily ratings. *J Affect Disord.* 1986;10:127–135.

66. Gallant SJ, Popiel DA, Hoffman DM, et al. Using daily ratings to confirm premenstrual syndrome/late luteal phase dysphoric disorder, II: what makes a "real" difference? *Psychom Med.* 1992;54:167–181.

67. Hammarback S, Backstrom T, MacGibbon-Taylor B. Diagnosis of premenstrual tension syndrome: description and evaluation of a procedure for diagnosis and differential diagnosis. *J Psychosom Obstet Gynecol.* 1989;10:25–42.

68. Parlee MB. Commentary on the Literature Review. In: Gold JH, Severino SK, eds. *Premenstrual Dysphorias: Myths and Realities.* Washington, DC: American Psychiatric Press; 1994.

69. Lyon KE, Lyon MA. The premenstrual syndrome. *J Reprod Med.* 1984;29:705–711.

70. Goei GS, Ralston JL, Abraham GE. Dietary patterns of patients with premenstrual tension. *J Appl Nutr.* 1982;34:4–11.

71. Rossignol AM, Bonnlander H. Prevalence and severity of the premenstrual syndrome: effects of food and beverages that are sweet or high in sugar content. *J Reprod Med.* 1991;36:131–136.

72. Boyd NF, Shannon P, McGuire V, et al. Effect of a low-fat high-carbohydrate diet on symptoms of cyclical mastopathy. *Lancet.* 1988;2:128–132.

73. Spellacy WN, Ellingson AB, Keith G, et al. Plasma glucose and insulin levels during the menstrual cycles of normal women and premenstrual syndrome patients. *J Reprod Med.* 1990;35:508–511.

74. Denicoff KD, Hoban MC, Grover GN, et al. Glucose tolerance testing in women with premenstrual syndrome. *Am J Psychiatry.* 1990;147:477–480.

75. Wurtman J, Brzezinski A, Wurtman RJ, Laferrere B. Effect of nutrient intake on premenstrual tension. *Am J Obstet Gynecol.* 1989;161:1128–1134.

76. Fernstrom J, Wurtman R, Hammarstrom-Wiklund B, et al. Diurnal variations in plasma concentrations of tryptophan, tyrosine, and other neutral amino acids: effect of dietary protein intake. *Am J Clin Nutr.* 1979;32:1912–1922.

77. Rapkin AJ, Edelmuth E, Li CC, et al. Whole blood serotonin in premenstrual tension. *Obstet Gynecol.* 1987;70:533–537.

78. Taylor DL, Mathew RJ, Ho BT, Weinman ML. Serotonin levels and platelet uptake during premenstrual tension. *Neuropsychobiology.* 1984;12:16–18.

79. Minton JP, Foecking MK, Webster DJ, et al. Responses of fibrocystic disease to caffeine withdrawal and correlation with cyclic nucleotides with breast disease. *Am J Obstet Gynecol.* 1979;135:157–158.

80. Rossignol AM. Caffeine-containing beverages and premenstrual syndrome in young women. *Am J Public Health.* 1985;75:1335–1337.

81. Rossignol AM, Zhang J, Chen Y, et al. Tea and premenstrual syndrome in the People's Republic of China. *Am J Public Health.* 1989;79:67–69.

82. Abraham GE, Rumley RE. Role of nutrition in managing the premenstrual syndrome. *J Reprod Med.* 1987;32:405–422.

83. Pearlstein TB, Rivera-Tovar A, Frank E, et al. Nonmedical management of late luteal dysphoric disorder: a preliminary report. *J Psychother Pract Res.* 1992;1:49–55.

84. Day JB. Clinical trials in the premenstrual syndrome. *Curr Med Res Opin.* 1979;6:40–43.

85. Abraham GR, Hargrove JT. Effect of vitamin B_6 on premenstrual symptomatology in women with premenstrual tension syndrome: a double-blind crossover study. *Infertility.* 1980;3:155–165.

86. Barr W. Pyridoxine supplements in premenstrual syndrome. *Practitioner.* 1984;228:425–427.

87. Williams MJ, Harris RI, Dean BC. Controlled trial of pyridoxine in premenstrual syndrome. *J Int Med Res.* 1985;13:174–179.

88. Hagen I, Hesheim BI, Turntland T. No effect of vitamin B_6 against premenstrual tension. *Acta Obstet Gynecol Scand.* 1985;64:667–670.

89. Kendall KE, Schnurr PP. The effects of vitamin B_6 supplementation on premenstrual symptoms. *Obstet Gynecol.* 1987;70:145–149.

90. Harrison WM, Endicott J, Rabkin JG, et al. Treatment of premenstrual dysphoric changes: clinical outcome and methodological implications. *Psychopharmacol Bull.* 1984;20:118–122.

91. Malmgren R, Collins A, Nilsson C. Platelet serotonin uptake and effects of vitamin B-6 treatment in premenstrual tension. *Neuropsychobiology* 1987;18:83–88.

92. Berman MK, Taylor ML, Freeman E. Vitamin B_6 in premenstrual syndrome. *J Am Diet Assoc.* 1990;90:859–861.

93. Dalton K, Dalton MJT. Characteristics of pyridoxine overdose neuropathy syndrome. *Acta Neurol Scand.* 1987;76:8–11.

94. Berger A, Schaumburg HH. More on neuropathy from pyridoxine abuse. *N Engl J Med.* 1984;311:986–987.

95. Leibman B. PMS: proof or promises? *Nutr Action Health Letter.* May 1990.

96. Schaumburg H, Kaplan J, Windebank A, et al. Sensory neuropathy from pyridoxine abuse: a new megavitamin syndrome. *N Engl J Med.* 1983;309:445–448.

97. Chakmakjian ZH, Higgins CE, Abraham GE. The effect of a nutritional supplement, Optivite for women on premenstrual tension syndromes II: effect on symptomatology, using a double-blind cross-over design. *J Appl Nutr.* 1985;37:12–17.

98. Stewart A. Clinical and biochemical effects of nutritional supplementation on premenstrual syndrome. *J Reprod Med.* 1987;32:435–441.

99. London RS, Bradley L, Chiamori NY. Effect of a nutritional supplement on premenstrual symptomatology in women with premenstrual syndrome: a double-blind longitudinal study. *J Am Coll Nutr.* 1991;10:494–499.

100. Mira M, Stewart PM, Abraham SF. Vitamin and trace element status in premenstrual syndrome. *Am J Clin Nutr.* 1988:47:636–641.

101. Thys-Jacobs S, Ceccarelli S, Bierman A, Weisman H, Cohen MA, Alvir J. Calcium supplementation in premenstrual syndrome: a randomized crossover trial. *J Gen Intern Med.* 1989;4:183–189.

102. Penland JG, Johnson PE. Dietary calcium and manganese effects on menstrual cycle symptoms. *Am J Obstet Gynecol.* 1993;168:1417–1423.

103. London RS, Murphy L, Kitlowski KE, et al. Efficacy of alpha-tocopherol in the treatment of premenstrual syndrome. *J Reprod Med.* 1987;32:400–404.

104. Steiner M, Haskett RF, Carroll B. Premenstrual tension syndrome: the development of research diagnostic criteria and new rating scales. *Acta Psychiatr Acad.* 1980;62:117–190.

105. Panganamala RV, Cornwall DG. The effects of vitamin E on arachidonic acid metabolism. *Ann NY Acad Med.* 1982;396:376–391.

106. Brush MSG. Abnormal essential fatty acid levels in plasma of women with PMS. *Am J Obstet Gynecol.* 1984;150:363–364.

107. Callender K, McGregor M, Kirk P, et al. A double-blind trial of evening primrose oil in premenstrual syndrome:nervous symptom subgroup. *Hum Psychopharmacol Clin Exp.* 1988;3:57–61.

108. Khoo SK, Munro C, Battistura D. Evening primrose oil and treatment of premenstrual syndrome. *Med J Aust.* 1990;153:189–192.

109. Stephenson MJ, Milner R, Lamont J, et al. Treatment of premenstrual syndrome with oil of evening primrose: a randomized controlled trial. In: Proceedings of the 16th Annual Meeting of the North American Primary Care Research Group, Ottawa, Ontario, Canada, 1988.

110. Timonen S, Procope BJ. Premenstrual syndrome and physical exercise. *Acta Obstet Gynecol Scand.* 1971;50:331–337.

111. Prior JC, Vigna Y. Conditioning exercise and premenstrual symptoms. *J Reprod Med.* 1987;32:423–428.

112. Lemon D. The effects of aerobic training on women who suffer from premenstrual syndrome. *Dissertat Abstracts Intl.* 1991;52:563.

113. Katz JL, Weiner H. The aberrant reproductive endocrinology of anorexia nervosa. In: Weiner H, Hofer MA, Stunkard AJ, eds. *Brain, Behavior and Bodily Disease.* New York, NY: Raven Press; 1981:165–180.

114. Baranowska B, Zgliczynski S. Enhanced testosterone in female patients with anorexia nervosa: its normalization after weight gain. *Acta Endocrinol.* 1979:90:328–335.

115. Lupton M, Simon L, Barry V, Klawans HL. Minireview. Biological aspects of anorexia nervosa. *Life Sci.* 1976;18:1341–1348.

116. Kurzer MS, Calloway DH. Effects of energy deprivation on sex hormone patterns in healthy menstruating women. *Am J Physiol.* 1986;251(Endocrinol Metab 14):E483–488.

117. O'Dea JPK, Wieland RG, Hallberg MC, Llerena LA, Zom EM, Genuth SM. Effect of dietary weight loss on sex steroid binding, sex steroids, and gonadotrophins in obese postmenopausal women. *J Lab Clin Med.* 1979;93:1004–1008.

118. Fichter MM, Pirke KM. Hypothalamic pituitary function in starving healthy subjects. In: Pirke KM, Ploog D, eds. *The Psychobiology of Anorexia Nervosa.* Berlin: Springer Verlag; 1984:124.

119. Pirke KM, Schweiger U, Lemmel W, Krieg JC, Berger M. The influence of dieting on the menstrual cycle of healthy young women. *J Clin Endocrinol Metab.* 1985;60:1174–1179.

120. Pirke KM, Schweiger U, Strowski T, et al. Dieting causes menstrual irregularities in normal weight women through an impairment of episodic luteinizing hormone secretion. *Fertil Steril.* 1989;51:263–268.

121. Pirke KM, Fichter MM, Lund R, Doerr P. Twenty-four hour sleep-wake pattern of plasma LH in patients with anorexia nervosa. *Acta Endocrinol.* 1979;92:193–196.

122. Frisch RE. Pubertal adipose tissue: is it necessary for normal sexual maturation? Evidence from rat and human female. *Fed Proc.* 1980;39:2395–2400.

123. Van Der Walt LA, Wilrnsen EN, Jenkins T. Unusual sex hormone patterns among desert dwelling hunter gatherers. *J Clin Endocrinol Metab.* 1978;46:658–663.

124. Warren MP. Effects of undernutrition on reproductive function in the human. *Endocr Rev.* 1983; 4:363–377.

125. Hartz AJ, Barboriak PN, Wong A, Katayama KP, Rimm AA. The association of obesity with infertility and related menstrual abnormalities in women. *Int J Obes.* 1974;3:57–61.

126. Grodstein F, Goldman MB, Cramer DW. Body mass index and ovulatory infertility. *Epidemiology.* 1994;5:247–250.

127. Bringon J, Hedon B, Giner B, Richard J-L, Jaffiol C. Influence of abnormal weight and imbalanced diet on female fertility. *Presse Med.* 1990;19:1456–1459.

128. Bates GW, Whitworth NS. Effect of body weight reductions on plasma androgens in obese infertile women. *Fertil Steril.* 1982;38:406–409.

129. Eden JA, Carter GD, Jones J, Alaghband-Zadeh J, Pawson M. Factors influencing the free androgen index in a group of subfertile women with normal ovaries. *Ann Clin Biochem.* 1988;25:350–353.

130. Nicolas MH, Crave JC, Fimbel S, Simean A, Pugeat M. Hyperandrogenism in hirsute and obese women. Effects of a low calorie diet. *Presse Med.* 1993;22:19–22.

131. Wild RA, Umstot ES, Andersen RN, Ranney GB, Givens JR. Androgen parameters and their correlation with body weight in 138 women thought to have hyperandrogenism. *Am J Obstet Gynecol.* 1983;146:602–606.

132. Siiteri PK, MacDonald PC. Role of extraglandular estrogen in human endocrinology. In: Green PO, Astwood E, eds. *Handbook of Physiology,* vol. 2. Washington, DC: American Physiological Society; 1973;615–629.

133. Zhang Y-W, Stern B, Rebar RW. Endocrine comparison of obese menstruating and amenorrheic women. *J Clin Endocrinol Metab.* 1984;58:1077–1083.

6

❧

Normal Nutrition in Premenopausal Women

Rachel K. Johnson

The premenopausal period conceivably represents the longest period of the life cycle for women. This phase, which lasts from about ages 19 to 50, bridges the adolescent and senior years. Nutrition plays an important role in promoting a woman's general health and well-being throughout this period. Also, the later incidence and severity of chronic diseases such as obesity, coronary heart disease, cancer, and osteoporosis are determined by life-style choices made during these years.

NUTRITIONAL NEEDS

Recommendations for fulfilling the nutritional needs of healthy premenopausal women can be obtained from two sources. The Recommended Dietary Allowances (RDAs) provide a guide for assessing the adequacy of nutrient intakes.[1] The dietary patterns advocated in the Food and Nutrition Board's report *Diet and Health*[2] can be used to evaluate whether a diet meets current recommendations for chronic disease prevention. Thus, the RDAs and the *Diet and Health* recommendations can be used together to ensure an optimal dietary pattern for the maintenance of good health.

Assessing Nutrient Adequacy

Energy

For women aged 19 to 50 years, the average energy allowance is 2200 kcal/day[1] (Table 6-1). However, the range of energy needs among premenopausal

The author thanks Theresa Masterson and Melissa Smith for their help with researching and editing this chapter.

Table 6-1 Recommended Dietary Allowances of Nutrients for Women Aged 19 to 50 Years

	Women	
	19–24 Yr	*25–50 Yr*
Weight (kg)[a]	58	63
Height (cm)[a]	164	163
Energy (total kcal)	2200	2200
Energy (kcal/kg)	38	35
Protein (g)	46	50
Vitamin A (μg RE)	800	800
Vitamin D (μg)	10	5
Vitamin E (mg α-TE)	8	8
Vitamin K (μg)	60	65
Vitamin C (mg)	60	60
Thiamin (mg)	1.1	1.1
Riboflavin (mg)	1.3	1.3
Niacin (mg NE)	15	15
Vitamin B_6 (mg)	1.6	1.6
Folate (μg)	180	180
Vitamin B_{12} (μg)	2.0	2.0
Calcium (mg)	1200	800
Phosphorus (mg)	1200	800
Magnesium (mg)	280	280
Iron (mg)	15	15
Zinc (mg)	12	12
Iodine (μg)	150	150
Selenium (μg)	55	55

[a]Weights and heights represent actual median weights and heights for females derived from national data collected by the National Center for Health Statistics.
RE, retinol equivalents; α-TE, α-tocopherol equivalents; NE, niacin equivalents.
Source: Reprinted with permission from *Recommended Dietary Allowances,* ed 10. 1989, by the National Academy of Sciences. Published by the National Academy Press.

women is broad, and individual needs depend on several factors including age, body weight, body composition, and customary activity level.[3] Unless levels of physical activity are exceptionally high, resting energy expenditure (REE) typically accounts for 60 to 75% of the daily total. Therefore, REE is used to estimate total energy needs.[3] To calculate REE, several formulas can be used[4-6] (Exhibit 6-1). REE can also be determined by indirect calorimetry.

Once REE is predicted, daily energy needs can be estimated using activity values (Table 6-2) that are weighted by the time engaged in each activity. The weighted activity factor is then multiplied by the predicted REE to derive the total daily energy needs (Exhibit 6-2).

Another method recently developed to assess energy expenditure is the doubly labeled ($^2H_2O_{18}$) water technique. Because of the high cost and limited availabil-

Exhibit 6-1 Equations for Predicting Resting Energy Expenditure (REE) in Women

---

World Health Organization equations[a]

Age
(years)

18–30	REE = (14.7 × wt in kg) + 496
30–60	REE = (8.7 × wt in kg) + 829

Mifflin-St. Jeor equation[b]

REE = 10 × weight (kg) + 6.25 × height (cm) − 5 × age (yr) − 161

Harris-Benedict equation[c]

REE (kcal) = 6.551 + 9.56(W) + 1.85(H) − 4.68(A)

(A = age; W = weight in kilograms; H = height in centimeters)

[a]Source: Reprinted from *Recommended Dietary Allowances,* ed 10, National Academy Press, 1989.
[b]Source: Reprinted from *American Journal of Clinical Nutrition (*1990;51:241–247).
[c]Source: Reprinted from *A Biometric Study of Basal Metabolism in Man,* by JA Harris and FG Benedict, Carnegie Institute of Washington, 1919.

Table 6-2 Approximate Energy Expenditure for Various Activities in Relation to Resting Energy Expenditure (REE)

Activity Category	Representative Value for Activity Factor per Unit Time of Activity
Resting	
Sleeping, reclining	REE × 1.0
Very light	
Seated and standing activities, driving, typing, cooking, ironing	REE × 1.5
Light	
Walking on level surface, 2.5–3 mph, carpentry, restaurant trades, housecleaning, child care	REE × 2.5
Moderate	
Walking 3.5–4 mph, weeding and hoeing, cycling, skiing, tennis, dancing	REE × 5.0
Heavy	
Walking with load uphill, basketball, climbing, football, soccer	REE × 7.0

Source: Reprinted from *Recommended Dietary Allowances,* ed 10, National Academy Press, 1989.

Exhibit 6-2 How to Calculate the Estimated Daily Energy Needs for a Moderately Active, 59-kg, 165-cm, 40-Year-Old Woman

---

Step 1: Resting Energy Expenditure (REE) calculated using the Mifflin-St. Jeor Equation

REE = $10 \times (59$ kg$) + 6.25(165$ cm$) - 5 (40$ yr$) - 161$
REE = 1260 kcal

Step 2: Derivation of activity factor

Activity as multiples of REE		Time spent in activity (hr)	Weighted REE factor
resting	1.0	8	8.0
very light	1.5	10	15.0
light	2.5	5	12.5
moderate	5.0	1	5.0
heavy	7.0	0	0.0
Total		24	40.5
Mean			1.69

Step 3: Calculations of energy need, kcal/day
Resting Energy Expenditure × Weighted Activity Factor = Total Energy Needs
　　　　　　　1260 × 1.69　　　　　　　 = 2169 kcal

---

ity of the stable isotope, this method is not suitable for large-scale epidemiologic studies. However, a few small studies have been conducted in premenopausal women and can provide insight into the energy requirements of this population group. Mean total daily energy expenditure, as measured by doubly labeled water, was 1839 kcal/day in 12 U.K. women[7] and 1985 kcal/day in six U.S. women.[8] It has been suggested that these unexpectedly low values were a reflection of life-style-related decreases in energy expended in physical activity. Lower than expected values of total energy expenditure were also found in young Swazi college women (1735 kcal/day).[9] Thus, energy needs for all these women were found to be lower than the current RDA of 2200 kcal/day. This emphasizes the need for a measure of physical activity to be used in the estimation of daily energy needs of women.

Evidence is accumulating that the traditional dietary intake methodologies, such as food frequency questionnaires, the 24-hour recall, and diet records have questionable validity for accurately determining energy intake.[10] Nutritionists must presume that bias is present and interpret dietary intake accordingly. Limited studies suggest that older women may underreport their food intake more than older men.[11] Also, body fatness is related to underreporting of intake in most age and gender groups.[12,13] Thus, nutritionists may want to use prediction equations, such as those presented here, to evaluate reported energy intakes against predicted energy requirements to give a rough assessment of whether dietary intake measures are biased.[14,15]

Calcium, Phosphorus, Vitamin D, and Iron

In the RDAs, premenopausal women are divided into two groups—women aged 19 to 24 years and women aged 25 to 50 years old. Because peak bone mass is not attained before age 25, the RDAs for calcium and phosphorus remain at the levels recommended for adolescents (1200 mg) through age 24. These levels promote the achievement of full bone mineral deposition. Recently, the National Institutes of Health sponsored a Consensus Conference on Optimal Calcium Intake.[16] Scientists reviewed available research to establish the ideal level of calcium intake for bone strength, as well as prevention of colon cancer, high blood pressure, and preeclampsia. The consensus was that the RDA for calcium is currently set too low. A calcium intake of 1000 mg (+200 mg over current RDA) per day was recommended for women aged 25 to 50. The RDA for vitamin D, which promotes calcium absorption, is maintained at 10 μg/day until the age of 25; thereafter, it falls to 5 μg/day.

During the reproductive years, women are at high risk for iron deficiency due to menstrual iron losses. Thus, the RDA for iron is set at 15 mg/day, the highest of any age/sex category except pregnant women. This level of intake should be adequate to replace iron losses for most healthy women.[1]

Reducing the Risk of Chronic Disease

Exhibit 6-3 lists the current dietary recommendations for risk reduction of diet-related chronic disease. Some of these diseases (coronary heart disease, cancer, obesity, and osteoporosis) are a major health threat for women.

Simple Dietary Screener for Women

Nutritionists can use screening tools to efficiently identify those women who are in need of nutrition intervention. Such a tool was developed for the Women's Health Trial (WHT) (see Chapter 18). The WHT was a feasibility study for a randomized trial of a low-fat diet for the prevention of breast cancer. Women selected for participation in the WHT needed to be consuming at baseline a diet with greater than 38% of energy from fat. The Simplified Fat Screener (Exhibit 6-4) was developed to screen women who met the eligibility criteria. This tool can be used by nutritionists for screening, monitoring compliance, and nutrition education. Also, the WHT had a Simplified Fiber/Fruit/Vegetable Screener (Exhibit 6-4). This tool can be used to identify women who should increase the amount of fruits, vegetables, and other fiber-rich foods in their diet.

Exhibit 6-3 Recommendations to Reduce Risk of Diet-Related Chronic Disease

- Reduce total fat intake to 30% or less of calories. Reduce saturated fatty acid intake to less than 10% of calories and the intake of cholesterol to less than 300 mg daily.
- Eat five or more servings of vegetables and fruits daily, especially green and yellow vegetables and citrus fruits. Also increase intake of starches and other complex carbohydrates by eating six or more daily servings of a combination of breads, cereals, and legumes.
- Maintain protein intake at moderate levels.
- Balance food intake and physical activity to maintain appropriate body weight.
- Alcohol consumption is not recommended. For those who drink alcoholic beverages, consumption should be limited to the equivalent of less than 1 ounce of pure alcohol in a single day. Pregnant women should avoid alcoholic beverages.
- Limit daily intake of salt (sodium chloride) to 6 g or less.
- Maintain adequate calcium intake.
- Avoid taking dietary supplements in excess of the RDA in any one day.

Source: Reprinted from *Diet and Health: Implications of Reducing Chronic Disease Risk,* by the Committee on Diet and Health with permission of the National Academy Press, © 1989.

DIETARY STATUS OF U.S. PREMENOPAUSAL WOMEN

To understand the nutritional issues confronting premenopausal women, it is necessary to know what they are eating. Key sources of information concerning the dietary status of U.S. women are obtained from government surveys. The most current data available are from the U.S. Department of Agriculture (USDA) Continuing Survey of Food Intakes by Individuals (CSFII) 1985–6 and 1989–91,[17,18] the USDA Nationwide Food Consumption Survey 1987–88 (NFCS 87–88),[19] and the National Center for Health Statistics (NCHS) National Health and Nutrition Examination Survey III (NHANES III 1988–94).[20,21] For a more detailed discussion of food intakes by women, see Chapter 4.

In the CSFII, participants provided six 24-hour recalls over a 1-year period. The NFCS 1987–88 includes dietary intake data, collected as one 24-hour recall followed by a 2-day food record. Estimates of nutrient intakes in NHANES III are obtained from one 24-hour dietary recall interview.

Vitamins

Vitamin intakes in NHANES III (1988–91) were higher than in NFCS 1987–88 (Table 6-3). Consequently, all averaged vitamin intakes across the population of women were greater than two-thirds of the RDA in the NHANES III.

Exhibit 6-4 Simplified Fat and Fiber/Fruit/Vegetable Screener

Food Questionnaire. Think about your eating habits over the past year or so. About how often do you eat each of the following foods? Mark an "x" in one box for each food.

	(0) Less than once per MONTH	(1) 2–3 times per MONTH	(2) 1–2 times per WEEK	(3) 3–4 times per WEEK	(4) 5+ times per WEEK	Points Score
Hamburgers or cheeseburgers	☐	☐	☐	☐	☐	
Beef, such as steaks, roasts	☐	☐	☐	☐	☐	
Fried chicken	☐	☐	☐	☐	☐	
Hot dogs, franks	☐	☐	☐	☐	☐	
Cold cuts, lunch meats, ham, etc.	☐	☐	☐	☐	☐	
Salad dressings, mayo (not diet)	☐	☐	☐	☐	☐	
Margarine or butter	☐	☐	☐	☐	☐	
Eggs	☐	☐	☐	☐	☐	
Bacon or sausage	☐	☐	☐	☐	☐	
Cheese or cheese spread	☐	☐	☐	☐	☐	
Whole milk	☐	☐	☐	☐	☐	
French fries	☐	☐	☐	☐	☐	
Potato chips, corn chips, popcorn	☐	☐	☐	☐	☐	
Ice cream	☐	☐	☐	☐	☐	
Doughnuts, pastries, cake, cookies	☐	☐	☐	☐	☐	

Meal/Snacks Score =

	(0) Less than once per WEEK	(1) About 1 time per WEEK	(2) 2–3 times per WEEK	(3) 4–6 times per WEEK	(4) Every Day	Points Score
Orange juice	☐	☐	☐	☐	☐	
Not counting juice, about how often do you eat any fruit?	☐	☐	☐	☐	☐	
Green salad	☐	☐	☐	☐	☐	
Potatoes	☐	☐	☐	☐	☐	
Beans, such as baked beans, pinto, kidney beans, or in chili	☐	☐	☐	☐	☐	
About how often do you eat any other vegetables?	☐	☐	☐	☐	☐	
High-fiber or bran cereal	☐	☐	☐	☐	☐	
Dark bread, such as whole wheat, rye	☐	☐	☐	☐	☐	
White bread, including french, italian, biscuits, muffins	☐	☐	☐	☐	☐	

Fruit/Vegetable/Fiber Score =

continues

Exhibit 6-4 (continued)

FAT SCORE

To score:

For each food, write the number that is at the top of the column you checked, in the box at the far right. Add up the numbers to get your total score. If your score is

- more than 27   Your diet is high in fat. There are many ways you can make your eating pattern lower in fat. You should look at your highest scores above to find areas in which to begin.

- 25–27   Your diet is quite high in fat. To make your eating pattern lower in fat, you may want to begin in the areas where you scored highest.

- 22–24   You are generally eating a typical American diet, which could be lower in fat.

- 18–21   You are making better low-fat food choices.

- 17 or less   You are making the best low-fat food choices! Keep up the great work!

If you scored 17 or less, you're doing well! This is the desirable score on this screener.

FIBER/FRUIT/VEGETABLE SCORE

To score:

For each food, write the number that is at the top of the column you checked, in the box at the far right. Add up the numbers to get your total score.

If your score is

- 30 or more   You are doing very well! This is the desirable score on this screener.

- 20 to 29   You should include more fruits, vegetables, and whole grains.

- less than 20   Your diet is probably low in important nutrients. You should find ways to increase the fruits and vegetables and other fiber-rich foods you eat every day.

Courtesy of Gladys Block, PhD, Block Dietary Data Systems, Berkeley, California.

Table 6-3 Mean Nutrient Intakes among Premenopausal Women from Two National
Surveys

	NHANES III 1988–91		NFCS 1987–88	
	mean	SEM	mean	SD
Energy (kcal)				
20–29 years	1957	34	1524	524
30–39 years	1883	35	1473	512
40–49 years	1764	34	1419	465
Protein (g)				
20–29 years	69	2	62	24
30–39 years	70	2	61	22
40–49 years	67	2	59	20
Fat (g)				
20–29 years	75	2	63	26
30–39 years	75	2	61	25
40–49 years	70	2	59	24
Carbohydrates (g)				
20–29 years	241	5	177	67
30–39 years	228	5	170	68
40–49 years	213	5	164	64
Vitamin A (IU)				
20–29 years	4626	291	4907	5323
30–39 years	6044	431	4798	4540
40–49 years	5594	423	5819	7252
Vitamin C (mg)				
20–29 years	87	4	72	52
30–39 years	99	5	73	57
40–49 years	88	5	82	59
Vitamin E (mg)				
20–29 years	8	<1	7	5
30–39 years	8	<1	7	5
40–49 years	8	<1	7	5
Thiamin (mg)				
20–29 years	1.4	0.04	1.1	0.5
30–39 years	1.4	0.04	1.1	0.5
40–49 years	1.3	0.04	1.1	0.4

continues

Table 6-3 Mean Nutrient Intakes among Premenopausal Women from Two National Surveys (continued)

	NHANES III 1988–91		NFCS 1987–88	
	mean	SEM	mean	SD
Riboflavin (mg)				
20–29 years	1.7	0.04	1.5	0.7
30–39 years	1.6	0.04	1.4	0.6
40–49 years	1.6	0.04	1.4	0.6
Vitamin B_6 (mg)				
20–29 years	1.5	0.04	1.2	0.5
30–39 years	1.5	0.04	1.2	0.6
40–49 years	1.4	0.04	1.2	0.5
Folate (µg)				
20–29 years	230	8	178	103
30–39 years	237	9	184	107
40–49 years	220	8	187	95
Calcium (mg)				
20–29 years	778	22	639	347
30–39 years	753	22	597	315
40–49 years	685	22	558	189
Magnesium (mg)				
20–29 years	240	6	188	73
30–39 years	261	6	200	77
40–49 years	251	6	200	75
Iron (mg)				
20–29 years	12	<1	10	5
30–39 years	13	<1	10	5
40–49 years	12	<1	10	5
Zinc (mg)				
20–29 years	10	<1	9	4
30–39 years	10	<1	8	4
40–49 years	9	<1	8	5

Source: Data from *Third National Health and Nutrition Examination Survey, Phase 1* (NHANES III), *1988–91* and *USDA Nationwide Food Consumption Survey* (NFCS), *1987–88.*

Mean vitamin E intakes were right at the RDA—an improvement since NFCS 1987–88. Epidemiologic evidence has suggested that intakes of vitamin E in excess of the RDA (as supplements) reduce the risk of coronary heart disease[22] and some cancers in women.[23] Concentrated sources of vitamin E in the U.S. diet are vegetable oils (Table 6-4). Primary sources of vitamin E in women's diets are grains, fruits and vegetables, fats, sweets, and beverages (Figure 6-1). Other than fortified cereals, it is difficult to recommend the addition of good food sources of vitamin E in the diet without increasing total dietary fat intake. Because epidemiologic studies cannot prove cause-and-effect relationships, randomized clinical trials to assess the effect of vitamin E supplements on the primary and secondary prevention of coronary heart disease are currently being conducted. Recommendations regarding the widespread use of vitamin E supplements need to await the results of these trials.

Mean daily folate intakes exceeded the RDA in both surveys, with average consumption at about 0.2 mg/day. The current RDA for folate is set at 0.18 mg/day for females aged 15 to 50, which is considerably lower than the 1980 RDA of 0.4 mg/day.[1] Substantial evidence has accumulated since the last RDA revision (1989), indicating that adequate intakes of folate before conception as well as during the early weeks of pregnancy can reduce the risk of neural tube defects (NTDs), a serious and debilitating birth defect.[24–26] On the basis of these studies, the U.S. Public Health Service concluded that folic acid, at a dose of 0.4 mg/day,

Table 6-4 Good Sources of Vitamin E

Food	Selected Serving Size	Percentage of U.S. RDA
Ready-to-eat cereals, fortified	1 ounce	+++
Wheat germ, plain	2 tablespoons	++
Nectarine, raw	1 medium	+
Peaches, canned, juice-pack	1/2 cup	+
Almonds, unroasted	2 tablespoons	+++
Safflower oil	1 tablespoon	+++
Corn oil	1 tablespoon	+++
Sunflower seeds	2 tablespoons	+++
Peanut butter	2 tablespoons	++
Chicken, turkey; braised	1/2 cup diced	+
Shrimp, cooked	3 ounces	++
Turnip greens, cooked	1/2 cup	+

+ 10–24% of the U.S. RDA for adults and children older than 4 years of age.
++ 25–39% of the U.S. RDA for adults and children older than 4 years of age.
+++ 40% or more of the U.S. RDA for adults and children older than 4 years of age.
Source: Reprinted from *Eating Right,* Fact Sheets, US Department of Agriculture, Human Nutrition Service, 1990.

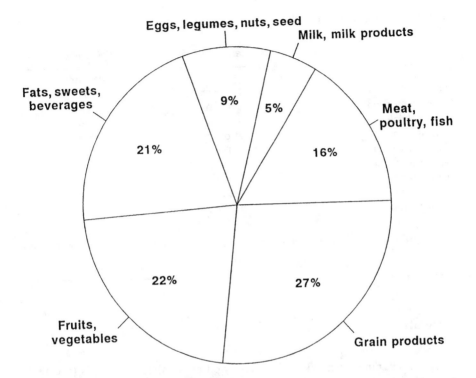

Figure 6-1 Where Do Women Get Vitamin E? *Source:* Data from *Continuing Survey of Food Intake by Individuals, 4 days,* US Department of Agriculture, Human Nutrition Service, 1985–1986.

will reduce the risk of NTDs in the United States by 50%.[27] As a result, the following was recommended:

> All women of childbearing age in the U.S. who are capable of becoming pregnant should consume 0.4 milligrams of folic acid per day for the purpose of reducing their risk of having a pregnancy affected with spina bifida or other NTDs.

Women who follow current dietary recommendations for fruits, vegetables, and grains are likely to consume at least 0.4 mg of folate daily because most folate in the diets of women comes from these food groups (Table 6-5; Figure 6-2). Increased folate intakes can also be achieved with supplementation (most multivitamin preparations contain 0.4 mg folate) or consumption of fortified cereals.

Table 6-5 Good Sources of Folate

Food	Selected Serving Size	Folate (mg)
Fortified breakfast cereal	1 ounce	100–400
Liver	3 ounces	204
Spinach, cooked	1 cup	164
Orange juice	1 cup	136
Wheat germ	1 ounce	118
Broccoli, cooked	1 medium spear	101
Romaine lettuce, raw	1 cup	98
Green peas	1 cup	77
Beans, kidney	1 cup	69
Tomato, raw	1 medium	53

Source: Reprinted from *Eating Right,* Fact Sheets, US Department of Agriculture, Human Nutrition Service, 1990.

Minerals

Unlike vitamins, mineral intakes were well below the RDA levels (see Table 6-3). Low intakes of calcium are associated with osteoporosis and poor bone health.[2] Because treatment for osteoporosis has not been fully successful,[28] attaining maximum bone mass and bone density during the premenopausal years is essential. Although dietary calcium intake seems to exert its greatest effect on bone mineral density during the bone-building years of childhood and early adulthood (up to age 24 years),[29] it is also necessary to achieve an adequate calcium intake during the adult years to avoid skeletal depletion.[30] In women, calcium intakes decrease with age. However, at all ages intakes were suboptimal compared with newer NIH recommendations.[16] Non-Hispanic blacks had lower intakes than other ethnic groups (range of means, 530 to 656 mg/day).[21] Calcium is concentrated in a limited number of foods (Table 6-6), with milk and dairy products providing the most bioavailable source. Almost half of women's calcium intakes comes from dairy products (Figure 6-3).

Although the intake of iron improved in the NHANES III survey, intakes were still below 80% of the RDA. Even lower intakes were seen in non-Hispanic blacks (mean, 11 mg/day for 30- to 49-year-olds).[20,21] Clearly, poor iron intakes increase the risk of developing iron deficiency, particularly among menstruating women.[31] This is of particular concern for female athletes, a population in which iron deficiency (with or without anemia) is a relatively common observation.[32]

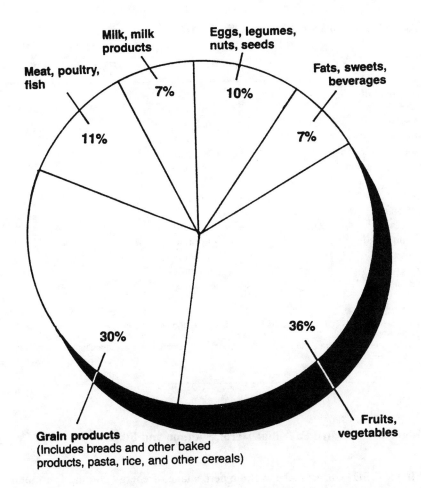

Figure 6-2 Where Do Women Get Folate? *Source:* Data from *Continuing Survey of Food Intake by Individuals, 4 days,* US Department of Agriculture, Human Nutrition Service, 1985–1986.

Good food sources of iron are shown in Table 6-7. More iron in women's diets is from nonheme iron in grain products than the more bioavailable iron in the meat group (Figure 6-4).

Women's average intakes of zinc were at 75% of the RDA for women 40 to 49 years old. Major dietary sources of zinc are animal products such as shellfish (especially oysters), meats, liver, poultry, eggs, and dairy products (Table 6-8). Women's lower energy intakes (in comparison with men) can make it difficult to meet their zinc needs, especially if animal products that provide 45% of the zinc in women's diets (Figure 6-5) are limited.

Table 6-6 Good Sources of Calcium Other Than Milk

Food	Selected Serving Size	Percentage of U.S. RDA
English muffin	1 muffin	+
Bran muffin	1 medium	+
Waffles, plain	2 4-inch squares	++
Broccoli, cooked	1/2 cup	+
Spinach, cooked	1/2 cup	+
Mackerel, canned	3 ounces	+
Salmon, canned	3 ounces	+
Tofu	1/2 cup cubed	++
Cheese		
swiss	1 ounce	++
parmesan	1 ounce	++
ricotta	1/2 cup	++
Ice cream	1/2 cup	+
Yogurt	8 ounces	++

+ 10–24% of the U.S. RDA for adults and children older than 4 years of age.
++ 25–39% of the U.S. RDA for adults and children older than 4 years of age.
Source: Reprinted from *Eating Right,* Fact Sheets, US Department of Agriculture, Human Nutrition Service, 1990.

Total Fat, Saturated Fat, Cholesterol, Sodium, and Fiber

In the USDA surveys, the average percentage of energy coming from total fat was 37%, well above the current recommended level of 30%. Mean percentage of calories from saturated fat was approximately 13%, also above the recommended 10%. Findings from the NHANES III update these national population estimates.[20] Women in NHANES III reported less energy consumed as fat and saturated fat, 34% and 12%, respectively. Although these downward trends indicate positive changes, intakes still remain higher than current recommendations. About 15% of premenopausal women in NFCS 87–88 met the recommendations for total fat and saturated fat (Table 6-9).

Mean intakes of cholesterol were below the recommendation of less than 300 mg and sodium intakes ranged from 2310 mg to 2500 mg, within the range of the recommendation to limit salt intake to 6 g (2400 mg of sodium). However, the sodium values reported in the USDA surveys do not include the use of discretionary salt, and thus actual mean sodium intakes likely exceed these figures. Fiber

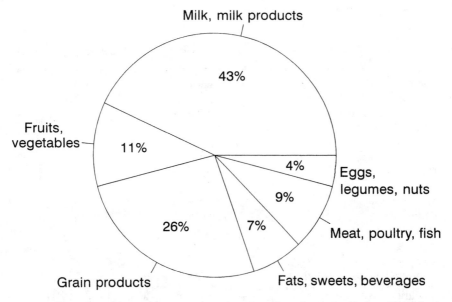

Figure 6-3 Where Do Women Get Calcium? *Source:* Data from *Continuing Survey of Food Intake by Individuals, 4 days,* US Department of Agriculture, Human Nutrition Service, 1985–1986.

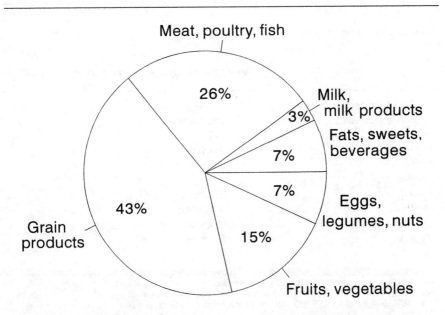

Figure 6-4 Where Do Women Get Iron? *Source:* Data from *Continuing Survey of Food Intake by Individuals, 4 days,* US Department of Agriculture, Human Nutrition Service, 1985–1986.

Table 6-7 Good Sources of Iron

Food	Selected Serving Size	Percentage of U.S. RDA
Bagel	1 medium	+
Oatmeal	2/3 cup	++
Ready-to-eat cereals	1 ounce	++
Apricots, dried	1/2 cup	+
Beans, lima	1/2 cup	+
Spinach, cooked	1/2 cup	+
Ground beef	1 patty	+
Liver, pork	3 ounces	+++
Turkey, dark meat	3 ounces	+
Clams	3 ounces	+++
Beans	1/2 cup	+

+ 10–24% of the U.S. RDA for adults and children older than 4 years of age.
++ 25–39% of the U.S. RDA for adults and children older than 4 years of age.
+++ 40% or more of the U.S. RDA for adults and children older than 4 years of age.
Source: Reprinted from *Eating Right,* Fact Sheets, US Department of Agriculture, Human Nutrition Service, 1990.

Table 6-8 Good Sources of Zinc

Food	Selected Serving Size	Percentage of U.S. RDA
Ready-to-eat cereals, fortified	1 ounce	+
Wheat germ, plain	2 tablespoons	+
Ground beef	1 patty	++
Pot roast	3 ounces	+++
Steak	3 ounces	++
Chicken leg	1 leg	+
Ham	3 ounces	+
Oysters	3 ounces	+++
Ricotta cheese	1/2 cup	+
Yogurt	8 ounces	+

+ 10–24% of the U.S. RDA for adults and children older than 4 years of age.
++ 25–39% of the U.S. RDA for adults and children older than 4 years of age.
+++ 40% or more of the U.S. RDA for adults and children older than 4 years of age.
Source: Reprinted from *Eating Right,* Fact Sheets, US Department of Agriculture, Human Nutrition Service, 1990.

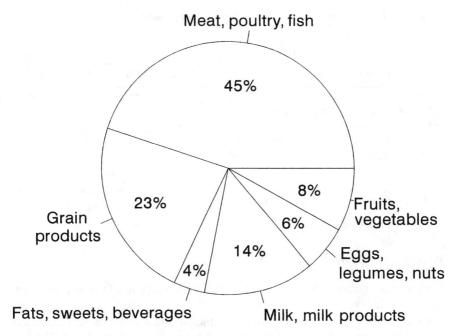

Figure 6-5 Where Do Women Get Zinc? *Source:* Data from *Continuing Survey of Food Intake by Individuals, 4 days,* US Department of Agriculture, Human Nutrition Service, 1985–1986.

intakes averaged approximately 12 g, which is about half of the recommended 25 g/day. Only 2% of women in NFCS 87–88 met the guidelines for fiber. Thus, with the exception of cholesterol, most women do not meet dietary recommendations outlined in the National Academy of Science's *Diet and Health* (Table 6-9).

FACTORS SHAPING WOMEN'S EATING PATTERNS

Knowledge of the factors that shape women's eating patterns can contribute to (1) an improved understanding of women's nutritional status, (2) an improved ability to anticipate trends in eating patterns, and (3) the development of better nutrition education and intervention programs designed to improve the nutrition and health status of U.S. women.

Greater employment of women, the increase in single female-headed households, increased accessibility to commercial food establishments, increased availability of convenience foods, and the use of tobacco by women are all factors that have been shown to influence women's eating patterns.[33]

Table 6-9 Percentage of Women Meeting Contemporary Dietary Recommendations

Recommendations	Age (yr)				
	30–39	40–49	50–59	60–69	≥70
≤30% of energy from fat	15	15	18	20	19
≤10% of energy from saturated fat	14	16	23	21	20
<300 mg cholesterol per day	72	75	70	74	81
>55% of energy from carbohydrate	16	18	13	17	23
25 g fiber per day	2	<1	5	1	2

Source: Reprinted with permission from *Journal of the American Dietetic Association* (1993;93:987–993), Copyright © 1993, American Dietetic Association.

Women's Employment

Women are entering the work force at unprecedented rates. Demographers predict that by the year 2000, approximately 50% of the work force will be women and 60% of all women will be at work.[34] Much of the increase in the numbers of women in the labor force has come from mothers becoming employed. The current rate of maternal employment for two-parent families with school-aged children is 73%.[35] The most impressive recent change in maternal employment rate, however, is among mothers of preschool children and infants. From 1960 to 1990, the share of all children younger than 6 years whose mothers were employed grew from 19 to 57%.[35]

When women enter the work force, they devote less time to family work.[36] The more hours women spend employed outside the home, the fewer hours they spend in meal preparation. Employed wives spend about 15 to 20 minutes less per day than nonemployed wives preparing meals.[37–41]

It is known that household consumption of prepared foods is increased when women are employed.[42] Whether the reduced amount of time spent in meal preparation and the increased consumption of prepared foods affects the diet quality of women and/or their families is not known.[37] Research has shown, however, that the diets of young children are not negatively affected by their mother's employment status.[38,39]

Single Female-Headed Households

Households headed by single women are a growing proportion of the total population. In 1970, female-headed households made up 12% of all family groups with children younger than age 18. By 1992, this percentage had increased to 26%.[43] Characteristics of female-headed households include high poverty rates and less formal education (Exhibit 6-5). In 1991, the majority (55%) of families maintained by single mothers fell below the poverty line (for their household size), compared with 14% of all families.[44]

The diet quality of female-headed families has been investigated. Using CSFII 1989–90, researchers examined (1) perceived food adequacy, (2) diet quality, (3) food expenditures, and (4) food shopping behaviors of 379 families maintained by single mothers and 1049 families maintained by married couples.[45] Single mothers viewed the food adequacy of their households less positively than married couples. As single mothers consumed significantly less fruits and vegetables and their children consumed less fruits, the quality of their diets supported this view. However, when noncash benefits such as food stamps and the Women, Infant, and Children Supplemental Food Program (WIC) were taken into account, expenditures on food were similar among single-parent families and their married-couple counterparts. Several reasons are proposed for the negative perception of food adequacy by these single mothers. They may have spent more for the same or lesser quality foods because they face time and transportation

---

Exhibit 6-5 Characteristics of Female-Headed Households

- High Poverty Rates
  55% of all families maintained by single mothers fell below the poverty line in 1991.

- High Proportion of Children
  60% of all children born today will spend some of their childhood in a single-parent household, mostly a female-headed household.

- Overrepresentation of Blacks
  Blacks represented 15% of all family groups with children in 1988; they accounted for 35% of all female-headed households.

- Overrepresentation of the Welfare and Food Assistance Population
  In 1988, female-headed households formed an estimated 50% of all households receiving food stamps and an estimated 33% of participants of the Women, Infants, and Children Program (WIC) lived in households with no adult male present.

- Less Formal Education
  In 1989 to 1990, 28% of single mothers did not graduate from high school in comparison with 11% of married mothers.

- Less Likely To Be Employed
  In 1989 to 1990, 52% of single mothers were employed in comparison with 66% of married mothers.

Source: Adapted from *Family Economics Review* (1994;7:1), USDA, Agricultural Research Service.

constraints in food shopping. They also shopped infrequently, which limits the purchase of perishable foods such as fruits and vegetables.

Eating Away from Home

There have been dramatic increases in the United States in the amount of food eaten away from home. The percentage of the food dollar spent on away-from-home food consumption increased from 27% in 1960 to 40% in the mid-1980s.[46] In NFCS 1987–88, 44% of the total sample consumed some food away from home on the days surveyed.

To determine personal and household characteristics related to eating away from home and the effect of eating away from home on diet quality, the dietary patterns of women who participated in the NFCS 1987–88 and the CSFII 1985 were examined.[47–49] Characteristics that increase the numbers of meals women consume away from home include (1) more income, (2) higher education, (3) single female-headed household, and (4) employment. When examining diet quality, women who participated in the NFCS had higher intakes of calories, fat, cholesterol, and sodium as the number of meals away from home increased.[47] Among women participating in CSFII 1985, extensive patronage of restaurants, fast-food places, and cafeterias led to significantly lower intakes of iron, calcium, vitamin C, and fiber and significantly higher intakes of total fat and saturated fat.[49] Others clustered women by eating patterns and confirmed that women who frequented restaurants had substantially higher calorie and fat intakes than women who ate most of their meals at home (42% total calories from fat for restaurant eaters versus 30% total calories from fat for home eaters).[48]

Convenience Foods

Economists have speculated that the increased time demands placed on women today should increase their expenditures for convenience foods in an effort to reduce time spent in food preparation.[42] Bureau of Labor reports have been used to examine the relationships between the use of prepared foods and various sociodemographic characteristics. Prepared foods included prepared flour and cake mixes, bakery products, and canned or frozen meats and dinners. Consumption of prepared foods was positively related to family income, women's employment, family size, the presence of children, and age of the woman. Interestingly, women with a college education used significantly less prepared foods. A possible explanation is that college-educated women are more nutrition-conscious and thus more selective of ingredients than is possible with many prepared food items.

How the increased use of convenience foods affects women's diet quality has not been examined. However, nutritionists need to understand the important role convenience foods may play in helping women balance their roles as both family provider and caregiver.

Tobacco Use

Cigarette smoking is the single most important health habit that contributes to preventable chronic disease in the United States.[50] Despite significant changes in the smoking and health environment in the United States in the past 25 years, in 1987 31% of U.S. women aged 25 to 44 and 29% of women aged 45 to 64 smoked.[51] Smoking prevalence rates among women aged 20 years and older have declined since 1974; however, the rates have declined more slowly than among men.[51] It is speculated that this reduced decline in smoking rates among women is in part due to the increasing tendency of cigarette manufacturers to target cigarette advertising and marketing toward women.[52]

Women who smoke have dietary patterns that tend to be less healthy than those of nonsmokers. In the CSFII 1985 and the 1987 National Health Interview Survey (NHIS), researchers found significant differences between the food intake and nutrient consumption of women smokers and nonsmokers.[53,54] Smokers had lower intakes of fruits, vegetables, whole grains/cereals, fiber, vitamin C, and carotenoids and higher intakes of meat, alcohol, fat, and cholesterol in comparison with nonsmokers (Table 6-10). Interestingly, the diets of former smokers more closely resembled those of never smokers than of current smokers.

It is interesting that the whole range of dietary recommendations, and not just a few selected ones, is in general less well adhered to by women who smoke. Tobacco

Table 6-10 Effect of Smoking on U.S. Women's Dietary Patterns

	More	*Less*	*Similar*
Food intake	Regular carbonated soft drinks Coffee Alcoholic beverages Eggs Sugars	Fruits Vegetables	
Nutrient intake	Cholesterol	Protein Dietary fiber Vitamin C Thiamin	Calories

Source: Reprinted with permission from *Journal of the American Dietetic Association* (1990;90:230–237), Copyright © 1990, American Dietetic Association.

use, in and of itself, is a major contributor to chronic disease risk and pregnancy complications in women. Research now suggests that smokers may be at additional risk from dietary intakes, which are further away from dietary recommendations than the diets of nonsmokers. Thus, nutrition educators should be cognizant that smokers generally have intakes of food or nutrients associated with chronic disease risk.

SPECIAL NUTRITION CONCERNS OF PREMENOPAUSAL WOMEN

Premenstrual Syndrome

Premenstrual syndrome (PMS) is a condition characterized by a group of psychological and physical symptoms that recur in some women each month between the time of ovulation and the beginning of menses. Symptoms may include tension, depression, fatigue, aggression, crying spells, headaches, and food cravings in almost any combinations.

Oral contraceptives have been used in the treatment of PMS as some studies report PMS symptoms are reduced in oral contraceptive users compared with nonusers.[55] Nutritional supplements have also been widely promoted as a treatment for PMS; however, scientific support for their use has been limited. Two studies found significant improvement in women with PMS receiving pyridoxine in doses of 500 mg/day and 50 to 200 mg/day, respectively.[56,57] However, the doses of pyridoxine used in these studies were well in excess of the RDA and approached levels reported to cause significant toxic effects (RDA for pyridoxine for women aged 25 to 50 = 1.6 mg).[58] Because toxic levels of pyridoxine can lead to neurologic disorders, caution is indicated and indiscriminate use of pharmacologic doses is not recommended.

Other researchers have found no evidence to support the hypothesis that PMS is caused by nutritional deficiencies.[59] Thus, science does not currently support a nutritional etiology of PMS. Despite this, some women may report relief of PMS symptoms after making dietary modifications. These may include the avoidance of caffeine, alcohol, and salt as well as supplementation with various vitamins and minerals. Nutritionists should note if these changes are causing serious restrictions of essential nutrients or leading to megadoses at potentially toxic levels and counsel women accordingly. See Chapter 5 for further discussion of PMS.

Vitamin and Mineral Supplements

The use of vitamin and mineral supplements is widespread among adults in the United States. In 1990, Americans spent 3.3 billion dollars on nutrition supplements.[60] Because supplements can have a substantial impact on the intake of vitamins and minerals for many individuals, it is important to know the demographic and personal characteristics of supplement users. Data from NHIS 1987 showed that women of all ages were more likely than men to consume supplements, 27% versus 19%, respectively.[61] Among these women, white women were more likely to use supplements than other races (Figure 6-6). Sociodemographic factors and health habits also influence supplement use (Table 6-11). Overall groups most likely to use supplements were (1) more educated, (2) at higher income levels, (3) nondrinkers and lighter drinkers, (4) never and former smokers, and (5) not morbidly obese. Multivitamins were the most commonly used supplement, followed by vitamin C, calcium, vitamin E, and vitamin A.[61] Women report taking supplements for several reasons, including compensating for perceived nutrient deficiencies, improving their sense of health and well-being, and promoting longevity.[62]

The NIH Consensus Conference on Optimal Calcium Intake recommended that women 25 to 50 years of age achieve a calcium intake of 1000 mg/day from food.[16] However, they do acknowledge that if a woman cannot get all her calcium from food, supplements or calcium-fortified foods can be used. Calcium supplements are available in several forms including oyster shell calcium, dolomite calcium, calcium carbonate, and calcium gluconate. Calcium-fortified foods on the market include milk, yogurt, and orange juice. Studies conducted to determine the bioavailability of various forms of supplements found that marked differences

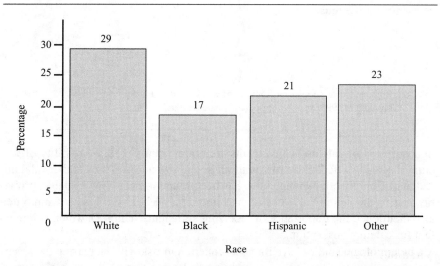

Figure 6-6 Percentage of Women, by Race, Reporting Daily Supplement Use *Source:* Reprinted with permission from *American Journal of Epidemiology* (1990;132[6]:1091–1101), Copyright © 1990, Society for Epidemiologic Research.

Table 6-11 Characteristics of Supplement Users

	Percentage Reporting Daily Supplement Use
Education	
0–8	18
9–11	20
12	23
Any college	27
Income (dollars)	
<5,000	16
5,000–24,999	22
25,000–49,999	24
≥50,000	27
Occupation	
White collar	25
Blue collar	16
Alcohol use (drinks/wk)	
Nondrinker	23
≤1–7	24
>7–14	23
>14	20
Cigarette smoking status	
Never	24
Former	26
Current	21
Body mass index (quartile)	
1	24
2	25
3	24
4	20

Source: Reprinted with permission from *American Journal of Epidemiology* (1990;132[6]:1091–1101), Copyright © 1990, Society for Epidemiologic Research.

in absorption of calcium supplements are not evident.[63,64] The solubility of calcium is greatly affected by pH, with an acidic pH necessary to ionize calcium. Calcium from fortified orange juice has been found to be highly available, probably due to the acidic nature of orange juice.[64] The NIH Consensus Committee also mentioned the importance of receiving sufficient vitamin D, which is important for calcium absorption.

Epidemiologic studies have found a reduction in risk with increasing intakes of various antioxidant vitamins for both heart disease and cancer. Female nurses taking vitamin E supplements had significantly less risk of developing coronary heart disease.[22] Enstrom et al.[65] examined data from the First National Health and Nutrition Examination Survey (NHANES I) Epidemiologic Follow-up Study (NHEFS) and found a reduction in risk for all causes of death associated with higher intakes of vitamin C. The reduction was stronger for the men than women. However, the women still showed a weakly inverse relationship between vitamin C intake and deaths from all causes as well as all cancers and all cardiovascular diseases.[65]

Other researchers have found that vitamin and mineral supplementation does not increase longevity in the adult population. Kim et al.[62] analyzed data from 10,758 people participating in the NHEFS and found no evidence that supplement use was associated with decreased mortality. This study examined the relationship between mortality and the use of supplements of all types and did not relate mortality to specific vitamins or minerals as did the aforementioned studies.

Based on this information, what kind of recommendations should nutritionists make to women regarding antioxidant supplement use? The fundamental issue is whether existing data are thorough enough to support the routine use of antioxidant supplements to lower the risk of chronic diseases that have been associated with oxidative cell damage. There are some strong animal and epidemiologic data that support the use of antioxidant supplements for chronic disease prevention. However, epidemiologic correlations alone do not establish causal relationships.[66] The known side effects from antioxidant supplement use are limited. However, there are no data on the long-term side effects of antioxidant therapy in humans, and it is not known if chronic usage of large doses is toxic.[66] Some groups have advised healthy women to increase their intake of selected antioxidant nutrients at levels 4 to 16 times higher than the RDA.[67] Federal agencies including the Food and Drug Administration (FDA) and the National Academy of Sciences (NAS) think these recommendations are premature.[67] They argue that if widespread use of a still largely unproven treatment is promoted, we must consider how many women will become careless in their adherence to better-established preventive measures for chronic disease, such as cholesterol-lowering diets, regular exercise, and smoking cessation. Several large, double-blind, clinical trials are currently in progress that should give nutritionists some badly needed answers regarding antioxidant supplementation. In the meantime, we can educate high-risk women about the *possible* benefits of antioxidant supplementation while at the same time continuing to emphasize the old adage of eating a wide variety of foods to ensure a nutritious diet.

FEDERALLY FUNDED FOOD AND NUTRITION PROGRAMS FOR WOMEN

Poverty in the United States is a persistent problem, and being a woman increases the chances of being poor by 60%.[68] If a woman is also black or Hispanic and has a work history of being poorly paid, her chances of falling below the government's poverty threshold are even higher.

The *feminization of poverty* refers to the growth in the proportion of the poverty population living in families headed by women. The United States has one of the highest proportions of single-parent families; nearly one child in four lives in a female-headed household.[69] In 1991, the poverty rate among children in female-headed families was 55%, more than five times the rate among married-couple families.[70]

Poverty is a vulnerability factor that contributes to health and nutritional risk. For example, the infant mortality rate is three times higher among poor families than it is among nonpoor families.[71] Poor families are more likely to have nutritionally inadequate diets than nonpoor families.[72] Housing and utility costs may use up the major portion of a poor family's resources, leaving them little income for food. Nutritionists can work to help women and their families achieve food security by ensuring that all eligible families are familiar with the federally funded programs such as food stamps, WIC, and the Cooperative Extension Expanded Food and Nutrition Education Program (EFNEP) (Table 6-12).

Food Stamp Program

The Food Stamp Program is the cornerstone of the nation's food assistance programs. The mission of the program is to help low-income people buy food to improve their diets. Initiated as a pilot program in 1961 and made permanent in 1964, the program operates in every county of the United States. The program issues monthly allotments of coupons that are redeemable at retail food stores. Eligibility and allotments are based on household size and income, assets, housing costs, work requirements, and other factors. The amount of benefits is based on the Thrifty Food Plan, a low-cost model diet plan based on the RDAs and food choices of low-income households.

The Food Stamp Program served an average of 25.4 million people per month in fiscal year 1992. Half of all food stamp participants are children and 87% are children, the elderly, or women. Average monthly benefits were $68.57 per person. The President's 1994 budget requested a total of $30.1 billion for the Food Stamp Program; the 1993 appropriation was $27 billion.[73]

Participants in the Food Stamp Program have dietary intakes that meet a significantly larger proportion of the RDAs than do eligible nonparticipants.[74] However, obstacles still remain. Four of five recipients fail to reach the RDAs on the average allotment of 70 cents per person per meal.[75] Government studies have found that bureaucratic obstacles prevent up to one-fourth of eligible households from receiving the coverage to which they are entitled.[76]

Table 6-12 Federally Funded Food and Nutrition Programs for Women

Program	Who Qualifies	Services/Benefits	Funding
Food Stamp Program	U.S. citizen, recognized refugee with visa status, or legal alien; households with low income and with resources (aside from income) of $2,000 or less with at least one elderly person (aged 60 or older); eligibility determined after formal application to local public assistance or social services	Coupons to purchase food at participating food markets	USDA
Special Supplemental Food Program for Women, Infants, and Children (WIC)	Pregnant women, postpartum women (6 months), breastfeeding women (up to 1 year), infants and children (up to 5 years); must be certified to be at nutritional risk; household income determined to be at or below 185% of poverty level	Monthly foods or coupons for milk, cheese, eggs, peanut butter or legumes, infant formula, and infant cereal; nutrition education	USDA
WIC Farmers Market	WIC participants	Coupons that can be used to purchase fruits and vegetables at authorized farmers' markets	USDA
Temporary Emergency Food Assistance Program (TEFAP)	Household with income at or below 150% of poverty level	Quarterly distribution: cheese, butter, rice, occasionally flour, cornmeal, and dry milk; emergency food available once per month: dairy products, rice, flour, cornmeal	USDA
Cooperative Extension Expanded Food and Nutrition Program (EFNEP)	Families with children younger than 19 years; income at or below 125% of federal poverty level; at nutritional risk	Education and training on food and nutrition for homemakers and youth	USDA

Source: Adapted from *Nutrition in Public Health: A Handbook for Developing Programs and Services* (pp 72–76) by M Kaufman, Aspen Publishers Inc, © 1990.

Special Supplemental Food Program for Women, Infants, and Children

WIC's goal is to improve the health of pregnant, breastfeeding, and non-breast-feeding postpartum women, infants, and children up to 5 years old by providing supplemental foods, nutrition education, and access to health services. Eligibility is determined by income (185% of poverty or below), and participants must be at nutritional risk, based on abnormal weight gain during pregnancy, iron-deficiency anemia, or related health risks. Participants receive nutrition education and vouchers that can be redeemed at retail food stores for specific foods that are rich sources of the nutrients frequently lacking in the diets of low-income mothers and children.

The WIC program has been shown to be highly cost-effective. A USDA report demonstrated that for every dollar spent on the prenatal component of the WIC program, the associated savings in Medicaid costs for illnesses beginning in the first 60 days after birth ranged from $1.92 to $4.21 for newborns and mothers and from $2.98 to $4.75 for newborns only.[77] Thus, on average every $1 spent on the prenatal component of WIC yields an average savings of about $3 in Medicaid. The greatest cost savings associated with WIC are recognized during the first year of life in the form of reduced medical costs.

WIC is not an entitlement program. Instead, there is a "cap" on the amount of federal money allocated, which limits the numbers of participants who can be served. A 1991 Government Accounting Office (GAO) report concluded that only 35% of pregnant women eligible for WIC participate.[77] The Better Nutrition and Health for Children Act of 1993 proposed full funding of the WIC program by the end of fiscal year 1996 and then remains at full funding levels.[77]

WIC Farmer's Market Nutrition Program

The WIC Farmer's Market Nutrition Program (FMNP) was established by Congress in 1992. The program provides WIC participants, or women and children on a waiting list for WIC services, with coupons that can be used to purchase fresh fruits and vegetables at authorized farmers' markets. The coupons are in addition to the recipient's regular WIC benefits. Congress appropriated $3 million for the program in 1994, the same amount that was available in 1993 and 1992.[73] States that choose to operate the FMNP must match federal funds by contributing at least 30% of the cost of the program. The Better Nutrition and Health for Children Act of 1993 proposes an increase of federal funding for the FMNP to $18 million by 1998 in an effort to more than double the number of participating states. In addition, it reduces the state match required for participation in the program from 30 to 25%.

Emergency Food Assistance Program

Responding to the paradox of reports of increased hunger at the time that agricultural surpluses were mounting in warehouses, Congress enacted the Temporary Emergency Food Assistance Program (TEFAP) of 1984. TEFAP distributes surplus commodities to needy households. TEFAP thus supplies a limited amount and variety of commodities to low-income households to act as a supplement to their purchased food. Although many low-income families rely on this program, it is not designed to provide well-balanced diets. Billions of pounds of food have been distributed since the program began, and surplus commodity supplies held in storage have been greatly reduced. Although some surplus is still distributed through TEFAP, since 1989 Congress has appropriated $120 million per year to purchase additional commodities for households. The program distributed more than $189 million worth of purchased and surplus food in fiscal year 1992.[73] The President's 1994 budget requests $209.5 million for TEFAP.

Expanded Food and Nutrition Education Program (EFNEP)

The Expanded Food and Nutrition Education Program (EFNEP) was authorized by the Smith-Lever Act of 1970 and is designed to teach low-income families, especially those with small children, the skills needed to choose and prepare an adequate, varied, and balanced diet. Women and children receiving food stamps and WIC have been targeted for special attention by EFNEP. In this program, nutrition education programs are conducted by trained paraprofessional nutrition aides, who are often members of the local community and are able to work well with women in their own homes. Evaluations of the program, including a Senate-mandated study completed in 1981, have shown that EFNEP improves the nutrition knowledge and food practices of the low-income women who participate.

NUTRITION EDUCATION

The primary goal of nutrition education for premenopausal women is to promote healthy eating behaviors. For nutrition education to be successful, educators need guides for teaching women how to choose a nutritionally adequate diet.

A self-test for women has been devised that can be used as a screening tool to assess overall nutritional risk (Exhibit 6-6). This tool can be used as a starting point to get women to think about some of their habits and feelings about nutrition.

Exhibit 6-6 Risk Profile Self-Test

	Yes	No
1. I am often too tired to eat	☐	☐
2. I often skip meals	☐	☐
3. I eat out frequently	☐	☐
4. I am combining two or more of the following:		
• job	☐	☐
• school	☐	☐
• child-raising	☐	☐
• working more than 40 hours per week	☐	☐
• competitive or recreational fitness activities	☐	☐
• active membership in charitable, professional, or social organizations	☐	☐
5. I do not like to cook	☐	☐
6. I have no time to eat	☐	☐
7. I am chronically dieting	☐	☐
8. I feel I have bad eating habits	☐	☐
9. I eat fewer than two servings from the milk group a day	☐	☐
10. I eat fewer than two servings from the meat group a day	☐	☐
11. I eat fewer than five servings from the fruit and vegetable group a day	☐	☐
12. I eat fewer than six servings from the grain group a day	☐	☐
13. I often eat fried food	☐	☐
14. I eat a lot of sweets	☐	☐
15. I drink four or more cups of coffee per day	☐	☐

*If you have two or more checks in the yes column, you may not be getting optimal nutrition for your health and well-being.

Source: From *Eating on the Run,* ed 1 (p 2) by E Tribole, Champaign Ill: Life Enhancement Publications. Copyright © 1987 by Evelyn Tribole. Reprinted by permission of Human Kinetics Publishers.

Food Guides for Women

The California Department of Health Services developed the Daily Food Guide for Women (Table 6-13) for use by nutrition educators to (1) assess the nutritional adequacy of women's diets in either a clinical or educational setting and (2) to teach women how to choose a nutritionally adequate diet.[78] Unlike other food guides, this guide was developed specifically to meet the nutritional needs of women during their reproductive years. The goal of the Daily Food Guide for Women is to ensure an average intake of protein, vitamins, and minerals that meets at least 90% of the 1989 RDA for nonpregnant, pregnant, and lactating women.

Table 6-13 Daily Food Guide for Women

Food Group	One Serving Equals		Recommended Minimum Servings		
			Nonpregnant		Pregnant/ Lactating
			11–24 yr	25+ yr	
Protein Foods Provide protein, iron, zinc, and B vitamins for growth of muscles, bone, blood, and nerves. Vegetable protein provides fiber to prevent constipation	**Animal Protein:** 1 oz. cooked chicken or turkey 1 oz cooked lean beef, lamb, or pork 1 oz. or 1/4 cup fish or other seafood 1 egg 2 fish sticks or hot dogs 2 slices luncheon meat	**Vegetable Protein:** 1/2 cup dry beans, lentils, or split peas 3 oz. tofu 1 oz. or 1/4 cup peanuts, pumpkin, or sunflower seeds 1¹/2 oz. or 1/3 cup other nuts 2 tbsp. peanut butter	5 A half serving of vegetable protein daily	5	7 One serving of vegetable protein daily
Milk Products Provide protein and calcium to build strong bones, teeth, healthy nerves and muscles, and to promote normal blood clotting	8 oz. milk 8 oz. yogurt 1 cup milk shake 1¹/2 cups cream soup (made with milk) 1¹/2 oz or 1/3 cup grated cheese (like cheddar, monterey, mozzarella, or swiss)	1 ¹/2–2 slices presliced American cheese 4 tbsp. parmesan cheese 2 cups cottage cheese 1 cup pudding 1 cup custard or flan 1¹/2 cups ice milk, ice cream, or frozen yogurt	3	2	3
Breads, Cereals, Grains Provide carbohydrates and B vitamins for energy and healthy nerves. Also provide iron for healthy blood. Whole grains provide fiber to prevent constipation	1 slice bread 1 dinner roll 1/2 bun or bagel 1/2 English muffin or pita 1 small tortilla 3/4 cup dry cereal 1/2 cup granola 1/2 cup cooked cereal	1/2 cup rice 1/2 cup noodles or spaghetti 1/4 cup wheat germ 14-inch pancake or waffle 1 small muffin 8 medium crackers 4 graham cracker squares 3 cups popcorn	7 Four servings of whole-grain products daily	6	7
Vitamin C-Rich Fruits and Vegetables Provide vitamin C to prevent infection and to promote healing and iron absorption. Also provide fiber to prevent constipation	6 oz. orange, grapefruit, or fruit juice enriched with vitamin C 6 oz. tomato juice or vegetable juice cocktail 1 orange, kiwi, mango 1/2 grapefruit, cantaloupe 1/2 cup papaya 2 tangerines	1/2 cup strawberries 1/2 cup cooked or 1 cup raw cabbage 1/2 cup broccoli, Brussels sprouts, or cauliflower 1/2 cup snow peas, sweet peppers, or tomato puree 2 tomatoes	1	1	1
Vitamin A-Rich Fruits and Vegetables Provide β-carotene and vitamin A to prevent infection and to promote wound healing and night vision. Also provide fiber to prevent constipation	6 oz. apricot nectar or vegetable juice cocktail 3 raw or 1/4 cup dried apricots 1/4 cantaloupe or mango 1 small or 1/2 cup sliced carrots 2 tomatoes	1/2 cup cooked or 1 cup raw spinach 1/2 cup cooked greens (beet, chard, collards, dandelion, kale, mustard) 1/2 cup pumpkin, sweet potato, winter squash, or yams	1	1	1
Other Fruits and Vegetables Provide carbohydrates for energy and fiber to prevent constipation	6 oz. fruit juice (if not listed above) 1 medium or 1/2 cup sliced fruit (apple, banana, peach, pear) 1/2 cup berries (other than strawberries) 1/2 cup cherries or grapes 1/2 cup pineapple 1/2 cup watermelon	1/4 cup dried fruit 1/2 cup sliced vegetable (asparagus, beets, green beans, celery, corn, eggplant, mushrooms, onion, peas, potato, summer squash, zucchini) 1/2 artichoke 1 cup lettuce	3	3	3

continues

Table 6-13 Daily Food Guide for Women (continued)

Food Group	One Serving Equals		Recommended Minimum Servings		
			Nonpregnant		Pregnant/ Lactating
			11–24 yr	25+ yr	
Unsaturated Fats Provide vitamin E to protect tissue	1/8 med. avocado 1 tsp. margarine 1 tsp. mayonnaise 1 tsp. vegetable oil	2 tsp. salad dressing (mayonnaise-based) 1 tsp. salad dressing (oil-based)	3	3	3

Note: The Daily Food Guide for Women may not provide all the calories you require. The best way to increase your intake is to include more than the minimum servings recommended.

Source: Reprinted with permission from Newman V and Lee D, Developing a Daily Food Guide for Women, *Journal of Nutrition Education* (1991;23:76–82), Copyright © 1991, Society for Nutrition Education.

USDA Food Guide Pyramid

The Food Guide Pyramid represents the first official attempt by the USDA to illustrate the dietary guidelines. Considerable research led the USDA to the conclusion that the pyramid graphic with fat and added sugars symbols and a black background was the most effective tool to communicate the key food guide concepts of (1) dietary variety, (2) moderation of fats, oils, and sugars, and (3) proportionality (the relative amount of food from each major food group as determined by the number of daily servings recommended for each specific food group).[79]

Women will need additional information about serving recommendations to make the pyramid work for them. Some women may think that all women should eat the smaller amounts of recommended servings. This is a misconception, especially for pregnant and lactating women. Others may conclude that dieters should eat the lowest numbers of servings in all food groups and women who wish to gain weight should eat the higher numbers. This may be an error as well, especially for the fruit and vegetable groups, which are low in calories yet nutrient-dense. Nutritionists can estimate a woman's total energy needs (See Exhibit 6-1, Table 6-2, and Exhibit 6-2) and then use Table 6-14 as an educational tool to accompany the Food Guide Pyramid.

SUMMARY

The RDAs and the dietary patterns advocated in the Food and Nutrition Board's *Diet and Health* can be used as standards to measure how well premenopausal women meet their nutritional needs. On average, with the possible exception of folate, U.S. women are meeting their nutrient requirements for vitamins. Average intakes of several minerals, including calcium, iron, and zinc, are low,

Table 6-14 Sample Diets for a Day at 3 Calorie Levels

	Lower (about 1,600)	Moderate (about 2,200)	Higher (about 2,800)
Bread group servings	6	9	11
Vegetable group servings	3	4	5
Fruit group servings	2	3	4
Milk group servings	2–3	2–3	2–3
Meat group (ounces)	5	6	7
Total fat (grams)	53	73	93
Total added sugars (teaspoons)	6	12	18

thus increasing U.S. women's risk of poor bone health, osteoporosis, and iron-deficiency anemia. Also, most U.S. women have intakes of fat, saturated fat, and sodium that exceed recommendations, thus increasing their risk for several chronic diseases.

The eating patterns of premenopausal women are shaped by many sociodemo-graphic factors including the increased employment of women, increase in single female-headed households, increased eating away from home, use of convenience foods, and tobacco use. Nutritionists need to be cognizant of how these factors affect food intake when designing contemporary nutrition education programs. Also, an increasing number of women and their children live in poverty. Poor families are more likely to have nutritionally inadequate diets than nonpoor families. Several federal food assistance and nutrition education programs exist to help low-income women and their families achieve food security.

Simple screening tools are available to assess women's fat intake and fiber, fruit, and vegetable intake. These tools can assist nutritionists in identifying women in need of nutrition intervention. The California Department of Health Services Daily Food Guide for Women and the USDA Food Guide Pyramid are other educational tools appropriate for healthy women. These food guides can be used to help women ensure an adequate intake of most essential nutrients while at the same time ensuring moderation in intakes of fat, sugars, and sodium. There are direct links between diet and the major chronic diseases such as heart disease, breast cancer, and osteoporosis that affect U.S. women. Nutritionists have the knowledge and the tools to educate premenopausal women about dietary changes they can make early in life to reduce their long-term risk of developing these diseases.

References

1. Food and Nutrition Board. *Recommended Dietary Allowances.* 10th ed. Washington, DC: National Academy Press; 1989.

2. Committee of Diet and Health, Food and Nutrition Board, Commission of Life Sciences, National Research Council. *Diet and Health, Implications for Reducing Chronic Disease Risk.* Washington, DC: National Academy Press; 1989.

3. Poehlman ET, Horton ES. The impact of food intake and exercise on energy expenditure. *Nutr Rev.* 1989;47(5):129–137.

4. *Energy and Protein Requirements.* Geneva: World Health Organization; 1985.

5. Harris JA, Benedict FG. *A Biometric Study of Basal Metabolism in Man.* Washington, DC: Carnegie Institution of Washington Publication; 1919.

6. Mifflin MD, St. Jeor ST, Hill LA, Scott BJ, Daugherty SA, Koh YO. A new predictive equation for resting energy expenditure in healthy individuals. *Am J Clin Nutr.* 1990;51:241–247.

7. Prentice AM, Davies HL, Black AE, et al. Unexpectedly low levels of energy expenditure in healthy women. *Lancet.* 1985;1:1419–1422.

8. Casper RC, Schoeller DA, Kushner R, Knilicka J, Gold ST. Total daily energy expenditure and activity level in anorexia nervosa. *Am J Clin Nutr.* 1991;53:1143–1150.

9. Huss-Ashmanre R, Goodman JL, Sibiya TE, Stein TP. Energy expenditure of young Swazi women as measured by the doubly-labelled water method. *Eur J Clin Nutr.* 1989;43:737–748.

10. Mertz W. Food intake measurements. "Is there a gold standard"? *J Am Diet Assoc.* 1992;92: 1463–1465.

11. Goran M, Poehlman E. Total energy expenditure and energy requirements in healthy elderly persons. *Metabolism.* 1992;41:744–753.

12. Livingstone MBE, Prentice AM, Strain JJ, et al. Accuracy of weighed dietary records in studies of diet and health. *Br Med J.* 1990;300:708–712.

13. Lichtman SW, Pisarska K, Berman ER, et al. Discrepancy between self-reported and actual caloric intake and exercise in obese subjects. *N Engl J Med.* 1992;327:1893–1998.

14. Goldberg GR, Black AE, Jebb SA, et al. Critical evaluation of energy intake data using fundamental principles of energy physiology: 1. Derivation of cut-off limits to identify under-recording. *Eur J Clin Nutr.* 1991;45:569–581.

15. Black AE, Goldberg GR, Jebb SA, Livingstone MBE, Cole TJ, Prentice AM. Critical evaluation of energy intake data using fundamental principles of energy physiology: 2. Evaluating the results of published surveys. *Eur J Clin Nutr.* 1991;45:583–599.

16. Porter D. Washington update: NIH Consensus Development Conference statement. Optimal calcium intake. *Nutr Today.* 1994;29(5):37–40.

17. *Nationwide Food Consumption Survey: Continuing Survey of Food Intakes by Individuals, Women 19–50 Years and Their Children 1–5 Years, 4 Days, 1985.* Hyattsville, Md: USDA, Human Nutrition Information Service; 1987. Report No. 85-4.

18. *Nationwide Food Consumption Survey: Continuing Survey of Food Intakes by Individuals, Women 19–50 Years and Their Children 1–5 Years, 4 Days, 1986.* Hyattsville, Md: USDA, Human Nutrition Information Service; 1988. Report No. 86-3.

19. Wright HS, Guthrie HA, Wang MQ, Bernardo V. The 1987–88 Nationwide Food Consumption Survey: An update on the nutrient intake of respondents. *Nutr Today.* 1991;26:21–27.

20. McDowell MA, Briefel RR, Alaimo K, et al. *Energy and Macronutrient Intakes of Persons Ages 2 Months and Over in the United States: Third National Health and Nutrition Examination Survey, Phase I, 1988–91.* Hyattsville, Md: National Center for Health Statistics; 1994. Advance data from Vital and Health Statistics no. 255.

21. Alaimo K, McDowell MA, Briefel RR, et al. *Dietary Intakes of Vitamins, Minerals and Fiber of Persons Ages 2 Months and Over in the United States: Third National Health and Nutrition*

Examination Survey, Phase I, 1988–91. Hyattsville, Md: National Center for Health Statistics; 1994. Advance data from Vital and Health Statistics no. 258.

22. Stampfer MJ, Hennekens CH, Manson JE, Colditz GA, Rosner B, Willett WC. Vitamin E consumption and the risk of coronary disease in women. *N Engl J Med.* 1993;328:1444–1456.

23. Smigel K. Vitamin E moves on stage in cancer prevention studies. *J Natl Cancer Inst.* 1992;84:996–997.

24. Czeizel AE, Dudas I. Prevention of the first occurrence of neural-tube defects by periconceptual vitamin supplementation. *N Engl J Med.* 1992;327:1832–1835.

25. Werler M, Shapiro S, Mitchell A. Periconceptual folic acid exposure and risk of occurrent neural tube defects. *JAMA.* 1993;269:1257–1261.

26. MRC Vitamin Study Research Group. Prevention of neural tube defects: results of the Medical Research Council Vitamin Study. *Lancet.* 1991;338:131–136.

27. Center for Disease Control. Recommendations for the use of folic acid to reduce the number of cases of spina bifida and other neural tube defects. *MMWR.* 1992;41:1–7.

28. McCarthy PE. Osteoporosis and its treatment. *N Engl J Med.* 1992;326:406–407.

29. Johnston CC, Miller JZ, Slemenda C, et al. Calcium supplementation and increases in bone mineral density in children. *N Engl J Med.* 1992;327:82–87.

30. Wardlaw GM. Putting osteoporosis in perspective. *J Am Diet Assoc.* 1993; 93:1000–1006.

31. Herbert V. Everyone should be tested for iron disorders. *J Am Diet Assoc.* 1992;92:1502–1507.

32. Clement DB, Sawchuk LL. Iron status and sports performance. *Sports Med.* 1984;1:65–74.

33. Kris-Etherton PM, Krummel DA. Role of nutrition in the prevention and treatment of coronary heard disease in women. *J Am Diet Assoc.* 1993;93:987–993.

34. Johnston WP, Packer AH. *Workforce 2000.* Washington, DC: Hudson Institute; 1987.

35. U.S. Bureau of the Census. *Statistical Abstract of the United States: 1990.* 110th ed. Washington, DC; 1990.

36. Ferree MM. Beyond separate spheres: feminism and family research. *J Marriage Fam.* 1990;52:866–884.

37. Goebel KP, Hennon CB. An empirical investigation of the relationship among wife's employment status, stage in the family life cycle, meal preparation time, and expenditures for meals away from home. *J Cons Studies Home Econ.* 1982;6:63–78.

38. Johnson R, Smiciklas-Wright H, Crouter A. The effect of maternal employment on the quality of young children's diets—the CSFII experience. *J Am Diet Assoc.* 1992;92:213–214.

39. Johnson R, Smiciklas-Wright H, Crouter A, Willitts F. Maternal employment and the quality of young children's diets—empirical evidence from the 1987–88 Nationwide Food Consumption Survey. *Pediatrics.* 1991;90:245–249.

40. Ortiz B, MacDonald M, Ackerman N, Goebel K. The effect of homemakers' employment on meal preparation time, meals at home, and meals away from home. *Home Econ Res J.* 1981;9(3):200–206.

41. Axelson ML. The impact of culture on food-related behavior. *Annu Rev Nutr.* 1986;6:345–363.

42. Redman BJ. The impact of women's time allocation on expenditure for meals away from home and prepared foods. *Am Agric Econ Assoc.* 1980;62:234–237.

43. Rawlings SW. *Household and Family Characteristics: March 1992. Current Population Reports, Population Characteristics.* Washington, DC: US Department of Commerce, Bureau of the Census. 1993.

44. *Poverty in the United States: 1991. Current Population Reports, Consumer Incomes.* Washington, DC: US Department of Commerce, Bureau of the Census 1992. Report no. 181:series P-60.

45. Lino M, Guthrie J. The food situation of families maintained by single mothers: expenditures, shopping behavior, and diet quality. *Fam Econ Rev.* 1994;7:9–21.

46. Putman JJ, Vandress MG. Changes ahead for eating out. *Natl Food Rev.* 1984;26:15–17.

47. Morgan KJ, Goungetas B. Snacking and eating away from home. In: *What is America Eating?* Proceedings of a symposium. Washington, DC: National Academy Press; 1986.

48. Haines PS, Hungerford DW, Popkin BM, Guilkey DK. Eating patterns and energy and nutrient intakes of US women. *J Am Diet Assoc.* 1992;92:698–707.

49. Guenther PM, Ricard G. Effects of eating at food service establishments on the nutritional quality of women's diets. *Top Clin Nutr.* 1989;4(2):41–45.

50. *Healthy People 2000. National Health Promotion and Disease Prevention Objectives.* Washington, DC: U.S. Department of Health and Human Services Public Health Services; 1991. DHHS Publication no. 91-50213.

51. Novotny TE, Fiore MC, Hatziandreu EJ, Giovino GA, Mills SL, Pierce JP. Trends in smoking by age and sex, United States, 1974–1987: the implications for disease impact. *Prev Med.* 1990;19: 552–561.

52. Davis RM. Current trends in cigarette advertising and marketing. *N Engl J Med.* 1987;316:725–732.

53. Larkin FA, Basiotis PP, Riddick HA, Sykes KE, Pao EM. Dietary patterns of women smokers and non-smokers. *J Am Diet Assoc.* 1990;90:230–237.

54. Subar AF, Harlan LC. Nutrient and food group intake by tobacco use status: the 1987 National Health Interview Survey. In: *Tobacco Smoking and Nutrition Influence of Nutrition and Tobacco-Associated Health Risks.* New York, NY: The New York Academy of Sciences; 1993:310–321.

55. Somer E. 3 Hot nutrition topics for women. *Idea Today.* 1993;6:55–62.

56. Abraham GE, Hargrove JT. Effect of vitamin B_6 on premenstrual symptomatology in women with premenstrual syndromes: a double blind crossover study. *Infertility.* 1980;3:155–165.

57. Williams MJ, Harris RI. Controlled trial of pyridoxine in the premenstrual syndrome. *J Int Med Res.* 1985;13:174–179.

58. Schaumburg H. Sensory neuropathy from pyridoxine abuse. *N Engl J Med.* 1983;309:445–448.

59. Mira M, Stewart PM, Abraham SF. Vitamin and trace element status in premenstrual syndrome. *Am J Clin Nutr.* 1988;47:636–641.

60. *1990 Overview of the Nutritional Supplement Market.* Washington, DC: Council for Responsible Nutrition; 1991.

61. Subar AF, Block G. Use of vitamin and mineral supplements: demographics and amounts of nutrients consumed. *Am J Epidemiol.* 1990;132(6):1091–1101.

62. Kim I, Williamson DF, Byers T, Koplan J. Vitamin and mineral supplement use and mortality in a US cohort. *Am J Public Health.* 1993;83:546–550.

63. Kohls KJ, Kies C. Calcium bioavailability: a comparison of several different commercially available calcium supplements. *J Appl Nutr.* 1992;44:50–61.

64. Schnepf M, Madrick T. The solubility of calcium from antacid tablets, calcium supplements and fortified food products. *Nutr Res.* 1991;11:961–970.

65. Enstrom JE, Kanim LE, Klein MA. Vitamin C intake and mortality among a sample of the United States population. *Epidemiology.* 1992;3:194–202.

66. Steinberg D. Antioxidant vitamins and coronary heart disease. *N Engl J Med.* 1993;328:1487–1489.

67. Voelker R. Recommendations for antioxidants: how much evidence is enough? *JAMA.* 1994;271:1148–1149.

68. Older women's league. The road to poverty: A report on the economic status of older women in America. Washington, DC: Older Women's League, 1988.

69. Hobbs F, Lippman L. Children's well-being: An international comparison. Washington, DC: U.S. Bureau of the Census; 1990.

70. U.S. Department of Commerce, Bureau of the Census. Poverty in the United States: 1991. Washington, DC: Government Printing Office; 1992.

71. Nersesian WS. Infant mortality in socially vulnerable populations. *Ann Rev Public Health.* 1988;9:361–377.

72. Kotch J, Shackelfor J. The nutritional status of low-income preschool children in the United States: A review of the literature. Washington, DC: Food Research and Action Center; 1989.

73. Food Program Facts, Food and Nutrition Service. U.S. Department of Agriculture; 1993.

74. Devaney B, Fraker T. The effect of food stamps on food expenditures: An assessment of findings from the Nationwide Food Consumption Survey. *Am J Agr Econ.* 1989;Feb:99–104.

75. Statement on the link between nutrition and cognitive development in children. Tufts University School of Nutrition, Center on Hunger, Poverty and Nutrition Policy; 1993.

76. United States Government. Food Stamp Program: Administrative Hindrances to Participation. General Accounting Office; 1988.

77. The Better Nutrition and Health for Children Act of 1993. *The Federal Register.* 1993: S14841–S14855.

78. Newman V, Lee D. Developing a daily food guide for women. *J Nutr Ed.* 1991;23:76–82.

79. Welsh S, Davis C, Shaw A. Development of the food guide pyramid. *Nutrition Today.* 1992;Nov/Dec:12–23.

7

ào

Nutritional Concerns during Pregnancy and Lactation

Cheryl A. Lovelady

The reproductive period of a woman's life is the most nutritionally demanding. Adequate nutrition is critical to support both fetal growth and maternal health. At this time, women are more likely to make dietary and behavioral changes to improve overall health. Dietitians and nutritionists must give pregnant and lactating women the proper guidance regarding nutrient intake during this period. This chapter focuses on healthy pregnant women by identifying the current issues in nutrition that affect maternal health.

Because many women are concerned about weight control, weight gain during pregnancy and weight loss in the postpartum period are reviewed. Recently, exercise programs for pregnant and postpartum women have increased; therefore, the nutritional needs of the exercising, pregnant, and lactating woman are discussed. Because many women are interested in preventing osteoporosis and have questions about the impact of pregnancy and lactation on the health of their bone mass, a section on calcium requirements is included. Common problems of nausea and anemia during pregnancy are reviewed, as well as a section on the controversial topic of nutrient supplementation. Research is continuing on many of these topics, and in some cases, specific recommendations may be made, whereas in other instances, there is still insufficient data for making recommendations for the professional to use in clinical practice.

DIETARY INTAKE

Over the past decade, few studies have measured the nutrient intakes of pregnant women.[1] In the Institute of Medicine's (IOM) report, "Nutrition during Pregnancy," daily energy intakes varied from 1500 to 2800 kcal/day. Protein, thiamin, riboflavin, niacin, and vitamins A, B_{12}, and C intakes were adequate in most of the studies. Intakes of vitamins B_6, D, E, and folate and iron, calcium, zinc, and magnesium were below the recommended dietary allowances (RDA).[2] However, these data should be interpreted cautiously because the RDAs have a safety net and are intended to meet the needs of most healthy, pregnant women.

Several factors affect dietary intakes of pregnant women. Calcium consumption varied by race; pregnant black, Hispanic, and Native-American women consumed low levels of calcium. Participation in the Special Supplemental Food Program for Women, Infants and Children (WIC) was associated with higher intakes of energy, protein, iron, calcium, magnesium, and vitamins C, B_6, B_{12}, thiamin, riboflavin, and niacin. There was a large variation in reported intakes of pregnant adolescents. Younger WIC participants consumed less energy, protein, and calcium. Adolescents receiving more nutrition education consumed an average of 400 kcal/day more than did those with little nutrition education.

Studies of dietary intake of lactating women published since 1976 were summarized in another IOM report, "Nutrition during Lactation."[3] Compared with pregnancy, there were even fewer studies of nutrient intake during lactation. Only 361 women were studied, and most of these were well-educated whites. Because of the small samples, there was large variation in reported intakes. However, the nutrients of most concern in these lactating women were vitamin B_6, folate, and zinc. One study of lactating adolescents reported mean dietary intakes that met or exceeded the RDAs.

It is important to determine the usual dietary intake of pregnant and lactating women as it is a major determinant of nutritional status. Intake should also be evaluated with respect to the time of gestation and the extent of lactation (whether the infant is partially or exclusively breastfed). The studies reviewed suggest that nutrition education and the WIC program enhance the quality and quantity of the dietary intake of low-income and adolescent pregnant women. Other groups of women who may also need special attention are vegans, women who diet to lose weight, and those who avoid dairy products.

Data from the few studies of dietary intake during pregnancy and lactation show that vitamin B_6, folate, and zinc are consumed in lower than recommended amounts during both pregnancy and lactation. Also, magnesium, calcium, iron, and vitamins E and D may be low in the pregnant woman's diet. The practitioner should assess intakes and then recommend food sources of these nutrients when counseling pregnant and lactating women.

ENERGY BALANCE

Energy Requirements during Pregnancy

The National Research Council (NRC) recommends an additional 300 kcal/day during the second and third trimesters for all pregnant women.[2] This recommendation is based on a total weight gain of 12.5 kg and does not take into account a woman's prepregnancy body mass index (BMI). However, there is a wide range of weight gain among women with healthy pregnancy outcomes. Data from the 1980 National Natality Survey showed that the 15th and 85th percentiles of weight gain were 16 and 40 lb for normal-weight women who delivered 3- to 4-kg babies at 39 to 41 weeks' gestation.[1] Considering the variability in weight gain, one would predict a wide variation in the energy requirement during the prenatal period.

When recommending energy requirements for individuals, it is important to consider the woman's prepregnancy BMI (as an indicator of energy stores) and current physical activity level. Normal weight and overweight women may need very little additional calories during pregnancy, especially if they reduce their physical activity. Studies measuring energy expenditure have reported a decrease in physical activity in some pregnant women in developed countries.[4,5] Under-weight women with limited food intake have been found to adapt to the energetic demands of pregnancy by reducing their basal metabolic rate/kg fat-free mass,[6] whereas normal-weight women with unlimited access to food increase their metabolic rate by approximately 8 to 9% over the entire pregnancy.[7]

The metabolic adaptations occurring in thin women with low energy intake may spare energy for fetal growth, but does it have functional consequences for the mother? When recommending energy intake levels during pregnancy, fetal birth weight should not be the sole criteria. It may be prudent to recommend a higher energy intake (e.g., greater than 300 kcal) for an active, leaner woman compared with a sedentary, fatter woman than to allow the reduction in metabolic rate to occur to support fetal growth. The practitioner should monitor the pregnant woman's food intake and weight gain, and recommend adjustments in energy intake when weight gain is not within the IOM's guidelines.

Weight Gain

The IOM's recommendations for weight gain during pregnancy are shown in Table 7-1.[1] These differ from past recommendations as they are based on prepregnancy weight for height and are divided into three different categories. The upper end of the range is recommended for young adolescents and black women; the lower end is recommended for short women (less than 157 cm or 62 in.). The rationale for black women gaining weight at the upper end of the range is based on reports of black infants who tended to be smaller than white infants for the same weight gain of the mother. The recommended gain for obese women (BMI greater than 29.0) is at least 6.0 kg (15 lb).

A recent retrospective study compared birth outcomes—small for gestational age (SGA), large for gestational age (LGA), and cesarean delivery—with the

Table 7-1 Recommended Weight Gains for Pregnant Women

	Recommended Gain	
Weight-for-Height Category	*kg*	*lb*
Low (BMI < 19.8)	12.5–18	28–40
Normal (BMI 19.8–26.0)	11.5–16	25–35
High (BMI 26.0–29.0)	7–11.5	15–25

Source: Data from *Nutrition During Pregnancy: Weight Gain and Nutrient Supplement, Pts 1 & 2* by the Institute of Medicine, Committee on Nutritional Status During Pregnancy and Lactation, National Academy Press, 1990.

IOM recommended weight gains.[8] Women with weight gains within the IOM guidelines had reduced risks of SGA, LGA, or cesarean delivery. However, low weight gain during pregnancy almost doubled the risk of delivering a SGA infant. Conversely, a high prenatal gain doubled the risk of having a LGA infant as well as increased the risk for a cesarean delivery by 20 to 30%, even after controlling for infant birth weight. Thus, both low weight gain and excessive weight gains are associated with negative infant outcomes.

Interesting results were also reported for obese women. Having a SGA infant was significantly associated with low maternal weight gain (i.e., less than 6 kg) and a LGA infant was marginally associated ($p = .06$) with high maternal gain (i.e., greater than 17 kg) among women with a prepregnant BMI greater than 29. Previous studies have reported no relationship between maternal weight gain and birth weight among obese women.[9] Further research needs to be done on the appropriate weight gain for obese pregnant women. However, in the light of this recent finding, the minimum weight gain of 7 kg for obese women should continue to be recommended.

Excessive weight gain during pregnancy may also result in greater postpartum weight retention. In a survey of 2000 women with a normal prepregnancy BMI,[10] those women gaining more than 35 lb during pregnancy retained significantly more weight (20 lb or more) during 10 to 24 months postpartum than those gaining less. Black women retained more weight than white women. Studies of body composition changes during pregnancy show that the amount of fat gained in normal-weight, healthy women ranged from a loss of 2 kg to a gain of more than 10 kg.[7] Also, there is a strong correlation between gestational weight gain and maternal fat gain ($r = .842$; $p < .001$); thus, large prenatal weight gain may increase the risk for obesity in the postpartum period.

Weight gain during pregnancy varies widely among women. Practitioners should use IOM recommendations (Table 7-1) as targets for identifying individuals with insufficient or excessive rates of gain. Women at risk for low weight gain (less than 6.8 kg or 15 lb) are unmarried women, black and Hispanic women, cigarette smokers, and women with low levels of education. These women need intensive nutritional care to ensure optimal outcomes for mother and infant.

Postpartum Weight Loss

Many women are anxious to lose weight during the postpartum period. The associations between parity and changes in adiposity over a 5-year period were examined in a large sample of women (680 white and 448 black women, 18 to 30 years old).[11] Women who remained nulliparous ($n = 925$) were compared with women who had a single pregnancy of at least 28 weeks' duration and who were at least 12 months postpartum at follow-up (primiparas, $n = 89$; multiparas, $n = 114$). Primiparous black women gained approximately 3 kg more weight during the 5-year period than did nulliparas; however, there were no significant differences in weight gain between black multiparas and nulliparas. Results were similar among the white women, with primiparous subjects gaining approximately 2 kg more than the nulliparas. It appears that women increase their body weight after a first pregnancy (and not later pregnancies) and that these increases persist until at least 12 months postpartum, the time in which most women would be expected to return to their prepregnancy body weight. Even though these weight changes were modest, measures to address postpartum weight retention in primiparas are recommended.

Theoretically, one would predict that lactation would promote weight loss. However, reports have been conflicting when comparing the rate of weight loss in lactating to nonlactating women in the postpartum period.[12–19] Many studies reporting no differences in weight loss have included subjects who only partially breast-fed or breast-fed for less than 6 weeks. None of these studies excluded women who were restricting their energy intake to lose weight. Dewey et al[20] compared weight loss between women who breast-fed for 12 months and those that did not breast-feed beyond the first 3 months postpartum. Subjects who intentionally dieted to lose weight at any time during the year were excluded, so that a normal pattern of weight loss during the postpartum period could be assessed. Weight loss was significantly greater in the lactating women than in nonlactating women in the first year postpartum (4.4 versus 2.4 kg, $p < .05$), with the greatest differences in weight loss from 3 to 6 months. Thus, prolonged lactation (i.e., greater than 3 months) enhanced postpartum weight loss.

Energy Requirements of Lactation

The 1989 RDA for energy intake during lactation is 2700 kcal/day, which represents an additional 500 kcal above the recommendation for nonpregnant women.[2] This is based on estimates that the average energy content of breast milk is 70 kcal/100 mL, and the efficiency of energy conversion into milk is about 80% (Table 7-2). Average milk production is estimated to be 750 mL/day during the first 6 months of lactation and 600 mL/day in the second 6 months. It is assumed that women will subsidize milk synthesis with about 100 to 150 kcal/day obtained from mobilization of fat stores deposited during pregnancy.

When estimating energy requirements during lactation, the NRC assumes that there is no change in resting metabolic rate (RMR) or activity levels from the prepregnancy state to the postpartum state. There have been conflicting reports regarding changes in RMR during lactation (Table 7-3). Two studies[21,22] found about a 5% increase in RMR above prepregnancy rates in lactating women at 2 months postpartum. By contrast, Illingworth et al[23] reported no differences in RMR during lactation in 12 women measured at 6 to 8 weeks postpartum and again 5 to 12 weeks after terminating breastfeeding. Similarly, Goldberg et al[24] found no differences in RMR at 4, 8, or 12 weeks postpartum. Rather, energy balance was achieved in these women by reducing physical activity and increasing caloric intake.[24]

Reported energy intakes of lactating women in the United States are generally below the RDA[25–34] (Table 7-4). This discrepancy may be due to inaccuracies in dietary intake measurements or lower than expected energy expenditure for physical activity. To validate dietary assessment methods, Lovelady et al[34] compared energy intakes (weighed food records) with measurements of energy expenditure using the doubly labeled water method. Energy intakes were in close agreement

---

Table 7-2 Energy Cost of Milk Production during Lactation

Energy content of milk	70 kcal/100 mL
Average milk production	750 mL/day
Efficiency of milk production	80%
Total energy cost	640 kcal/day

Source: Data from *Recommended Dietary Allowances,* ed 10, National Academy Press, 1989.

Table 7-3 Changes in Resting Metabolic Rate in Well-Nourished Women during Lactation

Reference	Weeks Postpartum	% Change in RMR
Sadurskis et al[21]	8	+5.2
	24	+7.5
Spaaij et al[22]	8	+4.5
Illingworth et al[23]	6–8	−1.1
Goldberg et al[24]	4, 8, and 12	+1.2

Table 7-4 Reported Dietary Intakes of Lactating Women in the United States

Reference	Number of Subjects	Energy Intake (kcal/day) mean (SD)
Blackburn and Calloway, 1976[25]	12	1800 (454)
Sims, 1978[26]	61	2124 (578)
Manning-Dalton and Allen, 1983[27]	27	2156 (576)
Moser and Reynolds, 1983[28]	23	1919 (110)
Stuff et al, 1983[29]	40	2028 (357)
Butte et al, 1984[30]	45	2186 (463)
Finley et al, 1985[31]	29	2158 (601)
Song et al, 1985[32]	26	2014 (620)
Strode et al, 1986[33]	14	2215 (256)
Lovelady et al, 1993[34]	9	2438 (225)

with the expenditure and weight loss data, which support the validity of the dietary intake measures. The mean intake of approximately 2400 kcal in these women losing an average of only 1.14 kg/mo was considerably below the RDA of 2700 kcal.

Because dietary intake measures have been validated, discrepancies between intake and weight loss could be due to differences in activity levels. Lactating women have been found to be more sedentary in the early postpartum period, as they were spending most of their time sitting to nurse.[35] As lactation progressed, energy expenditure increased from approximately 1900 kcal/day at 6 weeks postpartum to 2050 kcal/day at 12 weeks and remained there. The energy output in milk was the same at 6, 12, and 20 weeks postpartum (about 525 kcal/day). Thus, by 12 weeks postpartum, women were resuming their normal activity levels. Overall, total energy expenditure (including energy in breast milk) averaged approximately 2600 kcal/day at 12 and 20 weeks postpartum in these sedentary women who lost an average of 1.6 kg from 6 to 20 weeks postpartum. Again, this was below the RDA of 2700 kcal/day.

Table 7-5 summarizes the studies reporting energy expenditure (including the energy in the breast milk produced) during lactation. The average weight loss of women in these studies of approximately 14 weeks in duration was less than 2 kg. When counseling lactating women on energy intake, one should consider the decreased activity level in the early postpartum period. The recommendation of an additional 500 kcal/day may be an overestimate of energy needs and may be why weight loss during lactation is very slow or does not occur at all in many women.

To speed weight loss, some women restrict their caloric intake. The effect of low energy intake on lactation performance has been investigated in two intervention studies. Strode et al[33] compared milk volume production of 14 exclu-

Table 7-5 Total Energy Expenditure[a] during Lactation in Well-Nourished Women

Reference	Weeks Postpartum	Kcal/day	Kcal/kg
Dewey et al[35]	6	2419	36.1
	12	2592	39.3
	20	2593	39.4
Lovelady et al,[34b]	16	2954	45.6
Goldberg et al[24]	4	2647	45.0
	8	2704	45.9
	12	2669	45.5
Forsum et al[4]	8	3035	47.1

[a]Includes energy in breast milk.
[b]Half of these subjects were exercising 45 min/day, 5 days/wk.

sively breastfeeding women who reduced their energy intakes by 19 to 53% (average, 32%) for 1 week with that of a control group of eight women who did not change their intake. Women who consumed more than 1500 kcal/day during the diet week had no reduction in milk volume. However, women who consumed less than 1500 kcal/day had a 15% reduction in milk volume the week after the restrictive intake. Because a decrease in milk production can affect infant growth and hydration, hypocaloric diets (less than 1500 kcal/day) for weight loss cannot be recommended during lactation.

A longer study of energy restriction (10 weeks) was conducted to determine if adequate weight loss can be achieved without having a negative effect on lactation.[36] Twenty-two women restricted their normal energy intake (about 2300 kcal/day) by an average of 538 kcal, or approximately 25% of mean baseline intake. Thus, total energy intake was an average of 1800 kcal/day. Subjects met at least 90% of the RDA for calcium, iron, vitamin A, thiamin, riboflavin, niacin, and vitamin C. Average weight loss was 4.8 ± 1.2 kg. There was no decrease in milk volume or change in milk fat or protein, and infant growth was adequate during the study. Therefore, well-nourished women can safely lose weight at the rate of 0.45 kg/wk without compromising lactation performance.

Many women desire to lose weight during the postpartum period but are often advised not to restrict their energy intake by health care professionals because of the possible consequences of decreased milk production. Although more research needs to be done regarding weight loss during lactation, it seems prudent to recommend moderate dieting (more than 1500 kcal/day) for overweight women, once lactation is fully established, to achieve a weight loss of 2 kg/mo or less. However, lean women may be at risk for decreased milk production if they restrict their kilocalorie intake.

Very lean women may also need a higher percentage of energy intake from fat during lactation. In a study that evaluated milk lipid concentration, body composition, and dietary intake of exclusively breastfeeding women, there was a strong association between percentage body fat and milk lipid concentration ($r = 0.53$; $p = .002$).[37] Dietary fat (percentage of energy from fat) was not associated with milk lipid for mothers with more than 27% body fat but was positively correlated in women with less than 27% body fat. The mean percentage of kilocalories from fat ranged from 23 to 41% in the lean subjects. This was similar to the range of fat intake (20 to 41% of kilocalories) consumed by all subjects.

There is increased de novo fatty acid synthesis in the mammary gland of lactating women consuming a high-carbohydrate, low-fat diet. This results in a decrease in the energetic efficiency of breast milk synthesis and a higher kilocalorie requirement during lactation. Because the major source of energy to the breastfed infant is from milk lipid, it is critical to maintain adequate levels to support infant growth. Nutritionists must keep this in mind when counseling lactating women. The general recommendation of fat intakes at less than 30% of kilocalories from fat may not be appropriate for a lean, exclusively breastfeeding mother. This area needs further research.

Exercise

Many women continue to exercise during pregnancy. Benefits include prevention of excess weight gain, improved cardiovascular fitness, reduced incidence of cesarean section, shorter hospitalization, and decreased discomforts of pregnancy. These benefits may outweigh the risks of maternal hypoglycemia, chronic fatigue, and musculoskeletal injuries.[38] There is a paucity of studies investigating the nutrient intake of exercising pregnant women because most studies reporting the effect of exercise on pregnancy outcome do not measure dietary intake. Birth weight is often one of the outcome variables evaluated, and nutrient intake may be interacting with exercise to affect maternal weight gain and infant birth weight. If total energy expenditure is increased by the exercise program, energy intake may not be sufficient to support adequate fetal growth.

In a retrospective study,[39] pregnancy outcome was evaluated in three groups of women: (1) those who were sedentary before and during pregnancy ($n = 152$); (2) those who exercised before pregnancy but stopped exercising before the 28th week of gestation ($n = 47$); and (3) those who exercised before pregnancy and maintained exercise throughout gestation ($n = 29$). Women in the third group gained 4.6 kg less than those women who stopped exercising before 28 weeks' gestation and 2.4 kg less than the sedentary controls. Infant birth weight was approximately 500 g less in the women who exercised throughout pregnancy compared with the other two groups. Unfortunately, dietary intake was not measured in these subjects. Although much research needs to be done in this area, it is prudent to recommend increased energy intake if total energy expenditure is increased by participation in regular exercise.[40]

The effects of exercise on lactation performance have been investigated. Energy expenditure and intake and lactation performance (milk volume and composition) of eight sedentary and eight highly trained, exercising women who were exclusively breast-feeding were compared.[41] The trained women exercised an average of 88 min/day, and their energy expenditure was approximately 700 kcal/day higher than that of the sedentary women. The exercising women were significantly leaner, had a higher cardiovascular fitness level, and tended to have higher milk volume and milk energy output than the sedentary women. The women who exercised compensated for their higher energy expenditure by consuming approximately 700 kcal/day more than the sedentary women (Table 7-6). Exercising women also consumed a diet with the percentage of kilocalories from carbohydrates significantly higher and the percentage of kilocalories from fat significantly lower than the sedentary subjects.

An intervention trial to assess the effects of exercise on lactation performance of previously sedentary women was conducted.[35,42] At 6 weeks postpartum, exclusively breastfeeding women were randomly assigned to one of two groups: the exercise group who began an aerobic exercise program for 45 min/day, 5 days/wk for 12 weeks; and the control group who did not exercise more than once a week during the same 12 weeks. Energy expenditure for exercise was approximately 400 kcal/day. As reported previously, women in the exercising group consumed significantly more kilocalories than the control group. These studies suggest that women can perform aerobic exercise during the postpartum period and improve their cardiovascular fitness levels without jeopardizing breast milk

---

Table 7-6 Dietary Intake of Exercising and Sedentary Lactating Women

	Reference 41		Reference 35	
	Ex (n = 8)	*Sed (n = 8)*	*Ex (n = 18)*	*Sed (n = 15)*
Energy intake (kcal/day)	2739 ± 309*	2051 ± 335	2455 ± 120**	2089 ± 120
Percentage of calories from:				
Protein	16.4 ± 2.9	17.0 ± 2.4	15.6 ± 0.4	15.5 ± 0.5
Fat	25.5 ± 5.7**	40.0 ± 2.4	28.9 ± 1.1†	34.1 ± 1.3
Carbohydrate	59.1 ± 6.1**	42.6 ± 3.7	57.4 ± 1.1†	52.4 ± 1.1
Alcohol	1.8 ± 1.9	2.0 ± 3.5	0	0

Values reported are mean ± SD.
Ex, exercise; Sed, sedentary.
Significantly different from sedentary group: *$p < .01$; **$p < .001$; †$p < .05$.
Source: Data from *New England Journal of Medicine* (1994;330:449–453) and *American Journal of Clinical Nutrition* (1994; 59 [Suppl] : 446S–453S).

volume or composition. However, energy intake was increased by these women to compensate for the increased energy expenditure. Exercise alone, without restricting energy intake, did not increase the rate of postpartum weight or fat loss.

NUTRITIONAL ISSUES

Calcium

There is a large variation in calcium intakes during pregnancy and lactation but very few reports of calcium deficiency. Changes in absorption and metabolism of calcium during the reproductive period may result in an adaptation to the increased calcium requirements during pregnancy and lactation. The NRC recommends an additional 400 mg/day of calcium for pregnant and lactating women,[2] based on the estimate that approximately 200 mg of calcium per day is incorporated into the fetal skeleton during the third trimester and 240 mg/day is secreted into breast milk during full lactation. Prentice[43] has calculated the total calcium costs of a mother who has had two infants and breast-fed each for 3 months to be approximately 100 g.

Changes in calcium metabolism during pregnancy include increased absorption and increased excretion; however, overall calcium balance is positive.[44] Increases in bone turnover are greatest in the first and third trimesters. During lactation, calcium excretion is decreased, but calcium absorption does not change.[45,46] However, absorption is higher among women with low intakes (370 mg/day) compared with subjects with high intakes (1879 mg/day). Reports concerning changes in bone turnover have been conflicting, with some observing increased rates and others finding no change.[43]

Reports of changes in bone mineral density (BMD) during pregnancy have also been conflicting, possibly due to the differences of measuring techniques used and of the sites measured. Many studies begin measuring BMD during the second or third trimester and, therefore, may not detect changes during early gestation. Bone loss during lactation has been reported in some but not all studies. Recent studies have reported bone loss in early lactation, with increases in density after weaning.[43] Sowers et al[47] measured BMD in the femur and lumbar spine in 98 healthy women from 2 weeks to 12 months postpartum. Changes in BMD among women breast-feeding less than 6 months were not significant. Subjects lactating 6 months or longer lost approximately 5% of BMD. In those women who weaned between 6 and 9 months, the spine and femoral BMD levels had returned to baseline values by 12 months postpartum. The women that continued to lactate had lower BMD in the femoral and lumbar spine at 12 months postpartum compared with their baseline levels. There was no significant relationship between age, dietary calcium intake (mean intake was 1596 mg/day), or physical activity and the amount of change in BMD during 6 months postpartum. Thus, lactation of long duration was associated with short-term bone loss; however, there seems to be a return to baseline levels at 12 months postpartum.

There have been very few studies investigating the effect of calcium supplementation in women with low calcium intakes during pregnancy and lactation. One study in India reported increased bone densities of infants born to undernourished mothers given 300 and 600 mg of calcium per day during pregnancy.[48] Results from several studies suggest that 1 to 2 g of calcium in the form of calcium salts may reduce the incidence of pregnancy-induced hypertension.[43] Whether this may be achieved by increasing dietary calcium has not been investigated. The concentration of calcium in breast milk is not related to maternal calcium intake in women consuming moderate-to-high amounts of calcium. To date, there have been no reports on the effect of supplemental calcium in women with low intakes on breast milk concentrations. Current studies suggest that consuming higher levels of calcium than the current RDA of 1200 mg/day does not slow the bone loss that occurs during lactation.[43]

Iron

Normal physiologic changes occurring during pregnancy include an expansion of maternal plasma volume and an increase in red blood cell mass.[1] Red blood cell production is stimulated later than the increase in plasma volume, resulting in a decline in hemoglobin concentration and hematocrit during the first and second trimesters (Figure 7-1). Erythropoiesis is stimulated in the last half of pregnancy, and hemoglobin concentrations begin to rise in the third trimester. The risk of low birth weight, preterm birth, and perinatal mortality is greater among women with hemoglobin concentrations less than 10.0 g/dL.[1] Anemia is usually defined as a low hemoglobin concentration (Table 7-7). Whether the low hemoglobin levels among these pregnant women were caused by iron-deficiency anemia was not established. Iron-deficiency anemia is determined when low hemoglobin concentrations are accompanied with low iron stores, usually determined by serum ferritin levels (less than 12 µg/L), and inadequate delivery of iron to tissues, determined by a low transferrin saturation (15% or less).

The prevalence of anemia in women in the United States is estimated to be less than 5% for white women, 5 to 8% for Hispanic women, and 12 to 15% for black women in the first trimester, using data from the Pregnancy Nutrition Surveillance System.[49] Table 7-7 shows the Centers for Disease Control (CDC)[50] cutoff values for determination of anemia during pregnancy. Because smoking elevates hemoglobin and hematocrit levels, adjustments for the amount of cigarettes

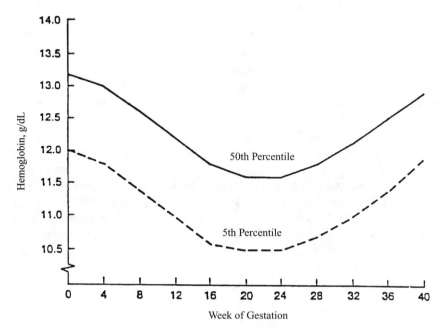

Figure 7-1 Normal Changes in Hemoglobin Concentration during Pregnancy *Source:* Data from *Nutrition During Pregnancy: Weight Gain and Nutrient Supplement, Pts 1 & 2* by the Institute of Medicine, Committee on Nutritional Status During Pregnancy and Lactation, National Academy Press, 1990.

smoked are included for diagnosing anemia. CDC also has adjustments for hemoglobin and hematocrit values for women living in higher elevations.

Scholl and Hediger[51] reviewed several large population studies examining anemia (hemoglobin, less than 11.0 g/dL and/or hematocrit less than 33%) and pregnancy outcome in women of many different ages, ethnic, and socioeconomic groups. They found when anemia is diagnosed early in pregnancy (i.e., first and second trimesters), it is associated with an increased risk of preterm delivery and low birth weight. However, anemia in the early part of the third trimester was not a risk factor for poor pregnancy outcome. Therefore, women with low hemoglobin concentrations in early gestation are true positives for anemia and women who test positive in the early portion of the third trimester have the physiologic anemia of pregnancy, due to hemodilution (see Figure 7-1).

Iron-deficiency anemia was investigated in low-income, predominantly minority teenage and mature pregnant women in Camden, New Jersey. Maternal iron-deficiency anemia diagnosed in the first two trimesters was associated with low dietary energy and iron, inadequate gestational weight gain, and twice the risk of preterm delivery and low birth weight. Diagnosis of iron-deficiency anemia in the

Table 7-7 Laboratory Values Indicating Anemia during Pregnancy, with Adjustments for Smoking

	Hb(g/dL)	*Hct (%)*
Trimester		
1st	<11.0	<33
2nd	<10.5	<32
3rd	<11.0	<33
Smoking		
1/2–1 pack/day	+0.3	+1.0
1–2 packs/day	+0.5	+1.5
>2 packs/day	+0.7	+2.0

Source: Reprinted from *Morbidity and Mortality Weekly Report* (1989;38:400–404), Centers for Disease Control and Prevention, 1989.

third trimester was associated with inadequate gestational gain only. Hence, iron-deficiency anemia may be the result of a poor diet, low in energy and other nutrients (e.g., zinc and protein), and supplements may not correct the true risk factor (i.e., the poor diet).

The current IOM[1] recommendation to prevent iron-deficiency anemia is 30 mg of ferrous iron per day for all women, beginning at approximately 12 weeks' gestation. For those with iron-deficiency anemia, treatment with 60 to 120 mg of ferrous iron per day is recommended until the hemoglobin concentration becomes normal for gestational stage. High doses of iron supplements (e.g., 200 mg/day) have been associated with constipation, diarrhea, nausea and upper abdominal pain, and interference with absorption of other nutrients (zinc in particular).[1] A review of the literature of longitudinal studies of iron supplementation in women without anemia during pregnancy by the IOM found that 30 or 65 mg of elemental iron per day was as effective as any of the higher doses in maintaining hemoglobin levels throughout pregnancy.

Supplements

The only supplement recommended routinely during pregnancy is 30 mg of ferrous iron per day, between meals or at bedtime, during the second and third trimesters.[1] This amount of ferrous iron is found in supplements containing 150 mg of ferrous sulfate, 300 mg of ferrous gluconate, or 100 mg of ferrous fumarate. Although the need for folate is increased during pregnancy, the IOM did not recommend routine supplementation of all pregnant women with folate. The role of folate in prevention of neural tube defects is discussed in Chapter 6. Since the critical period for neural tube formation is 17 to 30 days' gestation and most women do not realize they are pregnant at this time, the U.S. Public Health Service has recommended that "all women of childbearing age in the United States who are capable of becoming pregnant should consume 0.4 mg folic acid per day for the purpose of reducing their risk of having a pregnancy affected with spina bifida and other neural tube defects."[52] There is considerable debate among nutritionists regarding ways to increase the amount of folate consumed by women of childbearing age.[53]

The IOM recommends a daily multivitamin-mineral preparation beginning in the second trimester for "high-risk" pregnant women.[1] Examples of high-risk women include those consuming an inadequate diet, heavy cigarette smokers, abusers of drugs and alcohol, and women carrying multiple fetuses. The content of these supplements is shown in Table 7-8. The supplement should be consumed between meals or before bedtime to facilitate absorption.

Other women who may be in need of supplementation during pregnancy were also identified in the IOM report.[1] Women receiving more than 30 mg of iron per day may need supplementation with 15 mg of zinc and 2 mg of copper because large amounts of iron interfere with the absorption of these nutrients. Complete vegetarians need 2 μg of vitamin B_{12} and 10 μg of vitamin D each day. Women younger than age 25 whose daily calcium intake is less than 600 mg are advised to take 600 mg of calcium per day.

A second IOM report, "Nutrition during Lactation," recommended that women receive their nutrients from a well-balanced, varied diet rather than supplements.[3] However, special circumstances when a vitamin or mineral supplement may be appropriate were identified. Complete vegetarians need 2.6 μg of vitamin B_{12} and

---

Table 7-8 Multivitamin-Mineral Supplement Recommended by the Institute of Medicine for "High-Risk" Pregnant Women[a]

Nutrient	Amount Recommended/Day
Iron	30 mg
Zinc	15 mg
Copper	2 mg
Calcium	250 mg
Vitamin B_6	2 mg
Folate	300 μg
Vitamin C	50 mg
Vitamin D	5 μg

[a]See text for description of "high-risk" pregnant women.
Source: Adapted from Nutrition During Pregnancy: Weight Gain and Nutrient Supplement, Pts 1 & 2 by the Institute of Medicine, Committee on Nutritional Status During Pregnancy and Lactation, National Academy Press, 1990.

10 μg of vitamin D each day. Women with a low intake of calcium-rich foods are recommended to take 600 mg of calcium daily with meals. Those women consuming less than 1800 kcal/day may be advised to consume a balanced multivitamin-mineral supplement.

Management of Nausea

Nausea and vomiting are common complaints during the first 16 weeks of pregnancy among 50 to 80% of women.[54] General guidelines for controlling nausea are shown in Exhibit 7–1.[55] As early as the 1940s, supplemental doses of vitamin B_6 have been given to pregnant women to help control nausea. Most of the studies have not been controlled (i.e., placebos were not used or subjects were not randomized).

In a randomized, double-blinded study,[56] subjects with varying severity of nausea were given 25 mg of vitamin B_6 orally, every 8 hours for 72 hours. There was no symptomatic improvement with supplementation in women with mild-to-moderate nausea. However, those with severe nausea and vomiting had a significant reduction in their symptoms compared to the control group receiving a placebo with the same regimen.

While these data look promising, the safety of vitamin B_6 supplementation during pregnancy is unknown. One case has been reported in which a woman consuming 50 mg of pyridoxine hydrochloride, three or four times weekly for nausea, gave birth to an infant with convulsive seizures that responded to pyridoxine administration.[1] Oral doses greater than 100 mg/day for at least 6 months have resulted in sensory neuropathy in nonpregnant adults.[2] Consequently, the use of vitamin B_6 supplements greater than 50 mg/day should be avoided during pregnancy, until further studies are performed demonstrating the safety and efficacy of the vitamin in treating nausea.

Exhibit 7-1 General Guidelines for Controlling Nausea

- Drink soups and liquids between meals, instead of with meals, to avoid distending the stomach and causing vomiting.
- Avoid greasy or fried foods.
- Eat small amounts, every 2–3 hours.
- Eat bread or crackers before getting out of bed when feeling nauseated.
- Sip a carbonated beverage when nauseous.
- Get plenty of fresh air and rest.

Source: Adapted from *Nutrition During Pregnancy and the Postpartum Period* by the California Department of Health Services, 1990.

PROMOTION OF LACTATION TO IMPROVE MATERNAL HEALTH

Most health professionals recommend breastfeeding because it is the most appropriate milk for the developing infant. Benefits to the mother are rarely, if ever, discussed with the pregnant woman. Women should be made aware that lactation is the natural stage following pregnancy and that physiologic changes during pregnancy include development of mammary tissue to support lactation. Benefits of lactation to the mother include delayed ovulation, prolonged postpartum amenorrhea, and a more rapid return of the uterus to its nonpregnant state.[3] Another benefit that warrants further research is the possible link between decreased risk of breast cancer in women who lactate. A recent epidemiologic study of 5878 subjects with breast cancer and 8216 women with no cancer reported an approximately 20% lower risk of breast cancer before menopause for women who had lactated compared with those who had not nursed their infants.[57]

SUMMARY

Pregnancy and lactation are critical periods during the life cycle when one must consider the nutritional needs of the fetus and infant, as well as those of the mother. The large variation among individuals results in the need for continual assessment and monitoring of the nutritional status during this reproductive period. While pregnancy outcome (e.g., birth weight and general health of the infant) and breast milk volume and composition are important considerations when considering nutrient requirements, one must also consider the general well-being of the mother and the consequences of dietary intake during pregnancy and lactation on her future health status.

References

1. Institute of Medicine. *Nutrition during Pregnancy.* Washington, DC: National Academy Press; 1990.
2. National Research Council. *Recommended Dietary Allowances.* 10th ed. Washington, DC: National Academy Press; 1989.
3. Institute of Medicine. *Nutrition during Lactation.* Washington, DC: National Academy Press; 1991.
4. Forsum E, Kabir N, Sadurskis A, Westerterp K. Total energy expenditure of healthy Swedish women during pregnancy and lactation. *Am J Clin Nutr.* 1992;56:334–342.
5. Goldberg GR, Prentice AM, Coward WA, et al. Longitudinal assessment of energy expenditure in pregnancy by the doubly labeled water method. *Am J Clin Nutr.* 1993;57:494–505.
6. Poppitt SD, Prentice AM, Jequier E, Schutz Y, Whitehead RG. Evidence of energy sparing in Gambian women during pregnancy: a longitudinal study using whole-body calorimetry. *Am J Clin Nutr.* 1993;57:353–364.

7. King JC, Butte NF, Bronstein MN, Kopp LE, Lindquist SA. Energy metabolism during pregnancy: influence of maternal energy status. *Am J Clin Nutr.* 1994;59(suppl):439S–445S.

8. Parker JD, Abrams B. Prenatal weight gain advice: an examination of the recent prenatal weight gain recommendations of the Institute of Medicine. *Obstet Gynecol.* 1992;79:664–669.

9. Abrams B, Laros RK. Prepregnancy weight, weight gain and birth weight. *Am J Obstet Gynecol.* 1986;154:504–509.

10. Parker JD, Abrams B. Differences in postpartum weight retention between black and white mothers. *Obstet Gynecol.* 1993;81:768–774.

11. Smith DE, Caveny JL, Perkins LL, Burke GL, Bild DE. Longitudinal changes in adiposity associated with pregnancy. *JAMA.* 1994;271:1747–1751.

12. Ohlin A, Rossner S. Maternal body weight development after pregnancy. *Int J Obes.* 1990;14:159–173.

13. Greene GW, Smiciklas-Wright H, School TO, Karp RJ. Postpartum weight change: how much of the weight gained in pregnancy will be lost after delivery? *Obstet Gynecol.* 1988;71:701–707.

14. Dennis KJ, Bytheway WR. Changes in body weight after delivery. *J Obstet Gynecol Br Commonw.* 1965;72:94–102.

15. McKeown T, Record RG. The influence of reproduction on body weight in women. *J Endocrinol.* 1957;15:393–409.

16. Schauberger CW, Rooney BL, Brimer LM. Factors that influence weight loss in the puerperium. *Obstet Gynecol.* 1992;79:424–429.

17. Rookus MA, Rokebrand P, Burema J, Deurenberg P. The effect of pregnancy on the body mass index 9 months postpartum in 49 women. *Int J Obes.* 1987;11:609–618.

18. Potter S, Hannum S, McFarlin B, Essex-Sorlie D, Campbell E, Trupin S. Does infant feeding method influence maternal weight loss? *J Am Diet Assoc.* 1991;91:441–446.

19. Dugdale AE, Eaton-Evans J. The effect of lactation and other factors on post-partum changes in body-weight and triceps skinfold thickness. *Br J Nutr.* 1989;61:149–153.

20. Dewey KG, Heinig MJ, Nommsen LA. Maternal weight-loss patterns during prolonged lactation. *Am J Clin Nutr.* 1993;58:162–166.

21. Sadurskis A, Kabir N, Wager J, Forsum E. Energy metabolism, body composition, and milk production in healthy Swedish women during lactation. *Am J Clin Nutr.* 1988;48:44–49.

22. Spaaij CJK, van Raaij JMA, de Groot LCPGM, van der Heijden LJM, Boekholt HA, Hautvast JGAJ. Effect of lactation on resting metabolic rate and on diet- and work-induced thermogenesis. *Am J Clin Nutr.* 1994;59:42–47.

23. Illingworth PJ, Jung RT, Howie PW, Leslie P, Isles TE. Diminution in energy expenditure during lactation. *BMJ.* 1986;292:437–441.

24. Goldberg GR, Prentice AM, Coward WA, et al. Longitudinal assessment of the components of energy balance in well-nourished lactating women. *Am J Clin Nutr.* 1991;54:788–798.

25. Blackburn MW, Calloway DH. Energy expenditure and consumption of mature, pregnant and lactating women. *J Am Diet Assoc.* 1976;69:29–37.

26. Sims L. Dietary status of lactating women. I. Nutrient intake from food and from supplements. *J Am Diet Assoc.* 1978;73:139–146.

27. Manning-Dalton C, Allen LH. The effects of lactation on energy and protein consumption, postpartum weight change and body composition of well nourished North American women. *Nutr Res.* 1983;3:293–308.

28. Moser PB, Reynolds RD. Dietary zinc intake and zinc concentrations of plasma, erythrocytes, and breast milk in antepartum and postpartum lactation and nonlactating women: a longitudinal study. *Am J Clin Nutr.* 1983;38:101–108.

29. Stuff JE, Garza C, Smith EO, Nichols BL, Montandon CM. A comparison of dietary methods in nutritional studies. *Am J Clin Nutr.* 1983;37:300–306.

30. Butte N, Garza C, Stuff J, O'Brian Smith E, Nichols B. Effect of maternal diet and body composition on lactational performance. *Am J Clin Nutr.* 1984;39:296–306.

31. Finley DA, Dewey KG, Lonnerdal B, Grivetti LE. Food choices of vegetarians and nonvegetarians during pregnancy and lactation. *J Am Diet Assoc.* 1985;85:678–685.

32. Song WO, Wyse BW, Hansen RG. Pantothenic acid status of pregnant and lactating women. *J Am Diet Assoc.* 1985;85:192–198.

33. Strode MA, Dewey KG, Lonnerdal B. Effects of short-term caloric restriction on lactational performance of well-nourished women. *Acta Paediatr Scand.* 1986;75:222–229.

34. Lovelady CA, Meredith CN, McCrory MA, Nommsen LA, Joseph LJ, Dewey KG. Energy expenditure in lactating women: a comparison of doubly labeled water and heart-rate-monitoring methods. *Am J Clin Nutr.* 1993;57:512–518.

35. Dewey KG, Lovelady CA, Nommsen-Rivers LA, McCrory MA, Lonnerdal B. A randomized study of the effects of aerobic exercise by lactating women on breast-milk volume and composition. *N Engl J Med.* 1994;330:449–453.

36. Dusdieker LB, Hemingway DL, Stumbo PJ. Is milk production impaired by dieting during lactation? *Am J Clin Nutr.* 1994;59:833–840.

37. Lovelady CA, Nommsen MA, McCrory MA, Dewey KG. Relationship of human milk lipid concentration to maternal body composition and dietary fat intake. *FASEB J.* 1993;7:A200 (abstract).

38. Jarski RW, Trippett DL. The risks and benefits of exercise during pregnancy. *J Fam Pract.* 1990;30:185–189.

39. Clapp JF, Dickstein S. Endurance exercise and pregnancy outcome. *Med Sci Sports Exerc.* 1984;16:556–562.

40. Dewey KG, McCrory MA. Effects of dieting and physical activity on pregnancy and lactation. *Am J Clin Nutr.* 1994;59(suppl):446S–453S.

41. Lovelady CA, Lonnerdal B, Dewey KG. Lactation performance of exercising women. *Am J Clin Nutr.* 1990;52:103–109.

42. Lovelady CA, Nommsen-Rivers LA, McCrory MA, Dewey KG. Effects of exercise on plasma lipids and metabolism of lactating women. *Med Sci Sports Exerc.* 1995;27:22–28.

43. Prentice A. Maternal calcium requirements during pregnancy and lactation. *Am J Clin Nutr.* 1994;59(suppl):477S–483S.

44. King JC, Halloran BP, Huq N, Diamond T, Buckendahl PE. Calcium metabolism during pregnancy and lactation. In: Picciano MF, Lonnerdal B, eds. *Mechanisms Regulating Lactation and Infant Nutrient Utilization.* New York, NY: Wiley-Liss; 1992: 129–146.

45. Moser-Veillon PB, Vieira NE, Yergey AL, Nagey DA, Patterson KY, Veillon C. Fractional absorption and urinary excretion of calcium (Ca) stable isotopes in lactating and non-lactating women. *FASEB J.* 1989;3:A645(abstract).

46. Specker BL, Viera NE, O'Brien KO, et al. Calcium kinetics in lactating women with low and high calcium intakes. *Am J Clin Nutr.* 1994;59:593–599.

47. Sowers MF, Corton G, Shapiro B, et al. Changes in bone density with lactation. *JAMA.* 1993;269:3130–3135.

48. Raman L, Rajalakshmi K, Krishnamachari KAVR, Sastry KG. Effect of calcium supplementation to undernourished mothers during pregnancy on the bone density of the neonates. *Am J Clin Nutr.* 1978;21:466–469.

49. Kim I, Hungerford DW, Yip R, Kuester SA, Zyrkowski C, Trowbridge FA. Pregnancy Nutrition Surveillance System—United States, 1979–1990. *MMWR.* 1992;41:25–41.

50. Centers for Disease Control. CDC criteria for anemia in children and childbearing-aged women. *MMWR.* 1989;38:400–404.

51. Scholl TO, Hediger ML. Anemia and iron-deficiency and compilation of data on pregnancy outcome. *Am J Clin Nutr.* 1994;59(suppl):492S–501S.

52. U.S. Department of Health and Human Services, Public Health Service, Centers for Disease Control and Prevention. Recommendations for the use of folic acid to reduce the number of cases of spina bifida and other neural tube defects. *MMWR.* 1992;41(RR-14):1–7.

53. Rush D. Periconceptional folate and neural tube defect. *Am J Clin Nutr.* 1994;59(suppl):511S–516S.

54. Newman V, Fullerton JT, Anderson PO. Clinical advances in the management of severe nausea and vomiting during pregnancy. *J Obstet Gynecol Neonatal Nurs.* 1993;22:483–490.

55. California Department of Health Services, Maternal and Child Health Branch and WIC Supplemental Food Branch. Nutritional management of the pregnant woman. In: *Nutrition during Pregnancy and the Postpartum Period.* Sacramento, Calif: California Department of Health Services; 1990.

56. Sahakian V, Rouse D, Sipes S, Rose N, Niebyl J. Vitamin B_6 is effective therapy for nausea and vomiting of pregnancy: a randomized double-blind placebo-controlled study. *Obstet Gynecol.* 1991;78:33–36.

57. Newcomb PA, Storer BE, Longnecker MP, et al. Lactation and a reduced risk of premenopausal breast cancer. *N Engl J Med.* 1994;330:81–87.

8

✺

Vegetarianism for Women

Johanna T. Dwyer

For many American women, vegetarianism is a healthful choice. For others, it contributes significantly to ill health. This chapter reviews health pros and cons of vegetarian diets at various ages in women's lives and provides practical guidelines for vegetarian eating styles.

There is a distinction between *vegetarian eating styles,* which focus solely on dietary behavior,[1–3] and *vegetarianism,* which may base food choices on a particular belief system. A variety of vegetarian eating styles or diets exist (Table 8-1). Vegetarianism covers divergent beliefs and behaviors, including food choices and other life-style factors (such as nonsmoking) that affect health and nutritional status. Vegetarians may differ greatly or not at all from nonvegetarians in health attitudes and practices. Because many vegetarians also practice other healthy behaviors, including physical exercise and limited alcohol intake, it is often difficult to sort out the health impact of diet alone in vegetarianism.

WHO ARE VEGETARIAN WOMEN?

Prevalence

Vegetarian eating patterns are becoming increasingly popular. Approximately 7% of Americans or 12 million people considered themselves vegetarians in 1985. Only 4% claimed to be vegans (i.e., they eat no animal products at all);

Partial support from grant MCJ 8241, Maternal and Child Health Service, U.S. Department of Health and Human Services and grant NIH R01CA5439-03, "Estrogenic plant compounds in the etiology of breast cancer," was provided for preparation of this manuscript. The project has also been funded at least in part with federal funds from the U.S. Department of Agriculture, Agricultural Research Service, under contract no. 53-3K06-01. The contents of this publication do not necessarily reflect the views or policies of the U.S. Department of Agriculture, nor does mention of trade names, commercial products, or organizations imply endorsement by the U.S. government. The editorial assistance of Begabati Lennihan is acknowledged with thanks.

Table 8-1 Types of Diets and Foods Consumed

Type	Beef, Pork, Red Meat	Poultry	Fish	Eggs	Milk, Dairy	Vegetables, Fruits, Cereals, Breads, Nuts
Traditional "Omnivorous"	✔	✔	✔	✔	✔	✔
Semivegetarian		✔	✔	✔	✔	✔
Lacto-ovo-vegetarian				✔	✔	✔
Ovo-vegetarian				✔		✔
Lacto-vegetarian					✔	✔
Vegan						✔

Source: Reprinted from *Teddy Bears and Bean Sprouts* by B Ivens and WB Weil with permission of Gerber Products Co., © 1989.

40% reported consuming some animal products weekly, and a third even ate red meat on some occasions.[4] Other recent studies, conducted by the National Restaurant Association, reported that about 3% of the population of adults claimed that they never ate meat.[5] Therefore, vegetarians and semivegetarians today are probably no more than 3 to 7% of the population, but their numbers are growing.

Demographics

Americans who are vegetarians are slightly more likely to be female than male and tend to be older than age 60 or in their 30s and 40s, well educated, and in the Western part of the country, usually in cities.[5] They are generally mainstream in terms of their demographics and life styles, fairly affluent, and politically active and influential. They are apt to be concerned about the salt, saturated fat, and cholesterol content of their diets and often have reduced their animal food consumption accordingly. Among the 20% of adult Americans who seek out restaurants serving vegetarian dishes, health and personal taste preferences were the most important reasons given, whereas animal rights/animal welfare or religious concerns were cited by only half as many.[5]

Data are unfortunately not available on population-based samples of American vegetarians. Because vegetarians are very heterogeneous, it is important not to generalize from a few small studies; one group of vegetarians may differ greatly from another in motivations, attitudes, diets, and associated life styles. Therefore, each group must be evaluated separately. For example, in one small study, vegetarians were less educated and lower in their incomes than nonvegetarian age- and gender-matched controls; whereas in our own studies, vegetarians in the macrobiotic, yogic, and Seventh Day Adventist groups were more highly educated but had lower incomes than controls.[6,7]

SPECIAL CHALLENGES THAT VEGETARIAN EATING STYLES PRESENT TO WOMEN

The effects of vegetarian diets on women's nutritional status depend greatly on the specific type of diet and on the accompanying health-related practices. Table 8-2 shows some of the types of vegetarians and health practices that often distinguish them from omnivores. Vegetarian eating presents particular challenges to women. The nutrient needs of women vary more than do those of men across the life cycle because of altered requirements during adolescence, pregnancy, and lactation. Also, the nutrient density in women's diets must be greater than in men's, because women need less food (or, to be more exact, fewer calories) although their needs for specific nutrients are often the same or higher (Table 8-3).

These issues of nutrient density and nutrient sufficiency may present real risks with unplanned vegan diets (although they rarely become limiting on lacto-ovo-vegetarian diets).[8] Therefore, careful dietary planning is important for vegetarian women and mandatory for vegan women.

Vegetarian diets present a nutritional paradox for women. In some ways, they may be more risky and, in others, more beneficial. Consumption of animal foods

Table 8-2 Different Types of Vegetarian Eating Styles and Health Practices Commonly Associated with Them

Type of Vegetarian	Food Prohibitions	Health Practices and Comments
Vegan	Meat, fish, poultry, eggs, milk and milk products, dairy, often any animal products; often other types of prohibitions (such as against use of supplements, "processed" foods, etc.)	Physically active; abstain from tobacco, drugs, alcohol (with the exception of some macrobiotics and Rastafarians). Likely to rely on unconventional health care
Lacto-vegetarians	Meat, fish, poultry, eggs, may avoid "processed" or "non-organic" foods	Highly variable; often avoid tobacco, alcohol, drugs; often health-conscious; nutrient supplements and conventional medical care often acceptable
Lacto-ovo-vegetarians	Meat, fish, poultry	As for lacto-vegetarians
Semivegetarian	Meat (often include other flesh foods in small amounts in their diets)	Less highly linked to other life-style practices than among other vegetarian groups

Table 8-3 Recommended Dietary Allowances (RDA) Expressed by Nutrient Density in Women's versus Men's Diets

| Nutrients Required | Adult Males | | Adult Females | | | | | |
| | | | Nonpregnant | | Pregnant | | Lactating | |
	RDA	RDA Nutrient Density (/1000 kcal)	RDA	RDA Nutrient Density (/1000 kcal)	RDA	RDA Nutrient Density (/1000 kcal)	RDA	RDA Nutrient Density (/1000 kcal)
Energy (kcal)	2900.0	1000.0	2200.0	1000.0	2500.0	1000.0	2700.0	1000.0
Protein (g)	58.0	20.0	46.0	20.9	60.0	24.0	65.0	24.0
Fat-Soluble Vitamins								
Vitamin A (µg RE)[a]	1000.0	344.8	800.0	363.6	800.0	320.0	1300.0	481.5
Vitamin D (µg)[b]	10.0	3.5	10.0	4.5	10.0	4.0	10.0	3.7
Vitamin E (mg α-TE)[c]	10.0	3.5	8.0	3.6	10.0	4.0	12.0	4.4
Vitamin K (µg)	70.0	24.1	60.0	27.3	65.0	26.0	65.0	24.1
Water-Soluble Vitamins								
Vitamin C (mg)	60.0	20.7	60.0	27.3	70.0	28.0	95.0	35.2
Thiamin (mg)	1.5	0.5	1.1	0.5	1.5	0.6	1.6	0.6
Riboflavin (mg)	1.7	0.6	1.3	0.6	1.6	0.6	1.8	0.7
Niacin (mg NE)[d]	19.0	6.6	15.0	6.8	17.0	0.7	20.0	7.4
Vitamin B$_6$ (mg)	2.0	0.7	1.6	0.7	2.2	0.9	2.1	0.8
Folate (µg)	200.0	69.0	180.0	81.8	400.0	160.0	280.0	103.7
Vitamin B$_{12}$ (mg)	2.0	0.7	2.0	0.9	2.2	0.9	2.6	1.0
Minerals								
Calcium (mg)	1200.0	413.8	1200.0	545.5	1200.0	480.0	1200.0	444.4
Phosphorus (mg)	1200.0	413.8	1200.0	545.5	1200.0	480.0	1200.0	444.4
Magnesium (mg)	350.0	120.7	280.0	127.3	320.0	128.0	340.0	125.9
Iron (mg)	10.0	3.5	15.0	6.8	30.0	12.0	15.0	5.6
Zinc (mg)	15.0	5.2	12.0	5.5	15.0	6.0	19.0	7.0
Iodine (µg)	150.0	51.7	150.0	68.2	175.0	70.0	200.0	74.1
Selenium (µg)	70.0	24.1	55.0	25.0	65.0	26.0	75.0	27.8

[a]Retinol equivalents. 1 retinol equivalent = 1 mg retinol or 6 mg β-carotene.
[b]As cholecalciferol. 10 mg cholecalciferol = 400 IU of vitamin D.
[c]α-Tocopherol equivalents. 1 mg d-α tocopherol = 1 α-TE.
[d]1 NE (niacin equivalent) is equal to 1 mg of niacin or 60 mg of dietary tryptophan.
Source: Data from *Recommended Dietary Allowances*, ed 10, National Academy Press, 1989.

is the major (but not the only) way in which vegetarian diets differ from each other and from omnivorous diets. Animal foods are particularly rich sources of certain nutrients that women need for their own growth and also for optimal reproduction: protein, iron, calcium, zinc, vitamin B_6, and omega-3 fatty acids. They are unique sources of vitamins B_{12}, preformed vitamin A, and vitamin D. If a woman eliminates animal foods, she must get these nutrients from another source, or she risks adversely affecting not only her own nutritional status but that of her unborn or suckling infant as well.

However, animal foods are also concentrated sources of nutrients that are present in excess in many women's diets today: calories, total and saturated fat, cholesterol, and sodium. Reducing or eliminating animal foods may thus favorably influence nutritional health. Also, animal foods are devoid of potentially beneficial factors such as fiber, complex carbohydrates, and many biologically active substances (such as antioxidants and phytoestrogens) that are present in plant foods. Vegetarian diets have more of these beneficial substances than animal-based diets, at the same time as they have less of the harmful substances that animal foods have in excess.

FOOD GUIDANCE FOR VEGETARIAN WOMEN

Food Guides

For vegetarians, it is important as a starting point to follow general guidelines: use a wide variety of foods, minimize low-nutrient-density foods, use vitamin/mineral supplements, and complement plant proteins (i.e., use a vegetable protein high in certain amino acids to complement another that lacks those amino acids).[9] However, such general guidelines are not enough to ensure adequate nutrient intakes. Food guides are important for vegetarians, especially would-be vegetarians and those with little knowledge of nutrition. Professional guidance from a registered dietitian knowledgeable about vegetarianism is especially advisable for vegetarians with special health problems and for vegans (because vegans may need fortified foods to avoid nutrient deficiencies).

A variety of good food guides are now available. One of the most complete, a comprehensive guidance system designed for nutrition professionals by the Seventh Day Adventist Dietetic Association, includes a food guide and also adaptations for a variety of life situations and therapeutic vegetarian diets.[10] The Vegetarian Resource Group has also provided a helpful guide for vegans.[11] In Table 8-4, a food guide for lacto-ovo-vegetarians and vegans including pregnant and lactating women is presented.

Table 8-4 Daily Food Guide for Lacto-Ovo-Vegetarians and Vegans, Including Pregnant and Lactating Women, at Various Intake Levels

Food Groups	Lacto-Ovo-Vegetarians Daily Servings			Vegan Vegetarians Daily Servings		
	1600 kcal	2200 kcal	2800 kcal	1600 kcal	2200 kcal	2800 kcal
Breads, grains, cereals	6	9	11	8	10	12
Legumes	1	2	3	1	2	3
Vegetables, dark green and				dark green: 2	3	4
green leafy	3	4	5	green leafy: 2	2	2
Nuts and seeds	1	1	1	1	1	1
Milk, yogurt, and/or cheese	2–3	2–3	2–3	—	—	—
Milk alternatives[a]	—	—	—	2–3[b]	2–3[b]	2–3[b]
Eggs	1/2	1/2	1/2	—	—	—
Fats, oils (added)	2	4	6	2	4	6
Sugar (added tsp.)	3	6	9	3	6	9

Note: Provides approximately 30% of calories from fat.
[a]Tofu or soy milk fortified with calcium and vitamins D and B_{12}.
[b]Three servings for women who are pregnant, or breast-feeding, or for teenagers and young adults younger than age 24 years. If other foods are used, multivitamin and multimineral supplements may be needed.
Source: Data from *American Journal of Clinical Nutrition* (1994;59:1248S–1254S), American Society for Clinical Nutrition, 1994.

Several food guides for vegans do not meet all nutrient needs from food sources alone and would require adding appropriate nutritional supplements.[12] A vegan guide receiving a great deal of publicity recently is the New Four Food Groups—whole grains, legumes, vegetables, and fruits[13]—promoted by the Physicians' Committee for Responsible Medicine as a healthier replacement for the "old" omnivorous Four Food Groups (meat, milk products, breads and cereals, and fruits and vegetables). The problem is that the guide is not specific enough to ensure adequacy of all the essential nutrients. More specific and inclusive guides are therefore preferable: the Seventh Day Adventist Guide; a more recent guide to vegan eating prepared by a registered dietitian[11]; or others.[14,15] Good vegetarian cookbooks may further assist would-be vegetarians,[16,17] and vegetarian food models can assist professionals in counseling them.[18]

Other Sources of Information

The Vegetarian Nutrition Dietetic Practice Group of the American Dietetic Association provides balanced, objective information on planning vegetarian diets and is a referral service for registered dietitians specializing in vegetarian nutrition.[19] The *Vegetarian Times*, the largest periodical devoted to vegetarian life styles, carries news of particular interest to vegetarians and is unaffiliated with any particular vegetarian belief system. The Seventh Day Adventist Dietetic Association produces a variety of objective materials on vegetarian eating. State cooperative extension services and the Vegetarian Resource Group provide materials for vegetarians; the latter is especially helpful for vegans.[20] A variety of materials dealing with special issues is available from different sources.[21]

PLANNING AHEAD: LIFE CYCLE-RELATED CONCERNS

Women must consider the effects of their eating patterns not only on themselves but also on their offspring. The health of the infant at birth can be affected not only by the mother's diet during pregnancy but even by her diet during her growth years. Therefore, sensible dietary planning is important for young girls, whether vegetarian or not. Detailed consideration of the nutritional aspects of vegetarian diets during the reproductive years has recently been reviewed.[8]

Adolescence

Nutrient needs rise during adolescence, especially during the pubertal growth spurt. Vegetarian teenagers' dietary patterns need to be planned to provide enough calories, protein, calcium, phosphorus, iron, zinc, and vitamins D and B_{12}. Planning is especially important for vegan adolescents, because it is difficult to meet the needs for these nutrients from plant foods (unless the teenagers are willing to eat fortified foods). Intakes of other nutrients are usually adequate on most vegetarian diets. An advantage of vegetarian diets is that they are usually high in soluble dietary fiber and moderate or low in total fat, saturated fat, and cholesterol, which would decrease diet-related risks of high serum cholesterol and heart disease and set the stage for healthful eating in adulthood.

Bones grow most from birth to the later teens or early 20s in young women; even after they have stopped growing longer, they continue to increase in density, so that peak bone mass may occur in the later 20s (in some cases as late as the early 30s).[22,23] Bone density stays high until the menopause.[24,25] Because peak bone mass is achieved in early adulthood, calcium intake is especially critical during this time.

Preconceptional Period

Dietary guidance before pregnancy is prudent to ensure good nutritional status for the mother. Organogenesis occurs in the first several weeks of pregnancy, before many women even realize that they are pregnant. Thus, sound eating habits during the preconceptional period are critical. Anemia should be treated and corrected before pregnancy, because pregnancy makes large demands on iron stores, and the bioavailability of iron from plant sources is relatively low.

The menstrual cycle may be a day or two longer on some vegetarian diets, especially those that are low in fat, high in fiber, and high in some forms of soy products. These alterations in cycle length do not appear to decrease fertility. Much active research is now being done to determine whether these alterations have other effects on health, such as the risks for breast cancer.

Periconceptional Period

All women in the reproductive age group should consume at least 400 µg of folic acid per day, according to recent studies and the Surgeon General's 1993 report.[26] For women at high risk, those who have already had an infant with a neural tube defect, 4 mg/ day are recommended. For low-risk women, 400 µg/day is suggested. Good sources of folic acid are green leafy vegetables, citrus fruits, peanuts, fortified whole-grain cereals, and yeast extract. All women should include sources of folic acid in their diets to meet these recommendations; vegetarian women may tend to consume more of these folic-acid-rich foods than omnivores. The interconceptional period is also the ideal time to gain or lose weight to achieve a healthy level, to stop smoking, and to stop drinking alcohol. The immediate pre- or periconceptional period is not always ideal for losing weight, as a woman who uses an inadequate weight reduction diet during this period may enter pregnancy poorly nourished.

Pregnancy

The nutrient density of diets must rise during pregnancy regardless of eating style, because needs for vitamins, minerals, and protein increase more than do those for calories. Nutrients of special concern for vegetarians during pregnancy include iron, calcium, zinc, and vitamins B_{12} and D. Protein needs are usually easily met by increased intakes of milk and milk products, eggs, soy milk or tofu, cereals, nuts, and legumes. Iron needs increase dramatically because of the needs of the fetus. Levels of most nutrients are likely to be adequate if the diet is well planned. Guidelines for counseling vegetarians during pregnancy are available,[27] and other publications review the special issues of nutrition for pregnant vegetarians.[28,29] General dietary recommendations are shown in Exhibit 8-1.

It is difficult for both vegetarian and nonvegetarian women to meet their iron needs from food sources alone after the first trimester. For this reason, iron sup-

Exhibit 8-1 Dietary Guidance for Counseling Pregnant Vegetarians

- Ensure that dietary intakes preconceptionally adhere to the vegetarian food guide, that prepregnancy weight is within acceptable limits, and that folic acid intakes are at least 500 µg/day.
- Follow the vegetarian food guide, which ensures intakes approximating the Recommended Dietary Allowance.
- Include an iron supplement at doses prescribed by the physician.
- Monitor weight gain and adjust food intakes if necessary so that pregnancy weight gain is satisfactory.
- If diet-related diseases or conditions are present, obtain appropriate therapeutic dietary advice from a registered dietitian.

plements providing at least 30 mg elemental iron are recommended in addition to consumption of iron-rich food sources, such as whole-grain or iron-fortified cereals, legumes, green vegetables, and dried fruits. The iron in plant foods is best absorbed if taken with vitamin C-rich foods, such as citrus fruits and vegetables.[30]

Calcium needs also increase during pregnancy. During pregnancy, calcium absorption rises, and this helps to meet calcium needs if vitamin D nutrition is satisfactory. Milk and milk products such as yogurt and cheese are rich in calcium, and if these are included in amounts of two or three servings a day, calcium needs are met. Vegetable sources of calcium include green vegetables, almonds, sesame seeds, tahini, tofu, whole-grain and fortified cereals, and legumes. However, very large amounts of these plant sources of calcium must be eaten if no animal foods are included in the diet. There is a single report that suggests that low calcium intakes are associated with increased risks of pregnancy-induced hypertension.[31] However, it needs to be confirmed before deficiency of this nutrient can be linked to this disorder, which can arise from many causes. A large-scale trial is now in progress. In any event, there is no known benefit accruing from diets that fail to meet the Recommended Dietary Allowance (RDA) for calcium and every reason to assume that RDA levels should be met. If calcium intakes are very low (e.g., less than 600 mg daily if older than 25 years or less than 1000 mg daily at younger ages, and/or the woman is a vegan), a calcium supplement may be advisable.

Vitamin D intake is not usually a problem among lacto-ovo-vegetarians, but among vegans some source of 400 IU vitamin D (such as fortified soy milk or cod liver oil if vitamin D supplements are unacceptable) should be included. This is especially true in situations in which women are unlikely to form vitamin D from exposure to sunlight (e.g., in winter, in northern latitudes, in inclement weather, or if sunscreens are used).

Vitamin B_{12} sources for vegetarians include milk and milk products, eggs, and vitamin B_{12}-fortified nutritional yeast extract. Also, some brands of soy milks and other soy products are fortified with vitamin B_{12}. Supplements of the vitamin are also available. Regardless of which route is taken, it is critical that the RDA for this vitamin be met during pregnancy, lactation, and throughout the woman's life.

Pregnant lacto-vegetarian women differ little in nutritional status from their omnivorous peers. In both groups, iron status is not always satisfactory; thus, they should consume iron-rich food sources or use a prenatal iron supplement.

Pregnant vegans are more likely to experience inadequate intakes than other pregnant vegetarians, especially with respect to calcium, iron, and vitamin D. They often enter pregnancy at low weights and need to take particular care to ensure satisfactory weight gain. They also need to make sure that protein, iron, calcium, zinc, iodine, and vitamins B_6, B_{12}, and D intakes meet RDA levels, because in some studies, shortfalls and biochemical or clinical signs of deficiency have been reported in vegan women in other countries.[32] However, few studies have been done on the nutritional status of pregnant vegans following Western vegetarian diets. Individual assessment of a pregnant woman's dietary patterns is necessary. If she uses prenatal iron, calcium, and multivitamin supplements, diet planning is greatly simplified.

For the many vegetarians who avoid alcohol altogether, there is little need for concern about fetal alcohol effects. For those who do drink, they should be advised that abstinence is best and moderation is mandatory. Cigarette smoking is also rare among vegetarian women, but it too decreases birth weights. Those who smoke should be urged to stop, and those who cannot, to cut down.

Most vegetarian diets provide ample amounts of dietary fiber and water, which may help to decrease risks of constipation that commonly occurs in pregnancy owing to changes in gut motility. Additional resources for pregnant vegetarian women are provided in other publications.[33,34]

Lactation and Early Infancy

Breast feeding is common among vegetarians, with a duration of at least 4 to 6 months, as is currently recommended by health authorities. Among some vegetarians, it often continues into the second year of life. This is a healthful pattern as long as supplementary feeding is adequate. A recent publication provides detailed consideration of vegetarian diets during lactation.[35]

Dietary patterns during lactation need to be rich in protective nutrients such as protein, vitamins, and minerals as well as calories and fluids, because most women produce more than a quart of breast milk a day. Prolonged lactation can drain the mother's nutrient stores considerably.

A vegetarian eating pattern usually has little effect on the *volume* of milk produced, but it can influence the level of some *nutrients* in the milk, including vitamins D and B_{12} and other water-soluble vitamins.[36–38] Vitamin D is low in the milk of both vegetarians and nonvegetarians, providing less than 200 IU/L, and is especially low in the milk of vegans. The RDA for a 6-month-old infant is 400 IU, an amount unavailable in breast milk fed in usual quantities. For this reason, infants older than 4 to 6 months need supplemental vitamin D, especially vegan infants. Vitamin B_{12} concentrations (which depend on both the mother's dietary intake and her body stores) are low in the milk of vegan mothers, low enough to increase risks of vitamin B_{12} deficiency in her breastfed infant. For this reason, a supplement of 2.6 µg from a B_{12} supplement or from B_{12}-enriched nutritional yeast is suggested.

Iron status is satisfactory until 4 to 6 months in full-term infants because fetal hemoglobin stores are sufficient to sustain the infant until then. After that time, additional iron must be provided to meet the needs of growth and replacement of fetal hemoglobin. Because breast milk is a poor source of iron, some supplementary source of iron is recommended after 6 months of age on all dietary patterns. This is especially true on vegan diets, because the bioavailability of iron from plant sources is low, and many weaning foods lack iron. The nursing mother's food intakes should also emphasize rich iron sources, because maternal iron stores may already be decreased as a result of the pregnancy. If anemia is present, therapeutic iron supplements may be needed.

Sensible eating will help the mother preserve her own health as well as that of her infant. She should take calcium-rich foods or supplements in liberal amounts (at least RDA levels) to avoid maternal calcium depletion. Calcium absorption rises during lactation, but calcium intakes still need to be satisfactory. Exhibit 8-2 presents additional guidance for the breastfeeding mother.

The types of fatty acids in the mother's diet influence those found in breast milk to some extent. Although fatty acid composition has not yet been shown to be significant to the infant's health, it is another example of how maternal diets affect the suckling infant's intakes. Other minor differences in vitamins and minerals between vegetarians' and omnivores' breast milk are not known to be of health significance.

Adulthood

The large literature on the health effects of vegetarian diets can only be touched on here.[39–41] In brief, with appropriate dietary planning, there is no need for dietary deficiency disease to ensue, and there is every reason for vegetarian diets to be associated with excellent health. Well-planned vegetarian eating patterns can minimize the risks of several chronic degenerative diseases, especially coronary artery disease.[42] Vegetarians (and especially vegans) are also leaner than omnivores and less likely to be obese or to have high blood pressure, constipa-

Exhibit 8-2 Dietary Guidance for Vegetarian Mothers Who Are Nursing

- Enter lactation in good nutritional status; make sure to gain sufficient weight in pregnancy; take iron supplements to preserve your iron stores during pregnancy, and make sure that intakes of other nutrients meet recommended levels.
- Nurse frequently; at least 8 times a day at first, and 5 to 12 times a day after the first month, to make sure that the baby gets plenty of food. Check baby's weight gain and make sure it is adequate, remembering that although breastfed infants gain somewhat more slowly than bottle-fed, they too should gain weight and length.
- Eat a well-balanced varied diet with plenty of fluids to sustain good lactation. Avoid very rapid weight loss (i.e., more than 4 lb after the first month) to maintain good milk flow and avoid depletion of maternal reserves.

If you breast-feed more than 4 to 6 months:

- Start supplementary feedings as well as continuing to breast-feed, introducing solids only after 4 to 6 months, when the baby is developmentally ready, has doubled his or her birth weight, and weighs more than 13 lb.
- Gradually introduce solids (such as strained cereals first, then single fruits and vegetables). Remember that homemade baby foods are likely to be low in salt and nitrate. (Avoid foods such as spinach, beets, turnips, carrots, and collards that can cause methemoglobinemia in infants).
- Refrigerate homemade and commercial baby foods immediately after serving.
- Make sure supplementary feedings contain a good source of iron and vitamins D and B_{12}. Iron sources include iron-fortified formulas, iron-fortified baby cereals (after 4 to 6 months), and iron drops (1 mg/kg/day up to 15 mg). B_{12} sources include milk, cheese, yogurt, and eggs; seaweeds and other plant foods are not reliable sources of B_{12}. Commercial formulas provide Vitamin D, and vitamin supplements are also good sources. Check with your physician for supplements if you eat no animal foods at all.
- Keep track of your baby's weight gain and make sure it stays on track. Visit the physician to keep preventive measures up to date.
- Use soy or cow milk formula, not whole milk or soy milk, for liquids other than water and juices during the first year of the baby's life; whole milk may cause occult gastrointestinal bleeding. (Soy milk varies in nutrient content and is not recommended.) Avoid juice bottles before naps, because these may promote dental caries.
- Avoid high-bulk weaning foods; use high-protein, high-calorie, low-bulk weaning foods.

tion, type II (non-insulin-dependent) diabetes, lung cancer (due partly to vegetarians' lower rate of smoking but probably also due to their increased levels of β-carotene and other antioxidants), and possibly colon and breast cancer.[43-45] Associated health practices of many vegetarians, such as nonsmoking, may also have beneficial effects in reducing risks not only of lung cancers (and other well-recognized smoking-related cancers) but also of malignant degeneration of the bone marrow and its products, such as leukemia and myeloma.[45] Vegetarians' tendency to abstain from alcohol reduces alcohol-related health problems.

Many of the diet-related effects of vegetarian diets are linked to specific nutrients (and other biologically active compounds, such as cholesterol or fiber) that are high or low in vegetarian diets and not necessarily to the actual absence of animal foods. Nonvegetarians who have the same levels of these nutrients as vegetarians seem to enjoy the same health benefits. This finding is of practical importance, because it suggests that omnivores can have the health benefits of vegetarian diets if they boost their intake of these nutrients.[46] That is, if omnivorous diets are altered in a healthful direction, risks for chronic diseases can be reduced. (Careful planning would be needed to add these nutrient-rich foods without resulting in an excess of calories, because omnivores by definition would be adding these foods rather than substituting them for animal foods in their diets.)

However, there is growing evidence that plant foods may have some other constituents such as phytoestrogens that may be beneficial to health. Although data are preliminary, intakes of vegetables and fruits seem to be inversely (yet weakly) associated with decreased risks of colon cancer in several studies, and not all of the effects appear to be due to fiber.[47,48] If this proves to be true, vegetarian diets may offer advantages over omnivorous ones because they are usually higher in these foods. Omnivores can enjoy these health benefits by boosting their intakes of plant foods. However, there may also be toxic substances in plant foods, such as naturally occurring environmental contaminants and pesticides, that may have adverse effects on health. For this reason, it is important for federal agencies to monitor the food supply and for research to continue on both positive and negative biologic effects of various substances occurring in plants.

Vegetarians are not totally exempt from all diet-related health risks. Among the most common problems are iron-deficiency anemias (especially among vegan women in youth and in the childbearing years) and vitamin B_{12} deficiency (especially among vegans).[49] Good plant food sources of iron include dried beans, dark green vegetables, dried fruits, prune juice, blackstrap molasses, pumpkin seeds, sesame seeds, soybean nuts, and iron-fortified cereals, especially when they are consumed with foods high in vitamin C such as citrus fruits or juices, broccoli, tomatoes, or green pepper.[9]

Some vegetarians assume that they do not risk food poisoning, because they eat only organic foods or avoid the animal foods linked to food safety problems in recent years. But vegetarians should avoid raw or very lightly cooked eggs, even "free-range organic" eggs, because all eggs can contain *Salmonella,* and soft cheeses made from unpasteurized milks, because they may transmit tuberculosis, brucellosis, listeriosis, and other diseases.

Both vegetarian and nonvegetarian diets can promote bone health. All women, whether vegetarians or omnivores, need optimal intakes of calcium (and other nutrients needed for bone health) throughout the life cycle.

Calcium

Calcium is an important nutrient for all women. Since it is present in food sources of other nutrients, a low calcium intake is usually indicative of a diet that provides inadequate amounts of other nutrients. For example, omnivorous women with low calcium intakes also have low intakes of protein and several other vitamins and minerals.[50] Among omnivorous teenage girls, milk avoiders had lower intakes of calcium and also lower intakes of vitamins A, B_6, and B_{12}, folic acid, riboflavin, magnesium, and potassium than milk drinkers.[51] Similar nutrient intake studies are not available for vegetarians who used milk and milk products in contrast to those who obtained their calcium from supplements. Vitamin D intakes may also pose a problem for vegans. If calcium supplements are used, these should also contain vitamin D. Obtaining calcium from food rather than from supplements as much as possible is preferable, especially for pregnant, lactating, and elderly vegetarian women, because foods also supply other needed nutrients.

Overall, lacto-vegetarian diets have several advantages that make dietary planning easier for women than do vegan-vegetarian diets.[52] Milk and milk products provide not just calcium but also significant amounts of phosphorus, magnesium, and zinc, and so the inclusion of milk in the lacto-vegetarian pattern makes it easier to meet the RDA for these nutrients. Milk and some of the harder cheeses have a great surplus of calcium relative to protein, helping to overcome the calciuric effects of low-calcium protein foods. Also, the protein in milk is of high biologic value. Milk protein nicely complements the amino acid pattern of cereal proteins, which are low in the amino acid lysine, making the mixture of proteins higher in biologic value. Milk proteins are high in lysine, which favors calcium absorption, and low in the sulfur-containing amino acids such as methionine and cystine, which decreases calcium utilization. Finally, absorption of calcium is higher from milk and milk products than from the less bioavailable calcium in plant foods.

Those who do not use milk and milk products can get bioavailable (but often relatively expensive) calcium from calcium-fortified juices, tofu, soy milk, and breakfast cereals. Soy milks fortified with calcium should be used with caution, because they may not be fortified with vitamin B_{12}, and they may provide lesser amounts of phosphorus, riboflavin, and vitamin A than cow milk. However, some soy drinks now available overcome these disadvantages, so it is important to read nutrition labels before buying.

Zinc

About half the zinc in omnivorous American diets comes from zinc-rich animal products such as meats, poultry, seafood, egg, and dairy products. Zinc absorption is particularly good from animal foods. Plant foods, especially those based on whole grains and soy, also contain fiber, phytate, and oxalate (naturally occurring substances that bind zinc and reduce its bioavailability).[53] Vegetarians who limit or avoid animal foods need to plan their diets carefully to avoid a zinc deficiency. The need for zinc rises during disease and periods of cell replication and differentiation, such as in pregnancy and lactation, so special care is needed at these times.

Iron supplements, prescribed for most women during pregnancy, may interfere with zinc absorption (because of the competitive interaction between iron and zinc absorption). Thus, if iron supplements are greater than 30 mg/day, a zinc supplement of 15 mg is recommended[54] and should be taken at another time of day.

During lactation, zinc needs rise dramatically because of losses in breast milk. For breastfeeding women, an additional 7 mg zinc per day during the first 6 months postpartum and 4 mg zinc during the second 6 months should compensate for the losses in breast milk.[54] Older vegetarians may be at risk of zinc deficiency due to several factors: infection or surgery; reduced food intakes due to reduced energy needs; lowered zinc absorption due to gastrointestinal diseases or high-fiber foods; or treatment with drugs such as thiazides that increase zinc losses.

Vitamin D

Vitamin D occurs naturally only in animal foods such as milk and liver, although it is also added to fortified cereals, some soy milks, and other products. Those at risk of vitamin D deficiency include the infants of women who breastfeed for longer than 6 months and pregnant, lactating, and postmenopausal women.

Postmenopause and Aging

Changes in body composition during the menopausal years include increases in fat and decreases in lean body mass and bone mineral content.[55] Increases in body fatness at menopause are not inevitable but rather are determined largely by environmental influences, particularly physical inactivity and excessive food intake. Women should strive to keep their energy outputs high, emphasizing physical activity and exercise every day, aerobic exercise several times a week, and strength training to maintain muscle strength. The accumulation of abdominal fat is largely genetic, mediated by hormones. Hormone therapy can help prevent it, thus accounting in part for how hormone therapy lowers the risk of coronary artery disease (which is associated with abdominal fat).[56]

Older menopausal or postmenopausal women who are vegetarians have rarely been studied. The few data that do exist suggest that they are leaner than nonvegetarians.[57] Their diets are probably lower in fat and saturated fat and higher in nutrient density than that of omnivores (although in one study zinc, iron, and vitamin B_{12} intakes were lower than recommended levels,[58] and trace minerals may be low in some individuals).[59]

Iron Status

Iron needs fall after menopause because menstruation ceases. Even among postmenopausal women who lose blood due to cyclic estrogen replacement therapy, iron losses tend to be lower than premenopausally. In very old persons, atrophic gastritis (which decreases conversion of ferric to ferrous iron in the stomach) may decrease iron absorption. Also, blood loss from occult disease may be present. Therefore, anemia is always a cause for concern, and its etiology requires investigation.

Not only the amount of iron consumed but the type is important in determining iron status. Assuming equivalent amounts of iron are eaten and all other dietary factors are equal, it is well documented that those who have red meat as the predominant source of protein have higher iron status, probably because the bioavailability of heme iron is higher than plant-source iron. Although this disadvantage of plant sources of iron can be overcome by increased iron dose and by increased intakes of facilitators of iron absorption, it does remain an issue needing attention in vegetarian dietary planning.[60] Interestingly, lacto-ovo-vegetarians had higher iron status than did poultry or fish eaters, perhaps because the latter group's intakes of heme iron were lower, or because fish eaters, with very high intakes of omega-3 fatty acids, may have had increased bleeding tendencies, thus increasing iron losses.[61,62]

One other issue about iron deserves attention. Whereas vegetarians may run increased risks of iron-deficiency anemia without careful diet planning, they may be at lower risk of iron overload if they are among the 10% of the population who suffer from hemochromatosis.[63-65]

Bone Health

Increased vigilance is necessary for ensuring bone health in both older men and women. Women after menopause need to be especially concerned, because at menopause, estrogen production from the ovaries ceases. Estrogens enhance calcium absorption and slow calcium loss through the kidneys. Menopausal loss of estrogen changes the balance between mineralization and demineralization of the bones, causing a loss of 10% or more of total skeletal mass in the decade after menopause.[66] More gradual losses of bone occur among both men and women in the later decades of life owing to other hormonal changes, and after age 65, there is little difference between the sexes in rates of bone loss.

The effects of animal foods on bone health is not clear. In part, this is because animal foods vary not only in their protein content but also in their levels of calcium, phosphorus, vitamin D, zinc, and manganese (all nutrients known to affect bone health). Also, many dietary and life-style factors affect bone health; thus it is hard to separate out the effects of diet. Several studies of bone health in lacto-ovo-vegetarian women are now available. A very early report of elderly lacto-ovo-vegetarian women had suggested that the bone densities of vegetarian women were increased in old age over that of their nonvegetarian peers. Unfortunately, only an abstract of that study is available.[67] Among the subjects in three more recent studies, the lacto-ovo-vegetarians had similar calcium and phosphorus intakes, but lower protein intakes than the omnivores. Bone mineral densities of the two groups of women were similar, suggesting that the vegetarian dietary pattern provided no particular advantage or disadvantage from the standpoint of bone health. Also, very old women in both groups showed decreased bone density (as might be expected).[68–70]

Although not among vegetarians, one study paradoxically suggested that milk intakes were *negatively* correlated with bone density.[71] However, other reports among omnivores living in this country suggest *positive* correlations between childhood milk drinking and bone density measured postmenopausally.[72] Increased bone mass was also shown in middle-aged and elderly Chinese women, who had diets with varying calcium levels and very low amounts of animal foods (in comparison with Western countries). Chinese women living in counties where milk and milk products comprised a large proportion of the diet had large differences in bone density compared with those in areas where calcium intakes were very low. Those with calcium intakes less than 700 mg/day had increased risks of osteoporosis.[73,74] Studies on the differences in bone density between vegans and nonvegetarians are not available.

DISEASE PREVENTION

Osteoporosis

There is probably considerable disparity between different groups of vegetarians in their risks for osteoporosis; lacto-vegetarians usually have adequate bone density, whereas vegan vegetarians sometimes do not. Also, vegans may be at risk for osteoporosis because they lack good dietary sources of vitamin D, tend to be underweight, consume foods rich in calcium absorption inhibitors (such as dietary fiber, phytic, and oxalic acids), and have low calcium intakes. However, vegans are often physically active and abstain from smoking and drinking; these factors may decrease their risks of osteoporosis. Studies of older vegan women would help clarify their risk.

Protein

Protein adequacy is rarely an issue for adult vegetarian women; a more common issue is whether decreased protein intakes (or decreased animal protein intakes) are somehow beneficial to bone health. There is evidence that high-protein diets (e.g., diets far in excess of the RDA) increase urinary losses of calcium, particularly when these diets are very low in calcium. These data have been used to recommend moderation in protein intakes. However, there are also some data (less well established) that too little protein decreases both calcium absorption and losses in the urine.[75]

There is good evidence that the *amount* of protein is very important in determining urinary calcium excretion and net calcium retention, more so than the *type* of protein (e.g., plant versus animal).[76] Calcium and phosphorus intake levels are also important. It has been suggested that an excess of protein in animal food-rich diets leads to altered acid-base balance, mild acidosis, and leaching of calcium from bone, with the result that calcium requirements are higher on meat-rich omnivorous diets than on either milk product-rich vegetarian or plant product-rich vegan diets. The supposition is that the high animal protein stimulates an obligatory loss of calcium, which is uncompensated for by other dietary factors. However, these relationships are not simple. In a Japanese study, protein intake was positively, not negatively, correlated with bone density, perhaps because of the association of protein with some other substance (such as phytoestrogens in soy foods, a primary source of protein in Japanese diets).[77]

One rule of thumb for assessing calcium needs that takes into account the effect of the amount of protein is the calcium:protein ratio first suggested by Dr. Robert Heaney; that is, the ratio of the RDA for calcium (800 mg for adult women) versus the RDA for protein (50 g, for the reference woman in the current RDAs); or a ratio of 16:1 mg/g. The calcium:protein ratio was predictive of bone accretion rates in young women in the studies of Recker et al.[22] The average intake of calcium, especially of adult women, is much less than the RDA, whereas protein intakes are much higher (approximately 89 g for men and 63 g for women). Thus, the calcium:protein ratios are lower than what is thought to be optimal (probably about 9:10). Therefore, there is cause for concern about both calcium and protein intakes, especially among women. Calcium:protein ratios of 14:1 among young women consuming 1500 mg calcium per day (500 to 600 mg from dairy foods) and 107 g protein per day were associated with no deterioration in calcium balance from baseline levels before supplementation.[78] Lacto-ovo-vegetarians do not necessarily have more favorable calcium:protein ratios than do omnivores. Like omnivores, their protein intakes tend to be excessive.

Calcium

Calcium needs may rise with aging because vitamin D production and calcium absorption decrease.[79] There are many factors increasing calcium needs in the elderly by decreasing calcium absorption or increasing its excretion, including laxative use, physical inactivity, excess tobacco or alcohol use, gastrointestinal disorders, and renal insufficiency. Vegetarian women need to make sure to include ample amounts of calcium in their diets. They need to stay physically active and to include strength and resistance training, which increases bone mass. Estrogen replacement therapy may be indicated for those with a history of osteoporosis or its risk factors (including slight stature, fair coloring, and a history of smoking), although it should be considered with caution for those at risk for breast cancer.

For those who dislike or avoid food sources of calcium, the other option is to rely on calcium supplements, which provide bioavailable calcium when taken regularly. Calcium absorption levels appear to be similar from such common supplements as calcium carbonate and calcium lactate and milk and milk products.[80–82] However, milk and milk products have the advantage of also providing other nutrients.

Calcium supplements differ in the amount of elemental calcium (percentage of calcium) they contain. Calcium carbonate, which has a high amount of calcium per unit weight, requires fewer tablets to meet calcium needs than do some other supplements. It is also available in generic, nonbranded preparations, which are lower in cost, and in chewable forms for those who find swallowing pills difficult. Calcium citrate malate is a very highly bioavailable form of calcium, but it is not widely available in supplements.

Vitamin D

Aging decreases formation of provitamin D_3 in the skin and renal conversion of it into vitamin D.[83] Vitamin D nutritional status may be especially low among those with limited sun exposure (shut-ins, those in northern parts of the world, including the northern United States, and those using sunscreens because they are rightly concerned about skin cancer). Among such persons, supplementation with 400 IU of vitamin D increases spinal bone density, even in omnivorous women.[84]

A recent study found the mechanisms for the vitamin D-osteoporosis connection: it found that when vitamin D intakes were lower than 220 IU/day among postmenopausal women, parathyroid hormone secretion rose (especially during winter when there was little exposure to the sun), thus increasing risks of demineralization of bone.[85] Calcium retention fluctuates seasonally as blood levels of 25-OH vitamin D vary, especially among postmenopausal women with low calcium intakes. These women have lower rates of bone loss when more calcium is retained, thus indicating the importance of plasma 25-OH vitamin D.[86] Postmenopausal vegan women may be at particular risk of osteoporosis because their intakes of vitamin D-rich foods may be low. Therefore, older women probably would benefit from more than the 200 IU of vitamin D that is the current RDA; 400 IU are suggested especially for vegan women. Recently it was asserted that chronic, excessive amounts of vitamin D were associated with increases in both osteoporosis and atherosclerosis.[87] However, at present there is little data to support such a theory.

Among aging women (both vegetarian and omnivorous), adequate intakes of calcium and vitamin D are therefore important, as is the need for a physically active life, with weight-bearing, gravity-resisting exercises included in the daily routine. Light body weight is associated with lesser amounts of bone in post-menopausal women, so women should keep their weights at reasonable levels.[88] Apparently muscle rather than fat is responsible for this association between weight and bone mass, further emphasizing the importance of strength training.[89] Also, nonsmoking[90] is important because cigarette smoking greatly increases fracture risk. Moderation in alcohol consumption to no more than two or three drinks a day (less is better for a variety of reasons) also helps decrease risk, since high alcohol intakes increase risks of fracture.

Phosphorus

Phosphorus intakes also influence bone health, probably in a positive direction, although study results have been mixed. On diets containing meat and dairy foods (both are high in phosphorus), the calciuric effects of high protein intakes are blunted and calcium retention is encouraged, so that mixed diets containing meat and milk at protein intake levels of 95 g/day induce calcium balance at levels of 800 mg.[91] By contrast, much larger urinary calcium losses are observed when purified, low-phosphorus protein or egg albumin are fed by themselves.[92] These studies suggest that high intakes of both protein and phosphorus, such as are eaten on high-meat diets, reduce the effect of protein-induced hypercalciuria compared with changes in single nutrients.[93] However, other experts disagree that increased phosphorus neutralizes the effects of increased protein intakes, arguing that phosphorus' effect on decreasing urinary calcium excretion is countered by increasing calcium secretion into the gut, and via the gut to the feces, with a net neutral effect on calcium balance.[94] Others reported that calcium secretion into the gut was not significant; but the study was small, and precise measurement of fecal calcium (by radioisotope tracers) was not available then.[95,96] A reasonable conclusion is that intakes of milk and milk products are likely to have net positive effects on bone health for lacto-vegetarians.

Acid-Base Balance

Lacto-ovo and vegan diets often produce more neutral or alkaline urine than do meat-rich diets. Animal protein-rich foods are high in the sulfur-containing amino acids cystine and methionine. Such animal foods do cause greater urinary calcium losses than most (but not all) vegetable proteins, which are lower in these amino acids. The result is that an acid urine is produced. It has been suggested that such an acid urine increases calcium losses, explaining about half of the increased urinary calcium loss on meat-based as compared with plant-based diets.[97] The rest of the increased calcium loss on high-protein diets is thought to be due to protein-mediated increases in glomerular filtration and hormone shifts.

The amount of sulfur-containing amino acids in various animal and plant foods varies (Table 8-5). Vegetarian diets today may include processed soy products, some of which have the sulfur amino acids methionine or cystine added to them (while traditional soy foods such as tofu and tempeh do not). Therefore, it is difficult to predict what the alkalinity of the diet will be, simply by knowing if it is vegetarian or omnivorous. Although the acidosis theory of osteopenia is appealing theoretically, at present it lacks empirical data to support it.

Coronary Artery Disease

There is an impressive body of evidence that links dietary factors to heart disease.[98] Several reports summarize the evidence linking type and amount of dietary fat and cholesterol to serum lipid levels. Lower serum cholesterol is associated with decreased levels of total fat, saturated fat, and cholesterol, with possibly more minor effects from increased soluble fibers, antioxidant nutrients, and other dietary factors.[99–101] Vegetarian diets that are very low in fat and saturated fat and relatively high in polyunsaturated fats are associated with very low levels of serum cholesterol. No causal association has been found between very low serum cholesterol levels and deaths due to accidents, suicides, or homicides (as was indicated in an early and inadequate study), so there is no reason to assume that low serum cholesterol levels are harmful.[102]

Vegetarian diets may also have beneficial effects on other factors such as platelet aggregation and bleeding time. The end result is that vegetarians have a lowered risk of coronary artery disease.[103] Although omnivorous diets could theoretically attain these decreased coronary risk factors, low-fat lacto-ovo-vegetarian or vegan diets can do so much more easily from a practical standpoint. A physically active life also decreases risks of coronary artery disease, and vegetar-

---

Table 8-5 Sulfur-Containing Amino Acids in Various Plant and Animal Foods

Food	Sulfur-Containing Amino Acids (mg/g protein) (Produce acid when metabolized)
Chicken	46
Flank steak (beef)	38
Milk	34
Whole-wheat flour (cereal grains)	40
Tofu (soybean protein)	27
Broccoli (vegetable protein)	6

ians are often more likely to include healthy life-style factors such as physical exercise.[104]

Total Fat, Saturated Fat, and Cholesterol

Most vegetarian diets are low in fat, saturated fat, and cholesterol—all factors known to increase serum cholesterol levels if present in excess. The exception would be vegetarian diets that are based on full-fat dairy products and eggs or include very high amounts of fat. Therefore, it is not surprising that seven studies recently showed that vegans had serum cholesterol levels 45 to 50 mg/dL lower than nonvegetarians, after adjusting for differences in weight, smoking status, and intakes of calories, fat, and cholesterol (all factors that increase serum cholesterol levels, even among vegetarians).[105] Before adjusting for these factors, the vegans had 60 mg/dL lower blood cholesterol concentrations. Such differences in risk factors account for vegetarians' slightly lower death rates from heart disease observed in some studies.

Other Dietary Factors

Vegetarian diets appear to be more effective in treating hyperlipidemias than would be predicted solely from their content and type of fat and cholesterol. Other important factors include the type of protein, their higher fiber content (particularly soluble fiber), and possibly the presence of phytoestrogens such as the isoflavones (phenolic compounds structurally similar to steroid hormones).[106,107]

However, vegetarians may risk hyperhomocysteinemia, which has recently been suggested as an independent risk factor for vascular and coronary artery disease. One study showed that nonvegetarians with this condition had low serum levels of folic acid and vitamins B_{12} and B_6, associated with poor intakes of these vitamins. Vegetarians are more likely to be deficient in vitamin B_{12} and thus may have increased risk of hyperhomocysteinemia. This condition (possibly due to a deficiency of cystathionine-β synthase[108]) appears to be associated with subsequent risks of myocardial infarction.[109]

Hyperhomocysteinemia appears to be treatable by vitamin supplements; a vitamin supplement with generous amounts of these vitamins normalized levels of plasma homocysteine.[110] Whether it also reduces risks of heart disease remains to be determined. However, these preliminary observations suggest that folic acid and vitamin B_{12} and B_6 intakes must reach RDA levels in vegetarian as well as nonvegetarian women.

High Blood Pressure

Being overweight increases blood pressure and coronary heart disease risk.[111] When excess weight is lost, both systolic and diastolic blood pressure decrease in both hypertensive and normotensive persons.[112–114] Vegetarian women, often leaner than their nonvegetarian peers, are thus lower in this risk factor for heart disease.

High salt intakes, such as those among most omnivores of 100 to 200 mmol sodium per day (about 2500 to 5000 mg sodium, or 6 to 12 g salt), also increase risks of hypertension, as demonstrated by the very large INTERSALT population-based study.[115] In an analysis of more than 37,000 people in 24 different communities, differences of 100 mmol (2500 mg) in daily sodium intake were associated with systolic blood pressure differences ranging from about 5 mm Hg in teenagers, up to 10 to 19 mm Hg in the 60- to 69-year-old age group, with especially large differences seen among those who had high blood pressure.[116] Although the experimental studies have found somewhat smaller effects from reducing sodium chloride in the diet, clearly some effects are present.[117,118] Those vegetarians who have diets low in sodium (about 100 mmol, or 2500 mg sodium, or 6 g sodium chloride)—by avoiding highly processed foods and high-salt condiments such as soy sauce—may experience benefits in lowering blood pressure. Both the sodium and chloride ions appear to have significant effects.

Another blood pressure-lowering factor common among vegetarians is abstinence or moderation in alcohol use. There is good evidence that consumption of more than three drinks (40 g absolute alcohol or ethanol) per day on a long-term basis is associated with increased blood pressure. Because heavy use of alcohol is widespread in our society, as much as 5 to 7% of the prevalence of hypertension in the United States is due to excess alcohol intake.[119]

Other dietary characteristics that may further alter blood pressure, including calcium, magnesium, and omega-3 fatty acid content, are now being investigated. Present evidence suggests that their effects (if present at all) are less than the other factors already discussed. Finally, the physically active life styles of many vegetarians may account in part for their lowered blood pressures, because there is evidence from clinical trials that both systolic and diastolic pressures decline with low- to moderate-intensity exercise.[120]

Breast and Colon Cancer

Reproductive events and body fat exert similar effects on worldwide breast cancer incidence. This suggests that these factors are even more powerful determinants than diet.[121] Age-specific incidence rates of breast cancer across populations depend on factors that include menarche, age at menopause, occurrence and timing of full-term pregnancies, and body mass index. The rates jump higher after a woman's first childbirth and rise more slowly thereafter. Rates of breast cancer increase with age more slowly after menopause than before and increase quadratically with body mass index among all women.[122] Body composition affects sex hormone metabolism, because adipose tissue can convert androgens to estrogens. Diet affects sex hormone metabolism both by its influence on body composition[123] and by altering hormonal metabolic pathways.[124]

Several studies link diets high in fruits, vegetables, and dietary fiber and low in fat with decreased risks of certain cancers, including those of the breast and colon.[125,126] Other lines of evidence suggest that for breast cancer, a low-fat diet is key, that abstinence from alcohol is important, and that leanness is protective (at least for the postmenopausal forms of the disease). Therefore, health experts urge diets high in fruits and vegetables and low in fat to reduce risks of diet-related cancers.[46,127] Biologically active substances in foods, especially plant foods—such as dietary fiber or associated compounds, β-carotene, other antioxidants, and some nutrients (possibly vitamin D and calcium)—may be responsible for these beneficial effects.[128] Other beneficial plant-based substances associated with decreased cancer risk include the phytoestrogens, found in soy foods, which appear to act by inhibiting tyrosine kinase (an enzyme family needed in the carcinogenic process). Genistein, one of the phytoestrogens, also inhibits cancer-related enzymes, including those needed in signal transduction, angiogenesis,[129] and cell growth.[130,131] In addition to phytoestrogens, soy foods contain other protease inhibitors—such as the Bowman Birk Inhibitor—that appear to have potent anticancer effects. It remains unclear whether a high-plant food diet lowers cancer risks because these bioactive substances inhibit carcinogenesis or because it is lower in animal food-related substances that promote cancer growth (including fat and toxic substances such as pyrogens, chemical compounds produced by heat in broiled meat).

Protein and Kidney Disease

Well-planned vegetarian diets are rarely deficient in protein. Both the type and amount of protein consumed on most vegetarian diets is adequate if a variety of plant protein foods are eaten over the course of a day. Complementary proteins do not have to be combined at the same meal to balance out each other's amino acid profile.[132,133]

The association between dietary protein intakes and chronic renal disease, especially in older individuals, has recently received attention. The original hypothesis was that among individuals with previously damaged kidneys, high protein intakes accelerated the course of chronic renal failure and thus restriction of protein would slow the progression to end-stage renal disease. Although there is some support for this hypothesis among those with kidney disease, definitive evidence is currently lacking. Among individuals with normal renal function, there is little evidence that the usual protein loads reduce kidney function or accelerate its deterioration.

Vegetarian and omnivorous diets do not necessarily differ in their protein content; but when therapeutic diets must be very low in protein, this can usually be accomplished more easily by reducing animal protein. Vegetarian diets have recently been reported as effective for treating nephrotic syndrome.[107] However, it is unclear if this is a unique effect of the vegetarian diet or rather whether it is due to the combined factors of low fat, low saturated fat, low cholesterol, moderate protein, and relatively high content of phytoestrogens in vegetarian diets. The use of vegetarian diets in renal disease has been recently reviewed.[134]

Atrophic Gastritis and Pernicious Anemia

Dietary vitamin B_{12} deficiency usually takes years to develop, but in the presence of diseases of the gut, it can develop in a period of months. The mental changes associated with B_{12} deficiency are often wrongly attributed to advancing age. The elderly are more likely to suffer from gastrointestinal diseases that may compromise absorption of vitamin B_{12}, including pernicious anemia (lack of intrinsic factor causing malabsorption of vitamin B_{12}) and atrophic gastritis (a condition of decreased acid secretion in the stomach, which decreases the solubilization of food-bound forms of the vitamin). Therefore, vitamin B_{12} status should be carefully monitored in all elders. This is especially true in older vegans, especially those who have been vegans for many years and who do not use B_{12} supplements or B_{12} fortified foods.

CONCLUSIONS

Vegetarian and omnivorous women have similar physiologies, and their health concerns are more alike than dissimilar. Therefore, the usual considerations about nutrition that apply to all women also apply to vegetarians.[135] Women can enjoy good health on vegetarian diets, including reduced risks of several chronic degenerative diseases, provided that they are careful to get enough of certain nutrients, especially calcium, iron, and vitamins D and B_{12}. Vegan vegetarian women, who avoid milk and eggs as well as meat, need to be especially careful, as do pregnant, lactating, ill, or elderly women on any form of vegetarian diet. Supplements are a simple way to ensure that such women are receiving adequate levels of all the nutrients, but they do not eliminate the need for careful dietary planning. Those who wish to avoid supplements can still boost their intake of potentially deficient nutrients by consuming fortified foods and/or foods that are especially rich in these nutrients.

References

1. Douglas A. *The Beast Within*. London: Chapman Publishers; 1993.

2. Candland DK. *Feral Children and Clever Animals: Reflections on Human Nature*. New York, NY: Oxford University Press; 1993.

3. Center for Animals and Public Policy. Tufts University School of Veterinary Medicine. *The Animal Policy Report: A Newsletter on Animal and Environmental Issues*. Grafton, Mass; 1993.

4. Krizmanic J. Here's who we are: a new survey reveals some surprises about America: 12 million plus (and counting) vegetarians. *Vegetarian Times*. October 1992.

5. National Live Stock and Meat Board. *Vegetarianism: Definition, Scope and Impact on the Meat Industry*. Chicago: National Livestock and Meat Board; 1992. Research Report no. 100–3.

6. Freeland-Graves JH, Greninger SA, Young RK. A demographic and social profile of age and sex matched vegetarians and nonvegetarians. *J Am Diet Assoc*. 1986;86:907–913.

7. Dwyer JT, Miller LG, Arduino NL et al. Mental age and IQ of predominantly vegetarian children. *J Am Diet Assoc*. 1980;76:142–147.

8. Dwyer JT, Loew FM. Nutritional risks of vegan diets to women and children: are they preventable? *J Agricultural Environ Ethics*. 1994;7(1):87–109.

9. American Dietetic Association. *Eating Well: The Vegetarian Way*. Chicago, Ill; 1992.

10. Hodgkin G, Maloney S, eds. *Diet Manual: Including a Vegetarian Meal Plan*. 7th ed. Loma Linda, Calif: Seventh Day Adventist Dietetic Association; 1990.

11. Wasserman D, Mangels R. *Simply Vegan*. Baltimore, Md: The Vegetarian Resource Group; 1991.

12. Mutch PB. Food guides for the vegetarian. *Am J Clin Nutr*. 1988;48:913–919.

13. Physicians' Committee for Responsible Medicine. *PCRM Update*. May-June 1991.

14. Gregoire L, Pugh R, Dwyer JT. *A Guide to Planning a Healthy Vegetarian Diet throughout Life*. Tampa, Fla: Health Information Network; 1994.

15. Haddad E. Meeting the RDAs with a vegetarian diet. *Top Clin Nutr*. 1995;10:7–16.

16. Robertson L, Flinders C, Ruppenthal B. *The New Laurel's Kitchen*. Berkeley, Calif: Ten Speed Press; 1986.

17. Baird P. *Quick Harvest: A Vegetarian's Guide to Microwave Cooking*. New York, NY: Prentice Hall Press; 1991.

18. Nasco, 901 Janesville Avenue, P.O. Box 90, Fort Atkinson, WI 53538–0901.

19. American Dietetic Association, 216 West Jackson Boulevard, Chicago, IL 60606-6995, phone 1-800-366-1655.

20. The Vegetarian Resource Group/Vegetarian Journal, Box 1463, Baltimore, MD 21203.

21. Akers K. *A Vegetarian Sourcebook*. Arlington, Va: Vegetarian Press; 1989.

22. Recker RR, Davies KM, Hinders SM, Heaney RP, Stegman MR, Kimmel OB. Bone gain in young adult women. *JAMA*. 1992;268(17):2403–2408.

23. Anderson JJ, Tylavsky FA, Haliona L, Metz JA. Determinants of peak bone mass in young adult women: a review. *Osteoporosis Int*. 1993;suppl 1;S32–36.

24. Mazess RB, Barden HS. Bone density in premenopausal women: effects of age, dietary intake, physical activity, smoking and birth control pills. *Am J Clin Nutr*. 1991;53:132–142.

25. Recker RR, Lapper JM, Davies KM, Kimmel OB. Change in bone mass immediately before menopause. *J Bone Miner Res*. 1992;7:857–862.

26. Centers for Disease Control. Recommendations for the use of folic acid to reduce the number of cases of spina bifida and other neural tube defects. *MMWR*. 1992;41:1–7.

27. Johnson PK. Counseling the pregnant vegetarian. *Am J Clin Nutr.* 1988;48:901–905.

28. National Research Council. *Alternative Dietary Practices and Nutritional Abuses in Pregnancy: Proceedings of a Workshop.* Report of the Committee on Nutrition of the Mother and Preschool Child, Food and Nutrition Board, Commission on Life Sciences. Washington, DC: National Academy Press; 1982.

29. Institute of Medicine, Subcommittee on Nutritional Status and Weight Gain during Pregnancy. *Nutrition during Pregnancy. Part I: Weight Gain. Part II: Nutrient Supplements.* Washington, DC: National Academy Press; 1990.

30. Fairbanks VF. Iron in medicine and nutrition. In: Shils ME, Olson JA, Shike ME, eds. *Modern Nutrition in Health and Disease, I.* 8th ed. Philadelphia, Pa: Lea & Febiger; 1994:185–211.

31. Repke JT, Villar J. Pregnancy induced hypertension and low birth weight: the role of calcium. *Am J Clin Nutr.* 1991;54:237S–241S.

32. Dwyer JT. Vegetarian diets in pregnancy and lactation: recent studies in North Americans. *J Can Diet Assoc.* 1983;44:26–34.

33. Elliot R. *Vegetarian Mother and Baby Book.* New York, NY: Pantheon Books; 1986.

34. Vegetarian Resource Group. *The Vegan Diet during Pregnancy, Lactation, and Childhood.* Baltimore, Md: Vegetarian Resource Group; 1991.

35. Dwyer JT. Nutritional implications of vegetarianism for children. In: Suskind RM, Lewinter-Suskind L, eds. *Textbook of Pediatric Nutrition.* 2nd ed. New York, NY: Raven Press; 1993.

36. Specker BL, Miller D, Norman EJ, Greene H, Hayes KC. Increased urinary methylmalonic acid excretion in breast fed infants of vegetarian mothers and identification of an acceptable dietary source of vitamin B-12. *Am J Clin Nutr.* 1988;47:89–92.

37. Specker BL, Tsang RD, Ho M, Miller D. Effect of vegetarian diet on serum 1,25 dihydroxyvitamin D_3 concentrations during lactation. *Obstet Gynecol.* 1987;70:870–874.

38. Finley DA. Effects of vegetarian diets upon the composition of human milk. In: Hamosh M, Goldman AS, eds. *Human Lactation: Maternal and Environmental Factors, II.* New York, NY: Plenum Press; 1986.

39. Havala S, Dwyer JT. Position of the American Dietetic Association: vegetarian diets (technical support paper). *J Am Diet Assoc.* 1988;88:352–355.

40. Dwyer JT. Nutritional status and alternative life-style diets, with special reference to vegetarianism in the US. In: Reichigal M, ed. *CRC Handbook of Nutritional Supplements, I: Human Use.* Boca Raton, Fla: CRC Series in Nutrition and Food; 1980:343–410.

41. Dwyer JT. Health aspects of vegetarian diets. *Am J Clin Nutr.* 1988;48:712–738.

42. Millet P, Guilland JC, Fuchs F, Klepping J. Nutrient intake and vitamin status of healthy French vegetarians and nonvegetarians. *Am J Clin Nutr.* 1989;50:718–727.

43. Havala S, Dwyer JT. Position of the American Dietetic Association: vegetarian diets. *J Am Diet Assoc.* 1993;93:1317–1319.

44. Dwyer JT. Vegetarian eating patterns: science, values, and food choices—where do we go from here? *Am J Clin Nutr.* 1994;59(suppl):1255–1262S.

45. Mills PK, Newell GR, Beeson WL, Fraser GE, Phillips RL. History of cigarette smoking and risk of leukemia and myeloma: results from the Adventist Health Study. *JNCI.* 1990;82:1832–1836.

46. Committee on Diet and Health. *Diet and Health: Recommendations to Reduce Chronic Disease Risk.* Washington, DC: National Academy Press; 1989.

47. Steinmetz KA, Kushi LH, Bostick RM, Folsom AT, Potter JD. Vegetables, fruit, and colon cancer in the Iowa Women's Health Study. *Am J Epidemiol.* 1994;139(1):1–15.

48. Trock B, Lanz E, Greenwald P. Dietary fiber, vegetables and colon cancer: critical review and meta-analyses of the evidence. *JNCI.* 1990;83:650–661.

49. Dwyer JT. Nutritional consequences of vegetarianism. *Ann Rev Nutr.* 1991;11:61–91.

50. Barger-Lux J. Nutritional correlates of low calcium intake. *Clin Appl Nutr.* 1992;2(4):39–44.

51. Fleming KH, Heimbach JR. Consumption of calcium in the US: Food sources and intake levels. *J Nutr.* 1994;124(8):1426S–1430S.

52. National Dairy Council. *Bone Health and Vegetarians.* Chicago, Ill; 1993.

53. Freeland-Graves J. Mineral adequacy of vegetarian diets. *Am J Clin Nutr.* 1988;48:859–862.

54. Food and Nutrition Board, Subcommittee on the Tenth Edition of the RDAs. *Recommended Dietary Allowances.* 10th ed. Washington, DC: National Academy Press; 1989.

55. Compston JE, Bhambani M, Laskey MA, Murphy S, Khaw KT. Body composition and bone mass in post menopausal women. *Clin Endocrinol.* 1992;37(5):426–431.

56. Haarbo J, Marslew U, Gotfredsen A, Christiansen C. Postmenopausal hormone replacement therapy prevents central distribution of body fat after menopause. *Metab Clin Exp.* 1991;40(12): 1323–1326.

57. Melby CL, et al. Blood pressure and body mass index in elderly long term vegetarians and non-vegetarians. *Nutr Rep Intl.* 1988;37:47–55.

58. Brants HA, Lowi MR, Westenbrink S, Hulshof KF, Kistemaker C. Adequacy of a vegetarian diet at old age: Dutch Nutrition Surveillance System. *J Am Coll Nutr.* 1990;9:292–302.

59. Gibson RS, Anderson GM, Sabry JH, et al. The trace metal status of a group of post-menopausal vegetarians. *J Am Diet Assoc.* 1983;82:246–250.

60. Dallman PR. Iron. In: Brown ML, ed. *Present Knowledge in Nutrition.* 6th ed. Washington, DC: Nutrition Foundation; 1990:206–209.

61. Worthington-Roberts BW, Breskiin MW, Monsen ER. Iron status of premenopausal women in a university community and its relationship to habitual dietary sources of protein. *Am J Clin Nutr.* 1988;47:275–279.

62. Herold PM, Kinsella JE. Fish oil consumption and decreased risk of cardiovascular disease. *Am J Clin Nutr.* 1986;43:566–598.

63. Herbert V. Everyone should be tested for iron disorders. *J Am Diet Assoc.* 1992;92:1502–1509.

64. Lauffer R. *Iron Balance.* New York, NY: St. Martin's Press; 1991.

65. Herbert V, Show S, Jayatilleke E, Stopler KT. Most free radical injury is iron-related: it is promoted by iron, hemin, holoferritin and vitamin C, and inhibited by disferoxamine and apoferritin. *Stem Cells.* 1994;12:289–303.

66. Heaney RP, Recker RR, Saville PO. Menopausal changes in calcium balance performance. *J Lab Clin Med.* 1978;92:953–963.

67. Sanchez TV, et al. Bone mineral mass in elderly vegetarian females. Paper presented at the Fourth International Conference on Bone Mineral Measurement, Toronto; 1978.

68. Tesar R, Notelvitz M, Shim E, et al. Axial and peripheral bone density and nutrient intakes of postmenopausal vegetarian and omnivorous women. *Am J Clin Nutr.* 1992;56:699–704.

69. Hunt IF, Murphy NJ, Henderson C. Bone mineral content in postmenopausal women: comparison of omnivores and vegetarians. *Am J Clin Nutr.* 1989;50(3):517–523.

70. Lloyd T, Schaefer JM, Walker MA, et al. Urinary hormonal concentrations and spinal bone densities of premenopausal vegetarian and nonvegetarian women. *Am J Clin Nutr.* 1991;54:1005–1010.

71. Abelow BJ, Holford TR, Insogna KL. Cross-cultural association between dietary animal protein and hip fracture: a hypothesis. *Calcif Tissue Int.* 1992;50:14–18.

72. Sandler RB, Slemenda CS, LaPorte RE. Postmenopausal bone density and milk consumption in childhood and adolescence. *Am J Clin Nutr.* 1985;42:270–274.

73. Hu JF, Zhao XH, Jia JB, et al. Dietary calcium and bone density among middle aged and elderly women in China. *Am J Clin Nutr.* 1993;58:219–227.

74. Zhao XH, Chen XS. Diet and bone density among elderly Chinese. *Nutr Rev.* 1992;50:395–397.

75. Orwoll E, Ware M, Stribrska L, et al. Effects of dietary protein deficiency on mineral metabolism and bone mineral density. *Am J Clin Nutr.* 1992;56:314–319.

76. Yuan YV, Kitts DD. Effect of dietary calcium intake and protein source on calcium utilization and bone biomechanics in the spontaneously hypertensive rat. *J Nutr Biochem.* 1992;3:452–460.

77. Lacey JM, Nderson JJ, Fugita T, et al. Correlates of cortical bone mass among premenopausal and postmenopausal Japanese women. *J Bone Miner Res.* 1991;6(7):651–660.

78. Baran D, Sorenson A, Grimes J, et al. Dietary modification with dairy products for preventing vertebral bone loss in premenopausal women: a three year prospective study. *J Clin Endocrinol Metab.* 1990;70(1): 264–270.

79. Holick MF. Vitamin D requirements for the elderly. *Clin Nutr.* 1986;5:121–129.

80. Recker RR, Bammi A, Barger-Lux MJ, Heaney RP. Calcium absorbability from milk products, and imitation milk, and calcium carbonate. *Am J Clin Nutr.* 1988;47:93–95.

81. Lewis NM, Marcus MS, Behling AR, Greger JL. Calcium supplements and milk: effects on acid base balance and on retention of calcium, magnesium, and phosphorus. *Am J Clin Nutr.* 1989;49: 527–533.

82. Sheikh MS, Santa Ana CA, Nicar MJ, Schiller LR, Fordtran JS. Gastrointestinal absorption of calcium from milk and calcium salts. *N Engl J Med.* 1987;317:532–536.

83. Russell R. Micronutrient requirements of the elderly. *Nutr Rev.* 1992;50(12):463–466.

84. Dawson-Hughes B, Dallal GE, Krall EA, Harris S, Sokoll LJ, Falconer G. Effect of vitamin D supplementation on wintertime and overall bone loss in healthy postmenopausal women. *Ann Intern Med.* 1991;115:505–512.

85. Krall EA, Sahyoun N, Tannenbaum S, Dallal GE, Dawson-Hughes B. Effect of vitamin D intake on seasonal variations in parathyroid hormone secretion in postmenopausal women. *N Engl J Med.* 1989;321:1777–1783.

86. Krall EA, Dawson-Hughes B. Relation of fractional calcium 47 retention to season and rates of bone loss in healthy postmenopausal women. *J Bone Miner Res.* 1991;6(12):1323–1330.

87. Moon J, Bandy B, Davison AJ. Hypothesis: etiology of atherosclerosis and osteoporosis. Are imbalances in the calciferol endocrine system implicated? *J Am Coll Nutr.* 1992;11(5):567–583.

88. Harris S, Dallal GE, Dawson-Hughes B. Influence of body weight on rates of change in bone density of the spine, hip and radius in postmenopausal women. *Calcif Tissue Intl.* 1992; 50(1):19–23.

89. Aloia JF, McGowan DM, Vaswanian RP, Cohn SH. Relationship of menopause to skeletal and muscle mass. *Am J Clin Nutr.* 1991;51:1378–1383.

90. Krall EA, Dawson-Hughes B. Smoking and bone loss among postmenopausal women. *J Bone Miner Res.* 1991;6(4):331–338.

91. Linkswiler HM, Joyce CL, Anand CR. Calcium retention of young adult males as affected by level of protein and of calcium intake. *Trans NY Acad Sci.* 1974;36(2):333–340.

92. Allen LH, Oddoye EA, Margen S. Protein induced hypercalciuria: a longer term study. *Am J Clin Nutr.* 1979;32:741–749.

93. Shuette SM, Linkswiler HM. Calcium. In: Brown ML, ed. *Present Knowledge in Nutrition.* 5th ed. Washington, DC: The Nutrition Foundation, Inc.; 1984.

94. Heaney RP. Protein intake and the calcium economy. *J Am Diet Assoc.* 1993;93:1259–1260.

95. Spencer H, Spencer H, Kramer L, Osis D, Norris C. Effect of a high protein (meat) intake on calcium metabolism in man. *Am J Clin Nutr.* 1978;32:2167–2180.

96. Spencer H, Kramer L, Rubio N, Osis D. The effect of phosphorus on endogenous fecal calcium excretion in man. *Am J Clin Nutr.* 1986;43:844–851.

97. Zemel MB, Schuette SA, Hegsted M, Linkswiler HM. Role of the sulfur containing amino acids in protein induced hypercalciuria in men. *J Nutr.* 1981;111:545–552.

98. Chait A, et al. Rationale of the Diet-Heart statement of the American Heart Association. Report of the Nutrition Committee. *Circulation.* 1993;88:3008–3029.

99. *Second Report of the Expert Panel on Detection, Evaluation and Treatment of High Blood Cholesterol in Adults.* Bethesda, Md: U.S. Department of Health and Human Services, Public Health Service, National Institutes of Health; 1993. NIH Publication 93-3095.

100. National Cholesterol Education Program. *Report of the Expert Panel on Population Strategies for Blood Cholesterol Reduction.* Bethesda, Md: U.S. Department of Health and Human Services, Public Health Service, National Institutes of Health; 1990. NIH Publication 90-3046.

101. National Cholesterol Education Program. *Report of the Expert Panel on Blood Cholesterol Levels in Children and Adolescents.* Bethesda, Md: U.S. Department of Health and Human Services, Public Health Service, National Institutes of Health; 1991. NIH Publication 92-2732.

102. Davey Smith G, Pekkanen G. Should there be a moratorium on the use of cholesterol lowering drugs? *BMJ.* 1992;304:431–434.

103. Whitten C. Vegetarian diets and ischemic heart disease. *Top Clin Nutr.* 1995;10(2):27–33.

104. Powell KE, Thompson PO, Casperson CJ, Kendrick JS. Physical activity and the incidence of coronary heart disease. *Annu Rev Public Health.* 1987;8:253–287.

105. Smith RL. *Diet, Blood Cholesterol and Coronary Heart Disease: A Critical Review of the Literature, II.* Vector Enterprises; 1991.

106. D'Amico G, Gentile MG, Manna G, et al. Effect of vegetarian soy diet on hyperlipidemia in nephrotic syndrome. *Lancet* 1992;339:1131–1134.

107. Dwyer JT. Vegetarian diets for treating nephrotic syndrome. *Nutr Rev.* 1993;51:44–46.

108. Clarke R, Daly L, Robinson K, et al. Hyperhomocysteinemia: an independent risk factor for vascular disease. *N Engl J Med.* 1991;324:1149–1155.

109. Stampfer MJ, Malinow MR, Willett WS, et al. A prospective study of plasma homocyst(e)ine and risk of myocardial infarction in US physicians. *JAMA.* 1992;268:877–881.

110. Ubbink JB, Vermaak WJ, van der Merwe A, Becker PT. Vitamin B_{12}, vitamin B_6 and folate nutritional status in men with hyperhomocysteinemia. *Am J Clin Nutr.* 1993;57:47–53.

111. The Fifth Report of the Joint National Committee on Detection, Evaluation, and Treatment of High Blood Pressure (JNC-V). *Arch Int Med.* 1993;53:154–183.

112. The Trials of Hypertension Prevention Collaborative Research Group. The effects of non-pharmacological interventions on blood pressure of persons with high normal levels: results of the Trials of Hypertension Prevention Phase I. *JAMA.* 1992;267:1213–1220.

113. Stamler R, Stamler J, Gosch FC, et al. Primary prevention of hypertension by nutritional hygienic means: final report of a randomized controlled trial. *JAMA.* 1989;262:1801–1807.

114. Hypertension Prevention Trial Research Group. The Hypertension Prevention Trial: three year effects of dietary changes on blood pressure. *Arch Int Med.* 1990;150:153–162.

115. INTERSALT Cooperative Research Group. INTERSALT: an international study of electrolyte excretion and blood pressure: result for 24-hour urinary sodium and potassium excretion. *BMJ.* 1988;297:319–328.

116. Law MR, Frost CD, Wald NJ. By how much does dietary salt reduction lower blood pressure? Analysis of observational data among populations. *BMJ.* 1991;302:811–815.

117. Mascoli S, Grimm R, Launer C, et al. Sodium chloride raises blood pressure in normotensive subjects: the study of sodium and blood pressure. *Hypertension.* 1991;17(suppl):21–26.

118. Langford HG, Blaufox MD, Oberman A. Dietary therapy slows the return of hypertension after stopping prolonged medication. *JAMA.* 1985;253:657–664.

119. MacMahon S. Alcohol consumption and hypertension. *Hypertension* 1987;9:111–121.

120. Arroll B, Beaglehole R. Does physical activity lower blood pressure: a critical review of the clinical trials. *J Clin Epidemiol.* 1992;45:439–477.

121. Pathak D, Whittemore AS. Combined effects of body size, parity and menstrual events on breast cancer incidence in seven countries. *Am J Epidemiol.* 1992;135:153–168.

122. Whittemore AS, Henderson B. Dietary fat and breast cancer: where are we? *JNCI.* 1993;85:762–765.

123. Astrup A, Buemann B, Christensen NJ, et al. The contribution of body composition, substrates, and hormones to the variability in energy expenditure and substrate utilization in premenopausal women. *J Clin Endocrinol Metab.* 1992;74(2):279–286.

124. Adlercreutz H, Hamalainen E, Gorback SL, Goldin BR, Woods MN, Dwyer JT. Diet and plasma androgens in postmenopausal vegetarian and omnivorous women and postmenopausal women with breast cancer. *Am J Clin Nutr.* 1989;49:433–442.

125. Block G, Patterson B, Subar A. Fruit, vegetables and cancer prevention: a review of the epidemiologic evidence. *Nutr Cancer.* 1993;18:1–29.

126. Steinmetz KA, Potter JD. Vegetables, fruit and cancer, part 1: epidemiology. *Cancer Causes Control.* 1991;2:359.

127. Cancer. In: *Surgeon General's Report on Nutrition and Health.* Washington, DC: U.S. Department of Health and Human Services, Public Health Service; 1988.

128. Swarner J. The vegetarian diet and cancer prevention. *Top Clin Nutr.* 1995;10(2):17–21.

129. Fotsis T, Pepper M, Adlercreutz H, et al. Genistein, a dietary derived inhibitor of in vitro angiogenesis. *Proc Natl Acad Sci.* 1993;90:2690–2694.

130. Messina MJ, Barnes S. The role of soy products in reducing risk of cancer. *JNCI.* 1991;83:542–546.

131. Martin PM, Horwitz KB, Ryan DS, McGuire WL. Phytoestrogen interaction with estrogen receptors in human breast cancer cells. *Endocrinology.* 1978;103:1860–1867.

132. Young VR, Pellet PL. Protein intake and requirements with reference to diet and health. *Am J Clin Nutr.* 1987;45:1323–1343.

133. Pellet PL. Protein requirements in humans. *Am J Clin Nutr.* 1990;51:723–737.

134. Pagenkemper J. The impact of vegetarian diets on renal disease. *Top Clin Nutr.* 1995;10(2):22–26.

135. Abrams B, Berrin C. Women, nutrition and health. *Curr Probl Obstet, Gynecol Fertil.* 1993;16:13–61.

9

Nutrition for the Female Athlete

Louise M. Burke

During the past two decades, women's participation in sports has increased. Women have been a part of the fitness boom that has witnessed the growth of many new recreational sports and exercise activities. At the elite level of competitive sport, the professionalism and preparation of the female athlete now rivals that of her male counterpart. Consequently, in many sports the gender differences in exercise performance have narrowed considerably.

The nutritional needs of the female athlete reflect special dietary issues related to training and competition, as well as gender-specific considerations. Although many people think that sports nutrition is about pre-event and postevent eating, for many athletes it is the training period that produces the most extreme nutritional requirements. Nevertheless, meeting specific nutritional challenges before, during, and after competition is also part of achieving a winning performance. Female athletes differ from their male counterparts by having a smaller body size and muscle mass, and consequently, lower energy requirements. Greater care may be needed to meet nutrient needs with a lower energy intake, particularly for iron and calcium for which the requirements of females exceed those of males.

This chapter deals with the nutritional needs for sport, with special emphasis on issues that are of major concern to females. Most studies related to exercise physiology/biochemistry or nutritional strategies that might enhance sports performance are conducted on male subjects. Therefore, although recommendations for optimal nutritional practices are presented, it is not clear whether females respond similarly. Nevertheless, these guidelines remain the most current advice available.

GOALS OF THE TRAINING DIET

The training program largely determines the nutritional needs of most athletes, because it is the main influence on energy expenditure. At the elite level, training

The assistance of Elizabeth Broad in the preparation of this manuscript is gratefully acknowledged.

is a daily commitment, with some athletes undertaking two or more sessions a day and some sessions lasting in excess of 2 hours. Such a training program not only affects the athlete's energy and nutrient requirements but also has a large impact on social and life-style factors, including dietary practices. Specific nutritional needs and life styles vary among sports and individuals; however, there are some nutritional goals that are common to all female athletes (Exhibit 9-1).

Although the achievement of sports nutrition goals summarized in this chapter may require some modification of the dietary patterns typical in most affluent countries, this can be done without resorting to extreme dietary changes and the exclusion of all favorite foods. Moderation and variety are key elements in preserving not only nutritional adequacy but also the pleasures derived from food and eating. Many female athletes appear at risk of replacing dietary flexibility and enjoyment with dietary extremism and frustration. This problem arises most often in relation to body fatness goals and is discussed below. For many female athletes, however, the first step to improving nutrition is to affirm that food plays several essential functions and is important to our emotional as well as physical well-being.

In many countries, dietary guidelines not only address nutrient adequacy but also deal with long-term health and disease prevention.[1,2] Such guidelines recommend a reduced intake of fats and oils, increased intake of nutritious carbohydrate and fiber-rich foods, and moderate use of salt, sugar, and alcohol. These principles are congruent with what is recommended for optimal nutrition in athletes.

NUTRIENT INTAKES OF FEMALE ATHLETES

Dietary intake varies markedly between groups of athletes and, in some cases, within groups according to the time of the competitive year (Appendix 9-A).

Exhibit 9-1 Goals for the Training Diet

- To enjoy food and the pleasure of social eating opportunities
- To achieve and maintain an appropriate body weight and body fat level by balancing energy intake and exercise
- To achieve basic nutrient requirements, including any increase in requirements that arise from a strenuous exercise program
- To promote recovery and adaptation between training sessions by providing a suitable nutritional environment
- To incorporate nutritional practices that promote long-term health and reduce the risk of chronic diseases of affluent countries
- To experiment with intended competition practices so that beneficial strategies can be identified and familiarization and habituation can occur

Results must be interpreted cautiously due to limitations in dietary assessment methodologies,[3] especially the issue of validity (i.e., the extent to which the data reflect usual intake). In general, the results of these studies indicate that most groups of female athletes have adequate nutrient intakes and appear to eat better than sedentary women both in terms of macronutrient and micronutrient goals.[3] However, some groups and individuals, especially those who are focused on achieving or maintaining a low body fat appear to consume low total energy intakes, which may not meet the energy cost of their training program. Such low energy intakes predispose to nutrient intakes that do not meet Recommended Dietary Allowances (RDA) levels. Specific issues are discussed below.

ISSUES OF BODY FAT

It might sound incongruous that an athlete could be overfat, but in some situations, this is the case. Body weight and fatness are related to genetics that help determine athletic pursuits, as well as changes achieved through the conditioning effect of high-level training and diet. Three patterns of body weight and fatness found among sports have been suggested.[4] The first pattern involves sports that are essentially passive and based largely on skill (e.g., golf, archery, bowling). In these sports, performance is largely independent of body fatness. Because sports activity in these athletes, however lengthy, requires a low-to-moderate energy expenditure, it may not contribute significantly to energy balance. Both selection and conditioning factors tend to permit higher body fat levels in such athletes. Decisions to reduce body fat levels are often made for improvements in health, general fitness, and appearance rather than a direct improvement in performance.

The second category involves sports with specific weight divisions for competition, and includes weightlifting, lightweight rowing, and judo. Overall, competition weight divisions (commonly ranging from two to ten divisions) are intended to match opponents of similar size and strength to promote fair competition. However, in these sports, most competitors attempt to compete in a weight division that is below their typical training weight, trying to gain an advantage over a smaller, lighter opponent. Short-term weight loss is often achieved over the days leading up to the event, using techniques such as dehydration through forced sweating (e.g., saunas or exercise in heavy clothes), severe food restriction, and the use of diuretics and laxatives.

Weight fluctuations are often rapid, frequent, and large. These "making weight" practices have been well studied in male athletes[5-7] but rarely in females; nevertheless, they undoubtedly also occur in female weight-matched sports. Female body builders[8] practice similar techniques in "cutting up" immediately before competition. They believe that they will increase muscle definition by minimizing subcutaneous fat cover and by making dehydrated skin tissue appear "paper thin."

The final category involves sports in which low body mass, and in particular, low body fatness are considered necessary for optimum performance. The advantages of low body fat levels include physical and mechanical gains, whereby decreases in body fat cause an increased "power to weight" ratio, or simply a reduced amount of "dead weight" that must be moved by the athlete. This is a particular advantage in sports such as distance running, triathlons, and road cycling in which the athlete transports her own body weight and in hill cycling and jumping events in which the athlete must move vertically against greater gravity effects. However, low body fat levels are also important for values of aesthetics and appearance in sports such as diving, gymnastics, and figure skating. Some studies have reported that, within a certain sport, there is a strong negative correlation between body fatness and performance.[9]

The contribution of body fatness to performance varies according to the nature of the performance and the conditions in which it is undertaken.[10] What constitutes an "ideal" body physique remains a matter of speculation. However, it is generally assumed that those who excel in a sport will exhibit the characteristics that promote optimal performance. Thus, most of the information currently used to identify body fat and body weight goals for females in various sports is provided by anthropometric studies in elite female athletes.[11,12] However, there is a danger inherent in using this information to establish rigid body fat prescriptions for specific athletic groups and individuals. There is considerable variability in body characteristics and body fat levels between elite athletes in the same sport; moreover, statistical relationships between body fatness and performance do not always apply to individual athletes. Instead, it is preferable to use a range of acceptable values for each sport and then to monitor the health and performance of the individual athlete within this range. Sequential monitoring of body fat levels over several seasons should allow each athlete to determine her individual "optimal" body weight and body fat levels and even to set varying goals for different times of the training and competition season. The optimal body fat level for an athlete should be obtained from her individual history and should include criteria that consider both health and performance (Exhibit 9-2).

Exhibit 9-2 Criteria for Setting Ideal Body Fat Levels for Female Athletes

1. To be associated with (consistent) good performances
2. To promote good health in the athlete—including the absence of "underweight" or overtraining and the maintenance of a regular menstrual cycle
3. To allow the athlete to consume adequate energy and nutrients to achieve all other nutritional goals for good health and performance

Although some athletes easily achieve body composition that is suited to their sports, others may need to manipulate characteristics such as muscle mass or body fat levels through changes in diet and training. It is important that athletes identify suitable and realistic goals, take appropriate measures to achieve the desired changes in a reasonable time period, and have an appropriate means of measuring the results. Guidelines for facilitating loss of body fat are summarized in Exhibit 9-3. Measurements of body weight cannot distinguish between muscle mass or body fatness, yet many female athletes, like females in the general community, often judge the suitability of their size and body composition by this simple measure. Athletes might be advised that the only valuable use of scales is to determine short-term changes in hydration (e.g., to weigh before and after a training session) and thus estimate water losses from sweat that must be replaced.[13]

Much has been written about the pros and cons of the various methods of body composition assessment in athletes,[14–16] with the available techniques including underwater weighing (hydrodensitometry), determination of subcutaneous fat with calipers, bioelectrical impedance analysis, or dual energy x-ray absorptiometry. The criteria for choosing a technique include validity and reliability within the typical body composition ranges of the athlete, expense, ease of access within the athlete's life style, and the availability of normative-descriptive data to describe favorable characteristics in various sports. Sequential monitoring of the individual athlete should play an important role in determining the athlete's goals and observing her success in achieving them. Care should be taken with all techniques to maximize the reliability and validity of readings and to interpret the results carefully in the light of residual error.

Many athletes have problems in choosing safe and realistic targets for optimal body fatness. Athletes in "aesthetic" sports (e.g., gymnastics, diving, figure skating) frequently find a mismatch between their desired body fat levels and their energy expenditure; in these sports, very low body fat levels are considered necessary for optimal performance, yet training, although lengthy, involves only short bursts of high-intensity work. Even though athletes in high energy expenditure sports (e.g., distance running, cycling, triathlon, swimming) may be assisted by both their selection and training to achieve low body fat levels, many individuals still consider themselves overfat. At present, it is fashionable among some athletic groups to try to achieve minimum body fat levels. The pressure to set these goals may come from several sources. Athletes by nature can be compulsive and obsessive. The same traits that encourage good sports performance in many athletes—perfectionism, dedication, ability to set a narrow focus—may lead to false expectations and preoccupation with body fatness. Parents, peers, trainers, and coaches are often guilty of providing pressure and misguided expectations.[17,18] Female athletes are particularly vulnerable due to the general dissatisfaction of females with their body shape, as well as the biologic predisposition for higher levels of body fatness than similarly trained males.

Exhibit 9-3 Guidelines for Fat Loss for the Athlete

Identify individual "ideal" body fat and body weight targets that are consistent with good health and performance and are achievable.

In some sports, it may be sensible to organize different targets for different times of the sporting season.

If loss of body fat is required, plan for a realistic rate loss of about 0.5 kg/ wk.

If a substantial loss is to be undertaken, set both short-term and long-term goals.

Examine your current exercise and activity plans.

If your training is primarily skill- or technique-based or is based on brief sessions of very high-intensity exercise, then you may benefit from scheduling in some aerobic exercise activities that will encourage fat oxidation. This should always be done in conjunction with your coach and/or nutritionist. Look also for ways to increase energy expenditure in your daily life style (e.g., walking, using stairs, etc.). Many athletes are almost sedentary between training sessions.

Keep a food diary for a period (e.g., a week) so that you can take an objective look at what really goes into your mouth.

Many athletes who think that they "hardly eat anything" will be amazed at their actual food intake.

Reduce your typical energy intake by an amount that is appropriate to produce loss of body fat (e.g., 500–1000 kcal/day) but still ensures an adequate food and nutrient intake.

Do not decrease below 1200–1500 kcal/day unless supervised by a sports dietitian/nutritionist. Cut back on unnecessary energy intake. Do not skip meals; rather spread food intake over the day, particularly to allow for efficient refueling after training sessions.

Combat situations in which you generally overeat.

Make meals filling by choosing high-fiber forms of foods; fight the need to finish everything on your plate; spread food intake over the day so that you do not approach meals feeling extreme hunger.

Focus on opportunities to reduce intake of fats and oils.

Choose low-fat versions of nutritious protein foods; minimize added fats and oils in cooking and food preparation; and enjoy high-fat snacks and sweet foods as occasional treats rather than everyday foods.

Be prudent with alcohol and sugar.

These contribute calories but no micronutrients.

Focus on nutrient-rich foods.

You will need to meet your nutrient needs from fewer calories. Consider a broad-range low-dose vitamin/mineral supplement if you will be restricting your intake below 1500 kcal/day (6.4 MJ/day) for prolonged periods.

Be aware of inappropriate eating behavior.

This includes eating when bored or upset or eating too quickly. Redirect your stress or boredom to alternative activities.

Be wary of supplements that promise weight loss.

There are no special pills, potions, or products that produce safe and effective weight loss. If something sounds too good to be true, it probably is.

Consult a sports dietitian/nutritionist or a registered dietitian.

A dietitian can help if you are having difficulties with your weight loss goals or would like a supervised program. Expert advice is needed if you are struggling with an eating disorder or disordered eating behavior.

Cross-sectional surveys of the attitudes and self-reported practices of various groups of female athletes report that many are concerned about their weight and fatness and are dieting to reduce body fat levels.[19,20] These issues appear to be more common in sports in which weight and body fatness are important for performance. In addition to low-energy and fad diets, female athletes may resort to pathogenic weight loss techniques such as fasting, dehydration strategies, purging, and the use of diuretics and laxatives. Many studies report a higher prevalence of eating disorders or disordered eating behaviors and body perceptions among female athletes in weight/fatness-concerned sports than would be expected in the general community or than that observed in control groups.[19,20] It is difficult to determine the true prevalence of eating disorders among athletes; reports vary from less than 1 to 50% of athletic populations according to the type of athletes involved and the method used to assess eating disorders.[19]

The minimum "healthy" level of body fat remains somewhat nebulous and is better set at the individual level. Meanwhile, the female athlete should recognize the disadvantages of achieving (or trying to achieve) excessively low body fat levels. These include both direct consequences to the body (e.g., loss of body warmth and protective padding) as well as the indirect consequences of the strategies used to achieve the weight loss (e.g., chronic inadequate energy/nutrient intake, excessive training, psychological dysfunction). Evidence has accumulated for many years, both anecdotally and from dietary surveys, that a significant number of female athletes struggle to keep body fat levels low while reporting energy requirements that seem to be "less than they deserve."[21] Many dietary studies of female endurance athletes have reported an energy balance oddity—energy intakes that are too low to match energy expenditure from training.[22-24] Although this has been dismissed by some as an artifact of poor dietary survey methodology,[25] others have argued that the low intakes are often so striking and seem so consistent across studies that some attention to them is merited.[4]

In reviewing the weight control practices of athletes, Brownell and coworkers[4] discuss the setpoint theory of body fat maintenance.[26] They propose that female athletes may induce some complex metabolic changes when they reduce body fat below the natural level that their body wishes to defend or when there is loss of body fat from critical body stores (e.g., buttocks, thighs). They suggest that a decrease in metabolic rate and/or an increase in food efficiency could result from the chronic restriction of food intake and the maintenance of body fat below the natural or regulated level. There may be some implications for menstrual function. These theories[3] remain speculative and offer no cure for affected athletes other than a reassessment of goals. However, prevention of the problem would seem to be best served by safe and conservative methods of body fat loss. A more extensive review of issues of eating, body weight, and sports performance can be found elsewhere.[27]

NUTRIENT NEEDS

Carbohydrate

A goal for all athletes is to eat adequate carbohydrate to meet the fuel needs of their exercise program. Replacing muscle and liver glycogen stores between sessions is particularly challenging when there may be only 8 to 24 hours between training sessions. An athlete who is training intensively needs to follow a special food plan to meet carbohydrate needs for optimal recovery, because typical Western eating patterns may not provide adequate carbohydrate. Failure to consume sufficient carbohydrate to match the demands of training may lead to chronically depleted muscle and liver glycogen stores. This can interfere with optimal training performance and adaptation, although it is hard to find studies that consistently support this hypothesis.[28] Nevertheless, it remains prudent to promote high-carbohydrate eating for athletes, particularly those in heavy training.

Factors involved in the rate of muscle glycogen resynthesis after prolonged exercise[29,30] include the presence of muscle damage, the severity of glycogen depletion, and dietary carbohydrate intake. Eating carbohydrate soon after exercise may be a useful strategy in promoting recovery; the early provision of substrate to the depleted muscle hastens the restoration of muscle glycogen, and there is some evidence that the rate of glycogen storage is slightly enhanced during the first 1 to 2 hours postexercise.[31]

Nutrition guidelines for the athlete in general training recommend that carbohydrate intake should be increased above the levels currently typical of the Western diet (i.e., to above 55% of total energy intake) and that this should be achieved principally by increasing the consumption of nutritious carbohydrate and fiber-containing foods.[32] In the case of the endurance training athlete, carbohydrate intake guidelines have been set to maximize the capacity for daily glycogen restoration. These recommendations have been made both on the basis of absolute carbohydrate intake (8 to 10 g/kg body mass per day[33]) or as a contribution to total energy intake (65 to 70% of total energy[34]). Although an increased focus on carbohydrate-rich foods is important for athletes with heavy fuel requirements, in real life, absolute carbohydrate intakes of 8 to 10 g/kg (400 to 500 g/day) may not be feasible within the energy intake restrictions of many female endurance athletes. The mean carbohydrate intake of most groups of female athletes (see Appendix 9-A) is within the range of 250 to 400 g/day, or approximately 5 to 8 g/kg/day. However, some groups and individuals appear to be consuming less than 5 to 6 g carbohydrate/kg/day.

An increased intake of carbohydrate-rich foods should be promoted, particularly in athletes. The benefits of better training due to optimal glycogen stores may entice some female athletes to liberalize their total energy and carbohydrate intakes a little. The focus on nutrient-dense carbohydrate-rich foods may help athletes meet requirements for other nutrients simultaneously. Nevertheless, refined-carbohydrate foods offer the advantages of being compact and pleasant to eat and can provide a useful but smaller contribution to the athlete's total carbo-hydrate intake. These attributes may be appreciated most during or immediately postexercise. Guidelines for high carbohydrate eating are summarized in Exhibit 9-4, and sources of carbohydrate-rich foods are listed in Table 9-1.

Calcium and the Female Athlete Triad

Interest in the calcium status of female athletes has intensified, with recent studies reporting low bone density and stress fractures in various groups. The concern over reduced calcium status in athletes should include consideration of menstrual function and estrogen status of these athletes, because of the relation-ship between secondary amenorrhea and reduced bone density.[35] Surveys of the prevalence of secondary amenorrhea in female athletes vary due to differences in the definition of amenorrhea and differences in the caliber of athletes studied. However, it is generally agreed that young, intensively training athletes are at greater risk of developing amenorrhea and other disturbances of the menstrual cycle than sedentary women and that chronic exercise is either directly or indi-rectly responsible.[36]

Exhibit 9-4 Guidelines for a High-Carbohydrate Training Diet

Base meals and snacks around nutritious carbohydrate foods:
- whole-grain breads and breakfast cereals
- rice, pasta, noodles, and other grain foods
- fruits
- starchy vegetables (e.g., potatoes, corn)
- legumes (lentils, beans, soy-based products)
- sweetened dairy products (e.g., fruit-flavored yogurt, fruit smoothies)

These foods should occupy at least half of the room on your plate.

Use compact sugar and sugar-based foods wisely—add to a nutritious high-carbohydrate meal when energy needs are high, or consume when needed during and after exercise.

Eat a high-carbohydrate meal or snack within 15–30 minutes of lengthy training sessions to speed glycogen recovery.

Consume carbohydrate during lengthy training and competition sessions when additional fuel is needed. Sports drinks meet fluid and carbohydrate needs simultaneously.

Table 9-1 Carbohydrate-Rich Food Sources

Approximately 15 g of carbohydrate is supplied by the following foods:		
Cereals	Bread	1 thick slice (40 g) or 1/2 average roll (35 g)
	English muffin/bagel	1/2 average (35 g)
	Breakfast cereal	20 g = 1/2–2/3 cup flakes
	Rolled oats	1/4 cup (20 g)
	Untoasted muesli, granola	1/4 cup (20 g)
	Oatmeal, cream of wheat	3/4 cup cooked (180 g)
	Pancakes	30 g (= 1/2 average size)
	Whole meal cake/muffin	25 g = 1/2 to 1/3 average slice or muffin
	Crackers	25 g (4–6 crackers)
	Popcorn	20 g = 1 cup
	Rice	1/3 cup cooked (50 g)
	Pasta/noodles	1/2 cup cooked (60 g)
Vegetables	Potatoes	80 g cooked (1 medium or 1/3 cup mashed)
	Carrots/pumpkin/peas	300 g cooked (1/5 cup)
	Corn	70 g cooked (1/2 cup)
Legumes	Kidney/soy beans	1/3 cup cooked (80 g)
	Baked beans	3/5 cup (150 g)
	Lentils	1/3 cup cooked (80 g)
Fruit	Fresh fruits	100–150 g piece = medium apple or orange, small banana, 3/4 cup cherries/grapes
	Juice	120 mL sweetened
		180 mL unsweetened
	Dried fruit	20 g
	Canned fruit/fruit salad	1/2 cup sweetened
		1 cup unsweetened
Dairy products	Skim milk	300 mL
	Nonfat plain or fruit-flavored yogurt	100 g (1/2 carton)
	Low-fat ice cream/frozen yogurt	100 g
Sugary foods	Sugar	15 g (2 heaped teaspoons)
	Jam and honey	20 g (tablespoon)
	Candy	15–20 g
Drinks	Soda	150 mL
	Sports drinks	200–250 mL
	Liquid meal drinks	100 mL
	Fruit smoothies	100–150 mL
	Carbo-loader drinks	100 mL

Many causes of menstrual dysfunction in female athletes have been suggested (Exhibit 9-5). However, studies[37] have been unable to prove a consistent link with any factor across all sports. Many studies have also failed to demonstrate that low body fat levels per se or "critical body fat" levels are a universal cause of amenorrhea in athletes,[38–40] although there is an increased incidence of amenorrhea among groups of athletes who tend to be light and lean (e.g., runners and dancers). Other suggested causes are rapid changes in body fat or the depletion of specific body fat stores that are critical for the sustenance of pregnancy and lactation.[4] As noted, the body may adapt metabolically to defend some level of body fat. This hypothesis is supported by reports from dietary surveys that amenorrheic runners consume less energy per kilogram body mass than eumenorrheic runners or controls, often despite similar or greater training distances (Table 9-2). Whether these data reflect metabolic adaptations in amenorrheic runners or result from inadequate dietary data collection continues to be a topic of debate.

Generally, differences in the nutrient intakes of amenorrheic and normally menstruating athletes (see Table 9-2) can be explained by differences in energy intakes. However, vegetarianism[41] and eating disorders[42] per se stand out as strong dietary risk factors for disturbed menstrual function. Indeed, the term female athlete triad has been coined to describe the interrelation or concurrence of disordered eating, amenorrhea, and osteoporosis in female athletes,[43,44] and steps are being taken to promote recognition, prevention, and treatment of one or more of the medical disorders involved.[44]

The observations of reduced bone density in female athletes with menstrual dysfunction at first seems a paradox, because weight-bearing exercise is known as a potent stimulator for bone accretion.[45] However, it appears that in the pres-

---

Exhibit 9-5 Suggested Causes of Menstrual Dysfunction in Female Athletes

- Low body weight
- Low body fat levels
- Sudden decrease in body weight or body fat levels
- Loss of key body fat deposits
- Inadequate energy intake
- Excess fiber intake
- Low fat intake
- Vegetarianism
- Eating disorders
- Excess training or sudden increase in training intensity/frequency/duration
- Type of training
- Stress/emotional upsets
- Delayed age of menarche
- Prior menstrual irregularities before training

Table 9-2 Comparison of Dietary Intake in Amenorrheic and Eumenorrheic Runners

Study	Subjects	Body Mass Index	Dietary Method	Energy Intake (kJ)	CHO (g)	Protein (g)	Fat (g)
Eumenorrheic group							
Nelson et al[24]	17	20.3	3-day record	9430	263	55	84
Bruemmer and Drinkwater[113]	45	20.6	3-day record	8055	250	72	68
Marcus et al[23]	6	20.0	3-day record	7185	72		
Myerson et al[114]	10		6-day record	8105			
Drinkwater et al[22]	14	21.3	3-day record	8235	255	66	79
Weighted mean:		20.6		8200	254 (52%)	67 (14%)	75 (34%)
Amenorrheic group							
Nelson et al[24]	11	20.4	3-day record	7250	196	42	64
Bruemmer and Drinkwater[113]	30	19.8	3-day record	7020	237	69	51
Marcus et al[23]	11	18.7	3-day record	5330		49	
Myerson et al[114]	7		6-day record	7250			
Drinkwater et al[22]	14	19.7	3-day record	6800	222	66	57
Weighted mean:		19.7		6730	225 (55%)	61 (15%)	55 (30%)

Source: Reprinted with permission from Progress in Food and Nutrition Science (1987;11:307–361), Copyright © 1987, Elsevier Science Ltd.

ence of chronic hypoestrogenism, exercise cannot reverse the significant loss of calcium from trabecular bone, particularly in the spine. It is possible that while training may halt the loss or even increase the bone mineral density of trabecular sites that are directly exercised, there is significant loss of total body bone mineral density and of bone density at sites that are not directly involved in weight-bearing exercise.[46] Cortical bone seems better protected against loss of bone mineral.

Although dietary factors such as high intakes of phosphorus, alcohol, sodium, caffeine, and protein may promote increased calcium excretion, low calcium intake is an obvious problem.[47] Nutritional surveys of female athletes such as runners, gymnasts, and dancers have reported calcium intakes below the RDAs.[23,48–50] Thus, it seems probable that some amenorrheic athletes contribute to their loss of bone mass by consuming a diet that is inadequate in calcium intake. Dietary risk factors for inadequate calcium intake include low total energy intake, the presence of disordered eating, and poor dietary variety—particularly the exclusion of dairy products. Food strategies that promote calcium intake in conjunction with other dietary goals for the female athlete are presented in Exhibit 9-6.

It has been speculated that reduced bone density may have both short-term and long-term consequences on health and athletic performance. Whether reduced bone density is directly related to stress fractures in athletes remains a point of

---

Exhibit 9-6 High-Calcium Eating for the Athlete

The following represent low-fat, high-carbohydrate food ideas.

- Breakfast cereal and low-fat milk
- Fruit salad and low-fat yogurt
- Frozen yogurt and special ice-desserts (low-fat brands)
- Sardines on whole-meal toast (rinse oil from sardines)
- Whole-grain salad sandwich with salmon filling (include the bones!)
- Macaroni and cheese (sauce made with low-fat milk and reduced-fat cheese)
- Banana smoothie (low-fat milk with banana and low-fat ice cream/yogurt)
- Whole-grain toast with "creamy" vegetable soup (skim milk or skim milk powder added to soup)
- Stir-fried tofu and vegetables with rice
- Salmon or tuna casserole (include the bones) served with rice or noodles
- Calcium-fortified orange juice

Note: All cooking is done with minimal added oils or fat; many low-fat milks are fortified with extra calcium. Calcium-fortified orange juice and bread are good sources of low-fat, high-carbohydrate, calcium-rich foods.

controversy. Although bone strength is related to bone density, the incidence of stress fractures will also be influenced by the stress load or trauma experienced by the bones—making factors such as training load, biomechanical factors, training surfaces, and equipment (e.g., shoes) equally important. Indeed, a study of elite Australian athletes reported that the incidence of stress fractures was largely independent of bone mineral density.[51] However, this and other studies[23,52] have reported a significant correlation between stress fractures and amenorrhea among female athletes. The long-term consequences of reduced bone density in athletes is even more speculative in that its large-scale occurrence is too recent for any effect on aging and osteoporosis to be noted. However, it seems plausible that athletes who enter menopause with an already reduced bone density would be expected to reach the bone's "critical fracture threshold" earlier. Preliminary work suggests that the restoration of menstrual function in amenorrheic runners can lead to an increase in bone density[53] and that early intervention is important, because trabecular bone loss from untreated amenorrhea of long duration (as little as 3 years) may be irreversible.[54]

Stress fractures, reduced bone density, and amenorrhea must be viewed carefully, because they can occur both as separate or related problems in female athletes. The prevention and management of each issue must continue to be highly specific and individual, taking into account the mixed etiology of each problem. However, it is likely that menstrual dysfunction will underlie many cases of osteoporosis and that the problem of negative calcium balance in this situation is one of estrogen deficiency rather than a primary calcium deficiency. The cornerstone of management is either the restoration of menses (sometimes made possible by increasing body fat levels or reduction of training load) or estrogen replacement (oral contraceptives). Whether high-dose calcium supplementation is useful as an adjunct to hormone therapy in treating or preventing bone loss remains speculative; however, laboratory trials have reported that a daily intake of 1500 mg of calcium is needed to maintain calcium balance in an estrogen-deprived state of menopause.[55] Many female athletes need dietary counseling to ensure nutritional status that will maintain both menstrual and bone integrity. This may include advice to correct low energy intake, suboptimal intake of nutrients including calcium, and disordered eating behavior.

Iron Status and Sports Anemia

Iron status is crucially involved in exercise performance because of the role of iron in oxygen transport (myoglobin and hemoglobin) and aerobic energy production (cytochromes and other ferro-enzymes). Inadequate iron nutriture may therefore reduce exercise performance.[56,57] There is a lack of consensus among sports scientists on many issues related to iron—for example, the cut points for the hematologic/biochemical parameters of "optimal iron status," whether iron deficiency without anemia impairs exercise performance, and how to distinguish reduced iron status from exercise-mediated changes in iron metabolism. Nevertheless, it is believed that some athletes are at risk of low iron status due to increased iron requirements (to cover menstrual losses, growth, pregnancy), increased iron losses due to exercise (red blood cell trauma, sweat loss of iron, gastrointestinal blood loss), and poor dietary intake of bioavailable iron. In fact, females, particularly during adolescence and pregnancy, have increased iron requirements compared with males and represent a high-risk group for poor iron status. Iron losses resulting from heavy endurance training may increase daily requirements by a further 50 to 100%.[57]

The dietary iron intake of females is already lower than that of males by virtue of lower energy intake and will be clearly compromised in cases of long-term energy intake restrictions. Because the non-heme form of iron present in foods of plant origin is poorly absorbed, female athletes who are vegetarian or semivegetarian (i.e., those on very high-carbohydrate or Pritikin-style diets) may find that their diets are very poor sources of bioavailable iron.

The solution to this problem includes recognition of female athletes as a high-risk group for reduced iron status, with attention to chronic dieters, endurance athletes in heavy training, and adolescent and pregnant athletes as populations for special focus. Such groups should be monitored for early detection of reduced iron status.

Prevention or treatment may include iron supplementation, but this should be part of a clinical management decision for the individual athlete rather than a mass supplementation program. Management plans may also include strategies to reduce excessive iron losses and, most important, education to improve dietary iron intake. Iron-rich foods containing the better absorbed heme iron include red meat, shellfish, and the darker cuts of poultry. The nonheme iron in iron-fortified breakfast cereals, whole grains, legumes, and green leafy vegetables can be made more absorbable by consuming a food source of ascorbic acid at the same meal (e.g., red/green peppers, citrus fruits, berries) and by reducing absorption-inhibiting factors such as tannin (tea) and phytates (excess bran fiber). The most valuable dietary advice for the female athlete is that which ties together several nutritional goals. Exhibit 9-7 summarizes food ideas that provide a valuable source of absorbable iron while simultaneously achieving reduced fat (and kilocalories) and high-carbohydrate goals.

Supplements

Whether athletes have increased requirements for protein and micronutrients and whether increased intakes of these nutrients will improve athletic perfor-

Exhibit 9-7 Iron-Rich Eating for the Athlete

The following represent low-fat, high-carbohydrate food ideas.

Including heme iron sources
- Lean beef or lamb kebabs and rice
- Pasta and meat sauce (extra-lean ground beef)
- Meat lasagne (extra-lean ground beef, reduced-fat cheese)
- Pasta and marinara sauce (seafood including mussels, oysters)
- Chinese beef (lean) and vegetable stir-fry with noodles
- Lean roast beef and salad sandwich
- Chilli con carne (lean beef and kidney bean stew) with rice

Including nonheme iron sources complemented with vitamin C foods
- Breakfast cereal (iron-fortified brand) and low-fat milk + vitamin C fruit (e.g., berries, tropical fruit, citrus fruit)
- Baked beans on toast with glass of orange juice
- Pasta with tomato-based vegetable sauce, including kidney beans or other legumes
- Lentil burgers and salad (tomato, green/red pepper) with whole-grain roll
- Spinach omelet (made with egg substitutes or less egg yolk) with tomato and parsley and rice
- Fig bar cookies and glass of orange juice

mance continues to be a point of controversy between and among athletes and sports scientists. It is generally agreed that increased energy intake due to increased energy requirement, in conjunction with a variety of nutritious food choices, will provide the athlete with nutrient intakes well in excess of the RDAs. Female athletes at highest risk of inadequate nutrient intake are those with low energy intakes (e.g., those on chronic weight loss or maintenance diets) and those who limit their food variety (e.g., those with eating disorders, and those following vegetarian, fad, and other restrictive diets).

Comprehensive reviews of protein research[58,59] have identified the following major mechanisms by which protein requirements are increased by exercise:

- the contribution of protein catabolism to the fuel requirements of exercise
- a positive nitrogen balance during periods of heavy resistance training
- repair/recovery/adaptation needs after muscle damage, efflux of muscle enzymes, and production of new tissue compounds

Lemon[58] cites some evidence to support beneficial effects of very high protein intakes (greater than 2 g/kg/day) in strength athletes. However, estimates[25] and nitrogen balance studies[60,61] suggest that the protein requirements of heavily training athletes—both strength and endurance—are approximately 1.2 to 1.6 g/kg/day, provided that both carbohydrate and energy requirements are also met. Dietary surveys of a variety of athletic groups (see Table 9-2) show that with increased energy intakes and protein intakes of 12 to 15% of total energy intake, there seems little problem in reaching these targets.[62] Female athletes who chronically reduce their energy intakes are doubly at risk. Not only is total protein intake restricted by energy intake, but indirectly, inadequate energy intake and/or carbohydrate intake may increase protein requirements. A glycogen-depleted athlete will oxidize greater amounts of protein as a fuel substrate during prolonged exercise.[59] Also, as energy intake is reduced, greater protein intakes are required to maintain nitrogen balance.

The present consensus on vitamins is that studies have failed to support a beneficial effect of vitamin supplementation on athletic performance, except in the cases of a pre-existing vitamin deficiency.[63,64] Some female athletes may benefit from dietary counseling to increase energy intake and/or dietary variety and thus achieve the full nutrient intake potential from food sources. Nevertheless, problems remain for those who continue to be chronic low-energy consumers. In such cases, supplementation with a low-dose multivitamin/mineral supplement may be necessary.

Reviews of the supplementation practices of athletes show that approximately half the athletic population are current users of supplements including vitamins/minerals, special carbohydrate and multinutrient drinks, and products containing unusual substances such as ferulic acid, coenzyme Q10, free-form amino acids, and ginseng.[65,66] These products may be conveniently divided into two groups: dietary supplements that are concerned with meeting known nutritional or physiologic requirements, and nutritional ergogenic aids that propose a direct effect on exercise performance. Dietary supplements, which include products such as sports drinks, liquid meal supplements, and iron supplements, may provide a convenient or practical means for an athlete to achieve nutritional goals—particularly during and after exercise.[65] The case for sports drinks is discussed below. Although there is evidence of beneficial effects resulting from the use of caffeine, bicarbonate, and creatine in specific individuals or situations, research supporting the benefits of most of the nutritional ergogenic aids is limited.[66]

COMPETITION DIET

In addition to skill, success in sports performance may be determined by the capacity of the athlete to produce work or expend energy. An increasing understanding of the metabolism of exercise has allowed scientists to identify some of the factors that limit performance or cause fatigue. These factors may be seen as issues of impaired homeostasis (both at the cellular level and of the whole body) and of depletion of fuel substrates. Training produces several physiologic adaptations that allow the athlete to produce more work and to delay the onset of fatigue. Even so, the athlete should prepare for competition by understanding the factors that limit performance in her specific event and by taking steps to further reduce the effects of these factors.

In the next sections, dietary strategies for achieving the goals for optimal competition performance are discussed (Exhibit 9-8). These may include carbohydrate loading, pre-event eating, and fluid or food intake during an event. It is important that these strategies are practiced during the training phase, so that any problems can be identified and rectified before important competitions. Strategies such as eating and drinking during exercise may require plenty of practice in training to develop a successful plan and to become accustomed to the techniques. This will provide the athlete with confidence for competition and ensure better training performances. In some sports, athletes are aware of the importance of hydration and fuel needs in the competition setting but need encouragement to recognize these same needs in a training session.

Preparation for Competition

The normalization or recovery of liver and muscle glycogen levels between training sessions has already been set as a goal of everyday eating. Preparation for competition should extend this goal to ensure that body carbohydrate stores are able to match the anticipated fuel needs of the events. Normalized glycogen stores will be sufficient for most sports events, particularly "nonendurance"

Exhibit 9-8 Goals of the Competition Diet

1. To prepare adequate carbohydrate fuel stores in the precompetition phase
2. In weight-matched sports, to achieve the required competition weight division without sacrificing fuel stores or hydration level
3. During endurance events, to extend carbohydrate fuel availability by consuming additional carbohydrate during the event
4. To eat an appropriate pre-event meal
5. To prevent significant levels of dehydration, particularly by consuming fluids appropriately during the event
6. To avoid gastrointestinal discomfort during the event
7. To promote recovery after competition, particularly in sports involving events repeated over the same or successive days, or in events conducted on a weekly basis

sports, which are generally characterized as being of less than 60 minutes' duration of continuous exercise. This can be achieved by a high carbohydrate intake, in conjunction with an exercise taper, over the 24 to 36 hours pre-event. It may not always be possible to have adequate time between competitions or an adequate training taper in all competition situations.

An exercise-diet regimen known as glycogen loading (or carbohydrate loading) has been used by endurance athletes to increase glycogen availability before endurance exercise events (longer than 60 to 90 minutes of continuous high-intensity exercise). The original protocol, as described by Scandinavian researchers in the late 1960s, used extremes of diet and exercise to deplete then super-compensate glycogen stores. More recent work[67] has demonstrated that trained athletes need only to taper their training and ensure a high carbohydrate intake (e.g., 8 to 10 g/kg/day) over 72 hours to achieve similar increases in muscle glycogen. Because everyday training involves repeated depletion and repletion of muscle glycogen and increased glycogen synthase activity, the depletion phase of the "classical" carbohydrate loading regimen does not appear to be necessary in trained athletes. Dietary surveys have reported that many athletes undertaking carbohydrate-loading strategies may not have sufficient nutrition knowledge to ensure adequate carbohydrate intake.[68] A sample diet that might be used in carbohydrate loading is provided in Exhibit 9-9.

The goals and the practical challenges of the pre-event meal will vary between individual athletes, and factors such as the time of day of competition and the degree to which the athlete has prepared or recovered fluid and fuel status since the last exercise session must be considered. An athlete who is well tapered and has been consuming high-carbohydrate meals over the last days may only need to "top-up" liver glycogen stores after an overnight fast. Conversely, pre-event meals eaten 1 to 4 hours before exercise may promote a significant increase in muscle glycogen levels and carbohydrate availability if these are less than optimal due to inadequate preparation time.[69,70] Other goals of the pre-event meal are to ensure adequate hydration and to maintain gastrointestinal comfort.

A high-carbohydrate low-fat meal is generally advised, with reduced fiber and protein contents being an additional recommendation for those who experience gastrointestinal discomfort. Although athletes may be able to comfortably consume a larger meal or snack 3 to 4 hours before competition, those involved in early morning events may prefer to consume a smaller snack 1 to 2 hours before. If athletes experience difficulty in consuming solid foods before exercise, commercially available liquid meal supplements may be useful. Food ideas that are suitable for pre-event meals are presented in Exhibit 9-10.

Over the years, it has been recommended that athletes avoid consuming large amounts of carbohydrate, particularly simple sugars, the hour before strenuous exercise. This practice had been reported to cause lowered blood glucose levels with the onset of exercise and increased muscle glycogen use[71,72] and impaired

Exhibit 9-9 Sample "Carbohydrate Loading" Diet

These menu plans provide about 500 g of carbohydrate per day—providing the recommended carbohydrate intake of 9–10 g/kg body mass per day for a 50–55-kg athlete. They may need to be adapted for athletes outside this weight range. These menus are proposed for carbohydrate loading days only—although meeting carbohydrate intake goals, they do not meet all the nutrient requirements for everyday eating.

Day 1: (498 g CHO, 2620 kcal CHO = 75% of energy)

Breakfast:	1 cup Wheat Flake cereal + 200 mL skim milk
	1 cup sweetened canned peaches
	250 mL sweetened fruit juice
Snack:	2 thick slices toast + 2.5 g margarine + 15 g honey on each
	250 mL sports drink
Lunch:	2 bread rolls with vegetable salad with low-calorie dressing
	375-mL can of soft drink
Snack:	Large low-fat blueberry muffin
Dinner:	2 cups of boiled rice
	(made into "stir fry" with small amount of lean ham,
	peas, corn, and onion)
	250 mL sweetened fruit juice
Snack:	2 low-fat cookies

Extra water during day

Day 2: (501 g CHO, 2750 kcal CHO = 73% of energy)

Breakfast:	1 cup oatmeal + 200 mL skim milk
	1 banana
	250 mL sweetened fruit juice
Snack:	2 muffins + 2.5 g margarine + 15 g jam on each
Lunch:	Stack of two large pancakes + 60 mL maple syrup + small scoop frozen yogurt
	250 mL sweetened fruit juice
Snack:	50 g jelly beans
Dinner:	2 cups cooked pasta + 1 cup spaghetti sauce
	2 slices bread
	250 mL sports drink
Snack:	1 cup fresh fruit salad
	200 g carton low-fat fruit yogurt

Extra water during day

Day 3: The athlete may like to switch to a low-residue diet to reduce gastrointestinal contents and improve comfort during the event
- Use menus for Day 1 or 2, switching to white bread, white cereals, etc.
- From lunch on, replace some or all solid food with 500-mL snacks of commercial carboloader or liquid meal supplements

Exhibit 9-10 Suitable Pre-Event Foods (High-Carbohydrate, Low-Fat Ideas)

Choose one or more of the 10 selections according to the time of day.
The amount and timing of the pre-event meal will vary according to the event and the
  individual—experiment to find a plan that works for you.

1. Breakfast cereal with low-fat milk and fruit
2. English muffins or bagels with jam/honey
3. Pancakes with syrup
4. Baked beans on toast
5. Canned spaghetti on toast or muffins
6. Pasta with tomato/vegetarian sauce (low-fat)
7. Rice dish (e.g., "stir-fried" rice in nonstick pan or "rice pudding" made with low-fat milk)
8. Baked potato with low-fat filling
9. Fruit salad with low-fat fruit yogurt
10. Commercial liquid meal supplement or fruit smoothie

Note: many athletes may need to choose low-fiber versions (e.g., white bread or white rice
  rather than whole-grain varieties).

endurance performance.[73] These observations were attributed, at least in part, to
the hyperinsulinemia resulting from carbohydrate ingestion, which together with
the onset of muscle contraction produced a rapid decline of blood glucose. Also,
there was reduced availability of free fatty acids due to the antilipolytic effects of
insulin. However, more recent studies of pre-exercise carbohydrate ingestion have
failed to show these negative effects, and some have even observed enhanced performance.[74] It may be that any effects are short-lived or that the additional carbohydrate intake compensates for increased carbohydrate oxidation rates. Thus, it
may be necessary to revise the general caution about carbohydrate intake before
exercise, except in the case of individuals who have previously experienced negative side effects. In all aspects of precompetition eating, the athlete is advised to
experiment with various routines during training to define her optimal strategy.

Fluid and Food Intake

As much as 75% of the energy produced during exercise is released as heat
rather than mechanical work. Evaporation of sweat from the skin provides a
major mechanism of heat loss and thus the preservation of body temperature
homeostasis. Sweat rates are determined by factors such as the acclimatization of
the athlete, the intensity (and thus heat production) of exercise, and the environmental conditions and can be as high as 1.5 to 2.0 L/hr.[75] Although there is a need
for more studies to fully elucidate the effects of dehydration on exercise performance, reviews of literature summarize the following guidelines.[75–77]

- The athlete cannot adapt to chronic dehydration.
- Dehydration often impairs muscular endurance, but the effect on muscular strength and power and anaerobic exercise performance is variable.
- Dehydration impairs aerobic exercise performance, particularly prolonged exercise and exercise conducted in a hot climate.
- Although athletes consider that there is a certain degree of dehydration that can be tolerated and that performance is not significantly impaired until a critical level of dehydration has been reached (e.g., 3 to 5% loss of body weight as sweat), there is evidence to suggest that there is no such threshold. A study[78] reported that decrements in thermoregulation, heart rate, and perceived exertion were directly related to the degree of dehydration and that the closer the rate that fluid intake during exercise matches sweat loss, the better the exercise performance is in the heat.
- Dehydration also affects mental functioning. Therefore the effect of dehydration on sports which involve complex decision making and skill in addition to muscular work may be underestimated by the results of laboratory studies of work output.
- Dehydration is associated with a reduction in gastric emptying rate and an increased risk of gastrointestinal upset in athletes.[79] This may further compromise both exercise performance and ability to rehydrate during and after exercise.

It is difficult to produce guidelines for optimal fluid intake strategies for sport that take into account fluid needs (to match sweat losses) and opportunities to consume fluid during various sports. However, it is generally considered that in events longer than 30 to 60 minutes, there is a risk of impaired performance and even health damage due to dehydration, which may be eliminated or at least diminished through the provision of fluids to competitors during the event. Although this is not practical in every sport, as the duration of the sport increases and the environmental conditions become hotter, then fluid intake during the event becomes more important.

In terms of optimal fluid balance, the athlete might be advised to consume fluids to keep pace with sweat losses—or at least 80% of sweat loss rate. This may not be possible when sweat losses greatly exceed the general rate of gastric emptying (about 1 L/hr). From a practical sense, athletes who need to consume fluid during their event literally "on the run" (e.g., marathon runners, cyclists, cross-country skiers, triathletes) may need to balance their intake against the possibility of gastrointestinal discomfort or upset, as well as the time lost while eating/drinking (e.g., slowing down to approach an aid station or to handle fluids/food). Indeed, studies of the ad libitum fluid intakes of male endurance athletes in competition report that most do not, of their own accord, drink more than 400 to 600 mL/hr.[80] Although moderate levels of dehydration do not appear to be a concern to most athletes, this may not be consistent with optimal performance. Sports-specific studies need to be undertaken to ascertain present fluid balance issues in various sports and give clear guidelines for improved hydration practices. See Table 9-3 for general guidelines for fluid intakes during sports. Fluids consumed during exercise should be palatable to the athlete and served cold. Keeping beverages cool (e.g., 0 to 5°C) increases their palatability and may encourage greater intake.

During prolonged intense exercise (more than 60 to 90 minutes) fatigue may result from carbohydrate depletion, both through muscle glycogen depletion and through hypoglycemia. Even though competition preparation may have increased body glycogen stores, many endurance and ultraendurance events may challenge the athlete's carbohydrate reserves. Carbohydrate intake during such exercise may benefit performance, both by preventing hypoglycemia in susceptible individuals[81] and by supplying an additional fuel source for well-trained muscles, once muscle glycogen stores have become depleted.[82] Many studies have reported benefits to performance in prolonged exercise events when carbohydrate is consumed.[83–85] Factors that have been studied include the amount of carbohydrate that should be fed, timing of feedings, type and form of carbohydrate, and the effect of pre-exercise stores.[86]

In general, both solid foods and carbohydrate drinks have been used successfully to supply carbohydrate during exercise, although carbohydrate drinks are possibly favored because of the decreased risk of gastrointestinal side effects and the simultaneous consideration of fluid requirements. Whereas early studies warned against the inhibition of gastric emptying after intake of carbohydrate drinks greater than 2.5% in concentration,[87] there are now many studies that report that carbohydrate drinks of 5 to 7% concentration are emptied rapidly and do not compromise fluid replacement. Drinks of this concentration are easily able to provide 40 to 60 g of carbohydrate per hour to the exercising athlete. Although there may be substantial intraindividual and event-specific differences in the quantity of supplemental carbohydrate needed to maintain blood glucose availability during the latter stages of endurance exercise, these figures may provide a good starting point for experimentation.[86–88] High blood glucose levels must be available at the onset of muscle glycogen depletion if fatigue is to be delayed. If carbohydrate supplementation is withheld until the point of fatigue, a significant reversal of fatigue can only be achieved by a high rate of glucose infusion.[89] Therefore, carbohydrate intake should begin well in advance of muscle glycogen depletion and fatigue, and from the practical viewpoint might be ingested continuously throughout the exercise.[88]

The new commercial sports drinks use a combination of carbohydrate types (glucose, sucrose, glucose polymers) to achieve a palatable beverage of 5 to 7% carbohydrate. A moderate level of sodium is added (10 to 25 mmol/L) as a compromise between palatability and the positive effects of sodium on intestinal

Table 9-3 Guidelines for Fluid and Carbohydrate Requirements during Various Sports

Sports	Fluid Needs	CHO Needs (During the Event)	Comments
Weight-division sports (e.g., lightweight wrestling, boxing)	Variable	Generally not needed	The athlete is encouraged to "make weight" without resorting to severe dehydration and fasting. There may be some opportunity to top up fluid and fuel levels after the weigh-in. If the athlete is still dehydrated, extra care should be taken with fluid intake needs/opportunities during the event.
Brief events (e.g., sprints, throwing events)	Not applicable	Not applicable	There is generally no need or opportunity to replace fluid and carbohydrate during an event. For multiple events spread over the day, the athlete is encouraged to rehydrate and refuel between events with appropriate fluids and foods.
Nonendurance events (e.g., 5 to 10-km run)	Variable (e.g., minimal—1 L/hr)	Generally not needed	Sweat losses will vary with the length, intensity, and environmental conditions and events. The athlete should use opportunities during the event to keep fluid deficits below 1 L (approximately). Fluid replacement with water will generally be adequate; however, sports drinks are also suitable. Fluid deficits should be replaced after the event, and rapid fuel recovery can be assisted by immediate intake of carbo-containing foods and fluids.
Team events (e.g., basketball, football)	Variable (e.g., 500–1000 mL/hr)	May be useful in some sports (e.g., 50 g/hr)	Sweat losses will vary between players and sports, according to the length and intensity of individual play and the environmental conditions. In tournament conditions, there may be inadequate time for complete recovery of fluid and fuel needs between games. In this situation, aggressive intake of a carbo-containing fluid (e.g., sports drink) during the event will provide an advantage.
Endurance events >90 min (e.g., marathon, 80-km cycle, distance triathlon)	500–1000 mL/hr (more in extreme conditions)	Approximately 50 g/hr	Opportunities for regular intake of carbo-containing fluids (e.g., sports drinks) should be encouraged in these sports (e.g., aid stations, breaks in play). Sweat losses will vary as above; carbohydrate needs will vary according to pre-existing glycogen stores and the length and intensity of the event. The athlete is advised to keep pace with sweat losses as well as possible. Rehydrate fully and refuel after the event.

Table 9-3 Guidelines for Fluid and Carbohydrate Requirements during Various Sports

Sports	Fluid Needs	CHO Needs (During the Event)	Comments
Ultraendurance events >4 hr (e.g., Ironman Triathlon)	500–1000 mL/hr (more in extreme conditions)	Approximately 50 g/hr	As for endurance events, the sodium in sports drinks may be useful in reducing the risk of hyponatremia in susceptible athletes. Solid forms of carbohydrate may be eaten to prevent/alleviate hunger as well as to continue to supply additional fuel.

absorption.[86] An additional benefit of added sodium is observed during rehydration, because ingestion of water alone will cause a slower rate of recovery of plasma volume by lowering osmolality, thus reducing the "thirst" drive and stimulating urine production.[90] Thus sports drinks provide a practical way to achieve carbohydrate/fluid needs during exercise and rehydration after exercise. The athlete should experiment with carbohydrate intake strategies during training to perfect a competition plan. Guidelines to general carbohydrate intake requirements are summarized in Table 9-3.

Exercise has various effects on different parts of the gastrointestinal tract, and these effects appear to vary between individuals. It has been well acknowledged[91–93] that a significant number of athletes experience upper and lower gastrointestinal tract problems of mixed etiology during exercise. Factors that have been suggested to be involved in the cause of gastrointestinal problems include lack of training, extreme exercise intensities, inappropriate food and fluid intake before and during exercise, and dehydration.[94] Athletes who suffer from such problems may find relief by altering their pre-event meal and fluid/food consumption during event.

Recovery

In some sports, competition is conducted as a series of events or stages. Examples include track and field and swimming events in which athletes may compete in several brief events, or heats and finals, in one day. In events such as tennis tournaments and cycle tours, competitors may be required to undertake one or more lengthy bouts each day, with the competition extending for 1 to 3 weeks. The value of aggressive recovery between events is clear; and recovery strategies must consider the extent and type of nutritional stresses involved as well as the time interval between competition bouts. Even when athletes compete on a weekly basis, optimal recovery is desired to allow the athlete to undertake training between matches or races.

Refueling and rehydrating are important issues in the recovery phase and may necessitate a special postexercise plan of fluid and carbohydrate intake. When a single competition or competition sessions extend beyond a couple of days, the athlete must also consider overall nutrient goals such as requirements for protein, vitamins, and minerals. Although eating for optimal competition recovery may simply represent an extension of everyday nutrition patterns, it is important to remember the practical implications of the competition situation. Because athletes are often competing away from their home base, including overseas, some consideration may need to be given to ensuring access to suitable food supplies at the competition venue. The postevent phase is often a time of conflicting priorities, with the athlete being bombarded with requests for drug testing, equipment checks, travel, media interviews, and team activities. Athletes must be aware of the importance of recovery nutrition and that creative and practical ways of achieving this can be organized.

SUMMARY

Sound nutrition practices can help the female athlete optimize the adaptations and improvements achieved in her training program, as well as competition performance. This will include everyday eating strategies, as well as special tactics before, during, and after exercise. Many of the current nutrition guidelines for athletes have been formulated from studies using trained males or male athletes as subjects. There is a clear need for research to validate that females respond in a similar manner. Nevertheless, these guidelines remain the most up-to-date advice available. Body weight and body fat issues remain an important challenge to the nutritional status of some female athletes. Low energy intakes predispose the athlete to several nutrient inadequacies, including carbohydrate and minerals. Iron and calcium status of female athletes should be monitored in view of the conflict between increased requirements and low energy intakes in some athletes.

References

1. National Health and Medical Research Council. *Dietary Guidelines for Australians.* Canberra: Australian Government Publishing Service; 1992.
2. *Dietary Guidelines for Americans.* 3rd ed. Washington, DC: United States Departments of Agriculture and Health and Human Services; 1990. Home and Garden Bulletin no. 232.
3. Barr SI. Women, nutrition and exercise: a review of athletes' intake and a discussion of energy-balance in active women. *Prog Food Nutr Sci.* 1987;11:307–361.
4. Brownell KD, Steen SN, Wilmore J. Weight regulation practices in athletes: analysis of metabolic and health effects. *Med Sci Sports Exerc.* 1987;19:546–556.
5. Burke LM, Read RSD. Food use and nutritional practices of elite Olympic weightlifters. In: Truswell AS, Wahlqvist ML, eds. *Food Habits in Australia.* Melbourne: Rene Gordon; 1988:112–121.
6. King MB, Mezey G. Eating behavior of male racing jockeys. *Psychol Med.* 1987;17:249–253.

7. Steen SN, Brownell KD. Patterns of weight loss and regain in wrestlers: has the tradition changed? *Med Sci Sports Exerc.* 1987;22:762–768.

8. Wallberg-Rankin J, Edmonds CE, Gwazdauskas FC. Diet and weight changes of female body builders before and after competition. *Int J Sports Nutr.* 1993;3:87–102.

9. Wilmore J. Body weight standards and athletic performance. In: Brownell KD, Rodin J, Wilmore J, eds. *Eating, Body Weight and Performance in Athletes: Disorders of Modern Society.* Philadelphia, Pa: Lea & Febiger; 1992:315–329.

10. Burke LM. Sport and body fatness. In: Hill AP, Wahlqvist ML, eds. *Exercise and Obesity.* London: Smith-Gordon; 1994:217–231.

11. Withers RT, Whittingham NO, Norton KI, Ellis MW, Cricket A. Relative body fat and anthropometric prediction of body density of female athletes. *Eur J Appl Physiol.* 1987;56:169–180.

12. Telford RD, Egerton WJ, Hahn AG, Pang PM. Skinfold measures and weight control in athletes. *Excel.* 1988;5:21–24.

13. Stanton R. The overweight athlete. In: Burke LM, Deakin V, eds. *Clinical Sports Nutrition.* Sydney: McGraw Hill; 1994:104–123.

14. Kerr D. Kinanthropometry. In: Burke LM, Deakin V, eds. *Clinical Sports Nutrition.* Sydney: McGraw Hill; 1994:74–103.

15. Brodie DA. Techniques of measurement of body composition; part I. *Sports Med.* 1988;5:11–40.

16. Brodie DA. Techniques of measurement of body composition: part II. *Sports Med.* 1988;5:74–98.

17. Brownell KD, Rodin J, Wilmore J. An introduction. In: Brownell KD, Rodin J, Wilmore J, eds. *Eating, Body Weight and Performance in Athletes: Disorders of Modern Society.* Philadelphia, Pa: Lea & Febiger; 1992:3–14.

18. Dummer G, Rose L, Heusner W, Roberts P, Councilman J. Pathogenic weight control behaviors of young female swimmers. *Phys Sports Med.* 1987;15(5):75–84.

19. Brownell KD, Rodin J. Prevalence of eating disorders in athletes. In: Brownell KD, Rodin J, Wilmore J, eds. *Eating, Body Weight and Performance in Athletes: Disorders of Modern Society.* Philadelphia, Pa: Lea & Febiger; 1992:128–145.

20. Wilmore JH. Eating and weight disorders in the female athlete. *Int J Sports Nutr.* 1991;1:104–117.

21. Clark N, Nelson M, Evans W. Nutrition education for elite female runners. *Phys Sports Med.* 1988;16(2):124–136.

22. Drinkwater BL, Nilson K, Chestnut CH, Bremner WJ, Shainholtz SS, Southworth MB. Bone mineral content of amenorrheic and eumenorrheic athletes. *N Engl J Med.* 1984;311:277–281.

23. Marcus R, Cann C, Madvig P, et al. Menstrual function and bone mass in elite women distance runners. *Ann Intern Med.* 1985;102:158–163.

24. Nelson ME, Fisher EC, Catson PD, Meredith CD, Turksoy RN, Evans WJ. Diet and bone status in amenorrheic runners. *Am J Clin Nutr.* 1986;43:910–916.

25. Brotherhood JR. Nutrition and sports performance. *Sports Med.* 1984;1:350–389.

26. Keesey RE. A set-point theory of obesity. In: Brownell KD, Foreyt JP, eds. *Handbook of Eating Disorders: Physiology, Psychology and Treatment of Obesity, Anorexia and Bulimia.* New York, NY: Basic Books; 1986:63–87.

27. Brownell KD, Rodin J, Wilmore J, eds. *Eating, Body Weight and Performance in Athletes: Disorders of Modern Society.* Philadelphia, Pa: Lea & Febiger; 1992.

28. Sherman WM, Wimer GS. Insufficient dietary carbohydrate during training: does it impair performance? *Int J Sport Nutr.* 1991;1:28–44.

29. Robergs RA. Nutrition and exercise determinants of post-exercise glycogen synthesis. *Int J Sport Nutr.* 1991;1:307–337.

30. Ivy JL. Muscle glycogen synthesis before and after exercise. *Sports Med.* 1991;11:6–19.

31. Ivy JL, Katz AL, Cutler CL, Sherman WM, Coyle EF. Muscle glycogen synthesis after exercise: effect of time of carbohydrate ingestion. *J Appl Physiol.* 1988;65:1480–1485.

32. Burke LM, Read RSD. Sports nutrition: approaching the nineties. *Sports Med.* 1989;8:80–100.

33. Costill DL. Carbohydrates for exercise: dietary demands for optimal performance. *Int J Sports Med.* 1988;9:1–18.

34. American Dietetic Association and the Canadian Dietetic Association. Position stand: nutrition for physical fitness and athletic performance for adults. *J Am Diet Assoc.* 1993;93:691–696.

35. Martin AD, Bailey D. Skeletal integrity in amenorrheic athletes. *Aust J Sci Med Sport.* 1987;19(1):3–7.

36. Highet R. Athletic amenorrhea: an update on aetiology. *Sports Med.* 7:82–108.

37. Loucks AB, Horvath SM. Athletic amenorrhea: a review. *Med Sci Sports Exerc.* 1985;17:56–72.

38. Carlberg KA, Buckman MT, Peake GT, Riedesel ML. Body composition of oligo/amenorrheic athletes. *Med Sci Sports Exerc.* 1983;15:215–217.

39. Linnell SL, Stager JM, Blue PM, Oyster N, Robertshaw D. Bone mineral content and menstrual regularity in female runners. *Med Sci Sports Exerc.* 1984:16;343–348.

40. Sanborn CF, Albrecht BH, Wagner WW. Athletic amenorrhea: lack of association with body fat. *Med Sci Sports Exerc.* 1987;19:207–212.

41. Pirke KM, Schweiger U, Laessle R, Dickhaut B, Schweiger M, Waechtler M. Dieting influences the menstrual cycle: vegetarian versus nonvegetarian diet. *Fertil Steril.* 1986;46:1083–1088.

42. Gadpaille WJ, Sanborn CF, Wagner WW. Athletic amenorrhea, major affective disorders and eating disorders. *Am J Psychiatry.* 1987;144:939–942.

43. Yeager KK, Agostini R, Nattiv A, Drinkwater B. The female athlete triad: disordered eating, amenorrhea, osteoporosis. *Med Sci Sports Exerc.* 1993;25:775–777.

44. Nattiv A, Yeager K, Drinkwater B, Agostini R. The female athlete triad. In: Agostini R, ed. *Medical and Orthopedic Issues of Active and Athletic Women.* Philadelphia, Pa: Hanley & Belfus; 1994:169–174.

45. Bailey DA, Martin AD, Houston CS, Howie JL. Physical activity, nutrition, bone density and osteoporosis. *Aust J Sci Med Sport.* 1986;18(3):3–8.

46. Snyder AC, Wenderoth MP, Johnston CC, Hui SL. Bone mineral content of elite lightweight amenorrheic oarswomen. *Hum Biol.* 1986;58:863–869.

47. Nordin BEC. Calcium. In: Truswell AS, ed. *Recommended Nutrient Intakes: Australian Papers.* Sydney: Australian Professional Publications; 1990:201–206.

48. Berning J, Sanborn CF, Brooks SM, Wagner WW. Caloric deficit in distance runners. *Med Sci Sports Exerc.* 1985;17:242. Abstract.

49. Loosli AR, Benson J, Gillien DM, Bourdet K. Nutrition habits and knowledge in competitive adolescent female gymnasts. *Phys Sportsmed.* 1986;14(8):118–130.

50. Moffat JR. Dietary status of elite female high school gymnasts: inadequacy of vitamin and mineral intake. *J Am Diet Assoc.* 1984;84:1361–1363.

51. Carbon R, Sambrook PN, Deakin V, et al. Bone density of elite female athletes with stress fractures. *Med J Aust.* 1990;153:373–376.

52. Lloyd T, Triantafyllou SJ, Baker ER, et al. Women athletes with menstrual irregularity have increased musculoskeletal injuries. *Med Sci Sports Exerc.* 1986;18:374–379.

53. Drinkwater BL, Nilson K, Ott S, Chestnut CH. Bone mineral density after resumption of menses in amenorrheic athletes. *JAMA*. 1986;256:380–382.

54. Cann CE, Cavanaugh DJ, Schnurpel K, Martin MC. Menstrual history is the main determinant of trabecular bone density in women runners. *Med Sci Sports Exerc*. 1988;20(suppl):59. Abstract.

55. Heaney RP, Recker RR, Saville PD. Menopausal changes in calcium balance performance. *J Lab Clin Med*. 1978;92:953–963.

56. Newhouse IJ, Clement DB. Iron status: an update. *Sports Med*. 1988;5:337–352.

57. Haymes EM, Lamanca JF. Iron loss in runners during exercise: implications and recommendations. *Sports Med*. 1989;7:277–285.

58. Lemon PWR. Protein and amino acid needs of the strength athlete. *Int J Sport Nutr*. 1991;1:127–145.

59. Lemon PWR. Effect of exercise on protein requirements. *J Sports Sci*. 1991;9(special issue):53–70.

60. Tarnopolsky MA, MacDougall JD, Atkinson SA. Influence of body protein intake and training status on nitrogen balance and lean body mass. *J Appl Physiol*. 1988;64:187–193.

61. Meredith CN, Zackin MJ, Frontera WR, Evans WJ. Dietary protein requirements and body protein metabolism in endurance-trained men. *J Appl Physiol*. 1989;66:2850–2856.

62. Burke LM, Inge K. Protein requirements for training and bulking up. In: Burke LM, Deakin V, eds. *Clinical Sports Nutrition*. Sydney: McGraw Hill; 1994.

63. Van der Beek EJ. Vitamins and endurance training: food for running or faddish claims? *Sports Med*. 1985;2:175–197.

64. Williams MH. *Nutritional Aspects of Human Physical and Athletic Performance*. 2nd ed. Springfield, Ill: Charles C Thomas; 1985.

65. Burke LM, Read RSD. Dietary supplements in sport. *Sports Med*. 1993;15:43–56.

66. Burke LM, Heeley P. Dietary supplements and nutritional ergogenic aids in sport. In: Burke LM, Deakin V, eds. *Clinical Sports Nutrition*. Sydney: McGraw Hill; 1994:227–284.

67. Sherman WM, Costill DL, Fink WJ, Miller JM. Effect of exercise-diet manipulation on muscle glycogen and its subsequent utilization during performance. *Int J Sports Med*. 1981;2:114–118.

68. Burke LM, Read RSD. A study of carbohydrate loading techniques used by marathon runners. *Can J Sports Sci*. 1987;12:6–10.

69. Coyle EF, Coggan AR, Hemmert MK, Lowe RC, Walters TJ. Substrate use during prolonged exercise following a pre-exercise meal. *J Appl Physiol*. 1985;59:429–433.

70. Sherman WM, Brodowicz G, Wright DA, Allen WK, Simonsen J, Dernbach A. Effects of 4h pre-exercise carbohydrate feedings on cycling performance. *Med Sci Sports Exerc*. 1989;21:598–604.

71. Costill DL, Coyle EF, Dalsky G, Evans W, Fink W, Hoopes D. Effects of elevated plasma FFA and insulin on muscle glycogen usage during exercise. *J Appl Physiol*. 1977;43:695–699.

72. Hargreaves ML, Costill DL, Katz A, Fink WJ. Effect of fructose ingestion on muscle glycogen usage during exercise. *Med Sci Sports Exerc*. 1985;17:360–363.

73. Foster C, Costill DL, Fink WJ. Effects of pre-exercise feedings on endurance performance. *Med Sci Sports Exerc*. 1979;11:1–5.

74. Gleeson M, Maughan RJ, Greenhaff PL. Comparison of the effects of pre-exercise feeding of glucose, glycerol and placebo on endurance and fuel homeostasis in man. *Eur J Appl Physiol*. 1986;55:645–653.

75. Sawka MN, Pandolf KB. Effects of water loss on physiological function and exercise performance. In: Gisolfi CV, Lamb DR, eds. *Perspectives in Exercise Science and Sports Medicine III: Fluid Homeostasis During Exercise.* Carmel, Calif.: Benchmark Press; 1990:1–38.

76. Buskirk ER, Puhl S. Nutritional beverages: exercise and sport. In: Hickson JF, Wolinsky I, eds. *Nutrition in Exercise and Sports.* Boca Raton, Fla: CRC Press; 1989:201–231.

77. Williams MH. The role of water and electrolytes in physical activity. In: *Nutritional Aspects of Human Physical and Athletic Performance.* 2nd ed. Springfield, Ill: Charles C Thomas; 1985.

78. Coyle EF, Montain SJ. Benefits of fluid replacement with carbohydrate during exercise. *Med Sci Sports Exerc.* 1992;24(suppl):S324–330.

79. Rehrer NJ, Beckers EJ, Brouns F, ten Hoor F, Saris WHM. Effects of dehydration on gastric emptying and gastrointestinal distress while running. *Med Sci Sports Exerc.* 1990;22:790–795.

80. Noakes TD, Adams BA, Myburgh KH, Greeff C, Lotz T, Nathan M. The danger of an inadequate water intake during prolonged exercise. *Eur J Appl Physiol.* 1988;57:210–219.

81. Coyle EF, Hagberg JM, Hurley BF, Martin WH, Eheani AA, Holloszy JO. Carbohydrate feeding during prolonged strenuous exercise can delay fatigue. *J Appl Physiol.* 1983;55:230–235.

82. Coyle EF, Coggan AR, Hemmart MK, Ivy JL. Muscle glycogen utilization during prolonged strenuous exercise when fed carbohydrate. *J Appl Physiol.* 1986;61:165–172.

83. Coyle EF, Coggan AR. Effectiveness of carbohydrate feeding in delaying fatigue during prolonged exercise. *Sports Med.* 1984;1:336–458.

84. Lamb DL, Brodowicz GR. Optimal use of fluids of varying formulations to minimize exercise-induced disturbances in homeostasis. *Sports Med.* 1986;3:247–274.

85. Murray R. The effects of consuming carbohydrate electrolyte beverages on gastric emptying and fluid absorption during and following exercise. *Sports Med.* 1987;4:322–351.

86. Burke LM. Food and fluid intake during competition. In: Burke LM, Deakin V, eds. *Clinical Sports Nutrition.* Sydney: McGraw Hill; 1994:333–364.

87. American College of Sports Medicine. Position statement on prevention of heat injuries during distance running. *Med Sci Sports Exerc.* 1975;7:vii–ix.

88. Coyle EF. Timing and method of increased carbohydrate intake to cope with heavy training, competition and recovery. *J Sports Sci.* 1991;9(special issue);29–52.

89. Coggan ER, Coyle EF. Reversal of fatigue during prolonged exercise by carbohydrate infusion or ingestion. *J Appl Physiol.* 1987;63:2388–2395.

90. Nose H, Mack GW, Shi X, Nadel ER. Role of osmolality and plasma volume during rehydration in humans. *J Appl Physiol.* 1988;65:325–331.

91. Brouns F. Gastrointestinal symptoms in athletes: physiological and nutritional aspects. In: Brouns F, ed. *Advances in Nutrition and Top Sport: Medicine and Sport Science, 32.* Basel: Karger; 1991:166–199.

92. Brouns F, Saris WHM, Rehrer NJ. Abdominal complaints and gastrointestinal function during long-lasting exercise. *Int J Sports Med.* 1987;8:175–189.

93. Moses FM. The effect of exercise on gastrointestinal tract. *Sports Med.* 1990;9:159–172.

94. Brouns F, Beckers E. Is the gut an athletic organ? *Sports Med.* 1993;15:242–257.

95. Kleiner SM, Bazzarre TL, Litchford MD. Metabolic profiles, diet and health practices of championship male and female bodybuilders. *J Am Diet Assoc.* 1990;90:962–967.

96. Kleiner SM, Bazzarre TL, Ainsworth BE. Nutritional status of nationally ranked elite bodybuilders. *Int J Sport Nutr.* 1994;4:54–69.

97. Ellsworth NM, Hewitt BF, Haskell WL. Nutrient intake of elite male and female Nordic skiers. *Phys Sportsmed.* 1985;13(2):78–84,90–92.

98. Fogelholm M, Rehunen S, Gref C, et al. Dietary intake and thiamin, iron, and zinc status in elite Nordic skiers during different training periods. *Int J Sport Nutr.* 1992;2:351–365.

99. Clement DB, Asmundson RC. Nutritional intake and hematological parameters in endurance runners. *Phys Sportsmed.* 1982;10(3):37–43.

100. Deuster PA, Kyle SB, Moser PB, Vigersky RA, Singh A, Schoomaker EB. Nutritional survey of highly trained women runners. *Am J Clin Nutr.* 1986;44:954–962.

101. Grandjean AC, Lolkus LJ, Lind R, Schaefer AE. Dietary intake of female cyclists during repeated days of racing. *Cycling Sci.* 1992;Fall:21–25.

102. Faber M, Spinnler-Benade AJ, Daubitzer A. Dietary intake, anthropometric measurements and plasma lipid levels in throwing field athletes. *Int J Sports Med.* 1990;10:140–145.

103. Khoo C, Rawson NE, Robinson ML, Stevenson RJ. Nutrient intake and eating habits of triathletes. *Ann Sports Med.* 1987;3:144–150.

104. Green DR, Gibbons C, O'Toole M, Hiller WBO. An evaluation of dietary intakes of triathletes: are RDA's being met? *J Am Diet Assoc.* 1989;89:1653–1654.

105. Worme JD, Doubt TJ, Singh A, Ryan CJ, Moses FM, Deuster PA. Dietary patterns, gastrointestinal complaints, and nutrition knowledge of recreational triathletes. *Am J Clin Nutr.* 1990;51:690–697.

106. Cohen JL, Potosnak L, Frank O, Baker H. A nutritional and hematologic assessment of elite ballet dancers. *Phys Sportsmed.* 1985;13(5):43–54.

107. Short SH, Short WR. Four-year study of university athletes' dietary intake. *J Am Diet Assoc.* 1983;82:632–645.

108. Barry A, Cantwell T, Doherty F, et al. A nutritional study of Irish athletes. *Br J Sport Med.* 1981;15:99–109.

109. Steen SN, Mayer KV, Brownell KD. Dietary intake of female heavyweight rowers. *Med Sport Sci Exer.* 1990;22(2):S106.

110. Nowak RK, Knudsen KS, Schulz LO. Body composition and nutrient intakes of college men and women basketball players. *J Am Diet Assoc.* 1988;88:575–578.

111. Barr SI. Energy and nutrient intakes of elite adolescent swimmers. *J Can Diet Assoc.* 1989;50:20–24.

112. National Research Council. *Recommended Dietary Allowances.* 10th ed. Washington, DC: National Academy of Sciences; 1989.

113. Bruemmer BA, Drinkwater BK. Nutrient intake in amenorrheic and eumenorrheic athletes. *Med Sci Sports Exerc.* 1987;19(2):S37.

114. Myerson M, Guton B, Warren M, et al. Energy balance of amenorrheic and eumenorrheic runners. *Med Sci Sports Exerc.* 1987;19(2):S37.

Appendix 9-A

Dietary Intakes (per day) of Elite Female Athletes

Athlete Group	Energy (kJ)	Energy/kg (kJ/kg)	CHO g	CHO %E^a	Protein g	Protein %E	Fat g	Fat %E	Alcohol (g)	Vitamins	Minerals (mg)
Bodybuilding											
*(95) n = 8 precompetition 7-day record	9646	168	332	49	162	37	33	13			Calcium 293 Iron 24 Zinc 9
(8) n = 6 −28 to −26 day precompetition	6986	123	234	53.5	114	28.6	30	17		>100% RDA! A,C,B$_1$,B$_2$,B$_3$, folate,B$_6$,B$_{12}$	Calcium 667 Iron 14.4 Zinc 7.1
−9 to −7 days	6148	108	196	51	137	34.2	23	14.8		>100% RDA A,C,B$_1$,B$_2$,B$_3$, folate,B$_6$,B$_{12}$	Calcium 474 Iron 13.7 Zinc 6.8
−2 to −1 days	7882	138	386	78.3	74	16.6	13	6.4		>100% RDA A,C,B$_1$,B$_2$,B$_3$, folate,B$_6$,B$_{12}$	Calcium 280 Iron 18.1 Zinc 5.3
0 to +2 days postcompetition	12,874	243	445	51.3	114	14.7	123	34.5		>100% RDA A,C,B$_1$,B$_2$,B$_3$, folate,B$_6$,B$_{12}$	Calcium 1262 Iron 19.4 Zinc 12.3
+19 to +21 days	11,958	210	393	52.6	114	18.7	88	28.7		>100% RDA A,C,B$_1$,B$_2$,B$_3$, folate,B$_6$,B$_{12}$	Calcium 1047 Iron 19.4 Zinc 9.1
(96) n = 11 1 week precompetition 3-day record	6845	129	206	48	143	39	22	12		>100% RDA B$_1$,B$_2$,B$_3$,C,A,E	Calcium 418 Iron 16.5 Zinc 9.1
Nordic skiers											
(97) n = 14 4 x 3-day records	13,724	240	364	42	107	13	136	39	12.5	>100% RDA B$_1$,B$_2$,B$_3$,C	Calcium 1224 Iron 17.3
(98) n = 8 4 x 7-day records	12,087	208	438	58	99.5	14	93	30		>100% RDA B$_1$,B$_2$,C	Calcium 1310 Iron 21.1 Zinc 15.8

Dietary Intakes (per day) of Elite Female Athletes (continued)

Athlete Group	Energy (kJ)	Energy/kg (kJ/kg)	CHO g	CHO %E[a]	Protein g	Protein %E	Fat g	Fat %E	Alcohol (g)	Vitamins	Minerals (mg)
Distance runners											
(99) n = 17 7 day record	8683	252	46	74	14	87	39				Iron 12.5
(100) n = 51 3-day record	10,274	199	323	50	81	13	89	32			Calcium 1227 Iron 41.9 Zinc 14.2
Cyclists											
(101) n = 3 11-day race	11,286	193	343	52	106	16	96	32		<100% RDA B1,B2,B3,B6,C B12,A,folate	Calcium 1091 Iron 16 Zinc 11.4
Throwers											
(102) n = 15 7-day record	9285	112	269	46.4	94	17.2	91	38	1.4		
Triathletes											
Ultraendurance (103) n = 10 3-day record[b]	10,603	187	351	53	80	13	85	30	8	<100% RDA A,E,B1,B2,B3,B6, B12,C	Calcium 143% RDA Iron 565% RDA Zinc 189% RDA
(104) n = 34 2 x 3-day record	17,783	695	66	113.0	12	99	21	10			
Recreational											
(105) n = 21 3-day record	9058	153	290	51	84	16	73	30	9	<100% RDA A,C,E,B1,B2,B3,B6,B12 70–100% RDA folate	Calcium 1259 Iron 14.5 Zinc 10.6
Ballet dancers											
(106) n = 12 6-day record	7170		207	46	59	14	71	39		>100% RDA B1,B2,C,A 70–100% RDA B3, B12 <70% RDA B6, folate	Calcium 821 Iron 13
(107) n = 9 3-day record	8180		256	52	82	17	65	31		>100%RDA A,C,B1,B2,B3	Calcium 968 Iron 19

Dietary Intakes (per day) of Elite Female Athletes (continued)

Athlete Group	Energy (kJ)	Energy/kg (kJ/kg)	CHO g	CHO %E^a	Protein g	Protein %E	Fat g	Fat %E	Alcohol (g)	Vitamins	Minerals (mg)
Gymnasts											
(50) n = 13 2 x 3-day records	8242		222	43	74	15	82	39		<100% RDA B1,B12,C,A 70–100% RDA B1,B3,B6, folate	Calcium 707 Iron 11 Zinc 7
(49) n = 97 11–17 years old 3-day record	7880	183	220	49	71	15	74	36		No. consuming < 2/3 RDA B1 8,B12 10,A15,folate 68,B6 70,B3 11,C10,E50	No. consuming <2/3 RDA Iron 53 Calcium 40 Zinc 78
Various athletes											
(108) n = 21 3-day weighed record	11,800	208.5	338	45	108	15	133	40		>100% RDA B1,B2,B3,B6,C,B12,folate	Calcium 1416 Iron 14
Rowers											
Heavyweight (109) n = 16 5-day record	11,270	183	350	50	93	14	110	36		≥80% met 100% RDA for A,C,B1,B2,B3,B12 25% met RDA for Folate,B6	31% met RDA for iron
Crew (107) n = 24	10,025	148	272	46	96	16	96	36	7	>100% RDA A,C,B1,B2,B3	Calcium 1370 Iron 15
Basketball											
(107) n = 10 1-day record	11,270		320	45	92	14	111	36		>100% RDA A,C,B1,B2,B3	Calcium 1362 Iron 14
(104) n = 9 3-day record	13,890		379	46	108	14	145	40	5	>100% RDA A,C,B1,B2,B3	Calcium 1418 Iron 16
(110) n = 10 3-day record	7415	103	229	52	68	16	63	32	2	>100% RDA A,C,B1,B2,B3,B12 70–100% RDA C <70% RDA folate,B6	Calcium 903 Iron 10 Zinc 7

Dietary Intakes (per day) of Elite Female Athletes (continued)

Athlete Group	Energy (kJ)	Energy/kg (kJ/kg)	CHO g	CHO %E[a]	Protein g	Protein %E	Fat g	Fat %E	Alcohol (g)	Vitamins	Minerals (mg)
Lacrosse											
(107) n = 7 3-day record	9510		257	50	89	16	95	35		>100% RDA A,C,B_1,B_2,B_3	Calcium 798 Iron 14
Swimmers											
(107) n = 9 3-day record	17,090		425	40	133	13	198	43		>100% RDA A,C,B_1,B_2,B_3	Calcium 1771 Iron 16
(107) n = 4 3-day record	11,510		263	39	99	14	135	43	12	>100% RDA A,C,B_1,B_2,B_3	Calcium 1236 Iron 16
(107) n = 7 3-day record	9635		256	44	92	17	93	36	10	>100% RDA A,C,B_1,B_2,B_3	Calcium 828 Iron 13
(111) n = 10 3-day record	8636	139	284	54	89	17	69	30		>100% RDA A,C,B_1,B_2,$B_3$$B_6$,$B_{12}$,C	Calcium 1354 Iron 15.6 Zinc 9.3
Volleyball											
(107) n = 13 1-day record	8685		248	46	78	14	82	35		>100% RDA A,C,B_1,B_2 70–100% RDA B_3	Calcium 1075 Iron 10
(107) n = 11 3-day record	10,485		314	49	103	16	95	34	3.5	>100% RDA A,C,B_1,B_2,B_3	Calcium 1311 Iron 12
(107) n = 7 3-day record	7765		244	53	61	13	69	34	0	>100% RDA A,C,B_1,B_2,B_3	Calcium 1449 Iron 12

* Numbers in parentheses = references
I: RDAs (112)
[a] Percentage of total energy.
[b] Vitamin and mineral intakes reported **include** supplementation.

10

&

Nutritional Needs of Elderly Women

Ronni Chernoff

It is a well-known fact that at all ages older than 65, there are more women than men in the United States and that, although women live longer, they have more morbidity and disability than do older men. Recent data indicate that 70% of women older than age 75 are widows and that 85% of all nursing home residents are women.[1] Whereas older women have the same serious illnesses as older men, they often have additional burdens of chronic disease. Also well known is the continuing growth of the older segment of the American population. It has been projected that by the year 2020, there will be approximately 50 million people older than age 65 and more than 70% of them will be women.[2,3] Female longevity is well documented, particularly in developed countries.[4–6] There are likely many reasons why this is so. Perhaps the greatest contributor to the variance in gender-related mortality is premature cardiovascular disease mortality in men.[6] Also, mortality is linked to negative health behaviors, smoking being among the most important. Longevity must be tempered by acceptable health status, and efforts to extend and maximize the quality of life are, therefore, vital in developing approaches to health promotion for the future.

Because health care costs are highest during the last years of life and because it is anticipated that the greatest demands will not come until the "baby-boomer" generation comes of age between 2020 and 2040,[7] it is important to identify interventions that will contribute to the maintenance of health and the prevention of disease and disability now so that the potentially overwhelming demands on the health care delivery system can be controlled and minimized.

Many factors contribute to the maintenance of physical health in older persons, one of which has to do with psychological well-being. Although it may appear to be tangentially related to nutritional or health status, there appears to be a strong relationship between poor health and psychological factors such as depression, anxiety, and loneliness.[8–10]

There is evidence that older women maintain a relatively high level of psychological health despite greater social disadvantages and burdens. Nevertheless, depression, psychiatric morbidity, cognitive defects, and other mental health problems occur in older women. Health professionals should be aware of the signs of these psychological problems and be trained to do creative interventions when possible, particularly when the psychological problems affect health and nutrition status.[11,12]

Depression has been cited as a factor in appetite loss so there may be an association between emotional distress and health and nutrition. In elderly women, many factors may contribute to depression, including chronic disease conditions, bereavement, and institutionalization. In fact, in studies in which investigators have observed the dietary status and intake of elderly women, there was a lower intake of energy and nutrients in women who were institutionalized than in older women living independently or receiving home meal services.[13,14] These data indicate that in institutionalized people, the older the women's age, the lower the intake of energy and nutrients. Chronically decreased energy and nutrient intake will eventually lead to a subclinical malnutrition; when a traumatic event occurs, the usual consequences of malnutrition will appear and contribute to a more complicated outcome than might have been expected.

Even though there are many psychological reasons why energy intake is decreased in elderly women, there are also physiologic reasons why appetite is depressed and nutritional intake is depressed. The greatest challenge is recognizing when dietary intake is decreased to the level of risk for malnutrition.

Adequacy of Nutritional Intake of Elderly Women

Nutritional adequacy of dietary intakes in elderly women are summarized in Table 10-1. In three national surveys, the intakes of calcium and magnesium fell below the Recommended Dietary Allowances (RDA). On the other hand, the intakes of protein, vitamin B_6, vitamin B_{12}, vitamin C, vitamin A, and iron were adequate. However, many of the RDAs for the elderly, especially for protein, vitamin B_6, vitamin B_{12}, and calcium need further study as they may not promote optimal nutriture.

The current intakes of fat and saturated fat of elderly women (Table 10-2) do not meet the contemporary recommendations. However, the intakes of total fat and saturated fat in older elderly women (over 70 years) are closer to the recommended intakes than those of younger adult women (aged 20–59). Women of all ages meet the cholesterol recommendation of <300 mg/day.

ENERGY NEEDS

It is a well-known phenomenon that as people age, energy requirements decrease (Exhibit 10-1). It is likely that this is due to a reduction in the most met-

Table 10-1 Dietary Intakes of Selected Nutrients of Elderly Women in Major Surveys Relative to the 1990 Recommended Dietary Allowances (RDAs)

	% RDA		
Nutrient	NHANES I[a]	NHANES III[b]	NFCS (1987–1988)[c]
Protein[d]	106	122	119
Vitamin B$_6$[d]	—	100	87
Vitamin B$_{12}$[d]	—	195	225
Vitamin C	150	175	157
Vitamin A	—	191	170
Calcium[d]	62	84	70
Magnesium	—	89	77
Iron	92	129	115

[a]National Health and Nutrition Examination Survey I (1971–1974)
[b]National Health and Nutrition Examination Survey III (1989–1991)
[c]National Food Consumption Survey (NFCS 87–88)
[d]RDA may be too low

Table 10-2 Fat, Fatty Acids, and Cholesterol Intake of Women[a]

Age (yr)	Total Fat (%Kcal)	SFA (%Kcal)	MUFA (%Kcal)	PUFA (%Kcal)	Cholesterol (mg)
20–59	34.4	11.8	12.5	7.4	259
60–69	33.0	11.0	12.0	6.7	215
70–79	32.3	10.7	12.0	7.3	225

[a]Data from NHANES III

abolically active tissue, the total protein compartment. As lean body mass, and all the protein compartments, shrink with advancing age, the need for energy to maintain protein mass and protein constituents is decreased.[15] A second factor that contributes to a decrease in energy requirements is a reduction in either time spent or intensity of physical exercise.[16,17] A third cause for a reduction in energy requirements with advancing age is alterations in hormone production, particu-

Exhibit 10-1 Factors Contributing to the Decrease in Energy Requirements in the Elderly

1. Reduction in total protein compartment
2. Reduction in intensity and/or duration of physical activity
3. Alteration in testosterone and growth hormone production
4. Curtailment of physical activity

larly growth hormone and testosterone, both of which promote anabolism or lean tissue growth.[18] Another reason for a decrease in energy demands is the curtailment of physical activity related to the progression of chronic conditions such as cardiovascular disease, pulmonary conditions, musculoskeletal disease, obesity, and bone disease.[16]

Usually energy requirements are extrapolated from studies conducted on younger adults. This is not a very reliable process, and when metabolic studies are conducted, it is evident that there are factors that alter estimation of energy expenditure or demands in older versus middle-aged or younger women.[17,19–21] It is important to actually measure metabolic rate in older people if the resting metabolic rate (RMR) is an important factor in therapeutic plans; there is too much variability among individuals to rely on extrapolated data.

One method that may be used to ensure slower declines in energy and nutrient intake is institution of an exercise program. Studies show that exercise training is related to higher levels of energy and nutrient intake in elderly women.[22,23] This does not necessarily mean that there is an improvement in dietary quality, but there is a reconditioning of physical fitness, even through the very late years.[24] Exercise may contribute to a retention of lean body mass over time, or at least a slower decline than occurs in aging people who do not exercise regularly.[25] Fat distribution patterns change with exercise,[26] although exercise may or may not have a profound effect on bone density or muscle loss in elderly individuals.[27,28] Exercise may have many positive benefits beyond changes in body composition; including improvement of cardiorespiratory endurance, reduction of cardiovascular risk, control of blood pressure, prevention of obesity and osteoporosis, and elevation of basal metabolic rate.[29,30] The institution of an exercise program in aging individuals has been controversial; there is often a reluctance on the part of older women to participate in exercise programs,[31] but physical activity that begins at an early age and continues through life can only have positive effects as long as exercise regimens are not overdone to the point of injury.[32]

Nevertheless, energy requirements decrease with advancing age, but the alterations in macronutrient requirements do not decline at a parallel rate; in some cases, they may even be increased. This poses a challenge for the clinician to encourage the dietary inclusion of foods that are nutrient-dense but are lower in calories.

MACRONUTRIENTS

Whether or not the reason for the decrease in energy demands is described above or is as yet undiscovered, it is well known that total caloric intake is reduced in older people. The primary dietary sources of energy are fats and carbohydrates.

Fat

The need for dietary fat does not change significantly as individuals age. At least 10% of total energy intake should be from fat to provide an adequate amount of fat-soluble vitamins and essential fatty acids.[15,33] The adult American diet provides approximately 34% of energy from fat; the recommended fat content is 30% or less of total energy to reduce risk for heart disease.[34] Decreases in dietary fat, both saturated fat and cholesterol, decrease plasma cholesterol levels.[35–37] It appears that age does not alter this blood lipid response. However, some question the importance of plasma cholesterol as a risk factor for the elderly.[38–40]

Dietary fat has also been linked to the possible etiology of breast, colon, and endometrial cancer.[41–43] Decreasing dietary fat intake has been recommended to decrease the risk for cancer development; however, the value of this recommendation to prevent cancer in elderly individuals must be carefully examined. Cancer often takes many years to develop, and there is no evidence that dietary fat reduction has an impact on cancer risk in elderly persons. Fat adds mouth feel and flavor to foods. Reducing dietary fat may decrease the appeal of certain foods, which could adversely affect overall nutrient intake. Altering the diets of older adults requires compelling health promotion or disease prevention reasons because compliance is often poor and many elderly persons consume suboptimal diets that are low in essential nutrients.

Carbohydrates

The major role of dietary carbohydrate is to provide energy. Glucose can be used for energy by all tissues and is essential for brain and red blood cell energy production.[15] If there is an inadequate amount of dietary carbohydrate to meet energy demands, dietary or stored fat will be used as energy. Because fatty acids are incompletely oxidized, burning fat as fuel may lead to ketosis. To prevent this, at least 50 g of dietary glucose or complex carbohydrate equivalent is required per day to supplement glucose produced endogenously through gluconeogenesis. In general, the amount of dietary carbohydrate should approximate 55 to 60% of total dietary energy intake.

Fiber is another constituent of dietary carbohydrate that is important for older individuals. There are many effects of fiber, including improving glucose tolerance,[44] reducing incidence of constipation and diverticulosis,[45–47] and lowering serum lipids.[45] The potential benefits of fiber in the diets of older women support the efforts of health educators to increase dietary fiber in the American diet. As people age, the amount of dietary fiber tends to decrease, often due to the difficulty with chewing foods high in fiber or a perceived problem with digestion of high-fiber foods.[48] By limiting dietary fiber, there is also a risk of limiting the intake of nutrients found in high-fiber foods.[49] Although there are always suggestions for increasing dietary fiber, encouraging the incorporation of foods high in fiber, rather than fiber additives, will also increase the nutrient density of the diet.[49–51]

Protein

The decline in lean body mass that is associated with aging is a factor in total body protein turnover and distribution. As people age and experience a decrease in skeletal tissue mass,[52] the store of protein provided by skeletal muscle may be inadequate to meet the needs for protein synthesis, therefore making dietary protein intake more important to meet essential needs.[15,53] Protein requirements in adults have been determined in younger adults and do not compensate for the age-related changes in physiology or in the responses to stress, trauma, infection, injury, or chronic disease. Studies conducted in elderly subjects demonstrated that protein requirements per kilogram body weight do not decline with age[54] and that the RDA of 0.8 g protein per kilogram body weight as determined on younger adults is not adequate to maintain nitrogen equilibrium in elderly adults.[55]

The inability to maintain nitrogen balance with a dietary intake that meets the RDA may be a more significant factor in older adults than is first apparent. Protein-energy malnutrition has been noted in many different populations of elderly people,[56–60] and the slow, continual loss of protein may certainly be a contributing factor in the etiology of this condition. This chronic protein inadequacy may also result in depressed immune function, loss of muscle strength, poor wound healing, and pressure ulcer development in elderly individuals. New tissue cannot be made, ulcers cannot heal, and immune responses cannot be mounted without adequate dietary protein.

Indicators of dietary inadequacy of protein intake may be fasting plasma amino acids. Plasma amino acids may change in response to protein-energy malnutrition, protein malnutrition, a deficient intake of essential amino acids, or an imbalance in dietary protein.[61,62] Protein is a very important dietary component because of its essential need in the production of a vast array of physiologic compounds, including, for example, blood components (erythrocytes, leukocytes, platelets, etc.), hormones (epinephrine, insulin, etc.), enzymes (proteases, disaccharidases, lipases, etc.), smooth and striated muscle cells, epithelial tissue, and organ tissues.

Evaluating plasma proteins is a valuable tool in the nutritional assessment of older women. In general, women have smaller protein stores than men so that a decrease in this body compartment may contribute to increased frailty, muscle weakness, diminished ambulatory ability, and lower reserve capacity. The most valuable laboratory measure is serum albumin. Although it may be affected by various disease processes (cancer, renal failure, liver disease), serum albumin is generally not affected by age. Normal serum values range from 3.5 to 5 g/dL, although there may be variation in this range based on the methodology used in different laboratories. Serum albumin is the most reliable indicator of protein nutriture; other serum proteins often used in nutrition assessment (transferrin, urea nitrogen, total protein) are less reliable for a variety of reasons.[63] Gross estimates of body composition such as skinfold measures have not been derived from older adult populations and, therefore, are not valid indicators of body protein or fat stores.

Protein intake is important to assess. Protein-rich foods are often expensive, difficult to chew, and perceived to be high in fat or cholesterol. These foods (meat, fish, poultry, legumes, eggs, dairy products) are often voluntarily excluded from the diets of many older adults. These foods contain many essential nutrients, and inclusion in the diets of elderly women should be encouraged.

FLUID REQUIREMENTS

Fluid requirements are difficult to assess in older women. The problems associated with inadequate fluid intake in elderly people may be profound, but dehydration is difficult to prevent and often difficult to diagnose. Elderly persons are at risk for dehydration for a variety of reasons. First, as protein stores are reduced so is total body water, so it is easier to become depleted more rapidly.[64,65] Second, adaptation to water deprivation is inefficient because aging kidneys cannot concentrate urine rapidly.[66] Third, binding of antidiuretic hormone to renal receptors may decrease with advanced age, thereby contributing to difficulty in maintaining fluid volume.[67,68] Fourth, elderly people have a diminished thirst sensation due to a decrease in osmoreceptors, which are sensitive to blood concentration.[69–71] Fifth, many older adults voluntarily do not drink adequate amounts of fluid due to minor chronic problems with incontinence.[72]

To compound the problem of subclinical dehydration, identification of dehydration is often difficult because the presenting symptoms are frequently assumed to be associated with normal aging or they are signs that are expected in elderly people (Exhibit 10-2). If dehydration is identified as a problem, intervention may be simple but achieving compliance is difficult due to reduced thirst sensitivity and reluctance to consume large volumes of fluid due to the problem of chronic incontinence. Ironically, the treatment plan to manage incontinence includes consuming large volumes of fluid so that regularly scheduled voiding is reinforced because there is urine contained in the bladder.

Under usual conditions, fluid requirements approximate 30 mL/kg body weight, with a minimum volume of 1500 mL for small individuals.[73] Fluid may

Exhibit 10-2 Signs of Dehydration in Elderly People

- Dryness of mucosal tissue and skin
- Swollen, edematous tongue
- Sunken eyes
- Increased body temperature
- Decreased blood pressure
- Acute renal failure
- Decreased urine output
- Electrolyte disturbances
- Constipation
- Nausea and vomiting
- Mental confusion and depression

be taken as water, juices, carbonated beverages or ades, tea or coffee, gelatin or frozen desserts that are liquid at room temperature.

VITAMINS

Older adults generally are not at high risk for water-soluble vitamin deficiencies. Deficiencies, when they do develop, tend to be related to a poor diet rather than the elimination of a specific group of foods. Several water-soluble vitamins need attention in the evaluation of dietary quality, including vitamins B_6 and B_{12} and ascorbic acid.

Vitamin B_6

Elderly populations in many countries have been found to be deficient in vitamin B_6. For example, in one study conducted on older adults in Holland, 10 to 45% of the population, depending on the indicator used (aspartate aminotransferase activity coefficient or plasma pyridoxal phosphate level), were classified as vitamin B_6 deficient.[74] The RDA for vitamin B_6 is the same for adults regardless of age; it is based on a ratio of 0.16 mg of vitamin B_6 per gram of dietary protein. Therefore, there is a different allowance for men and women (2.0 mg and 1.6 mg, respectively). However, a depletion-repletion study demonstrated that once depleted, elderly subjects required several periods of repletion to bring their urinary xanthurenic acid excretion after a load of tryptophan back to baseline levels.[75] The conclusion was that the RDA for vitamin B_6 for adults may be too low for elderly people and should be re-examined in this population.

This vitamin is important in older subjects; a vitamin B_6 deficiency has been shown to impair specific measures of cell-mediated immunity. Both lymphocyte proliferation and interleukin-2 production are depressed in vitamin B_6 deficiency in elderly persons.[76] An adequate vitamin B_6 intake should be a major goal of modified diets for the elderly. The primary source of vitamin B_6 in free-living elderly is from fruits and vegetables. Therefore, these foods should be encouraged to provide B_6 as well as other nutrients.[77]

Vitamin B_{12}

Based on low serum levels there is a relatively high prevalence (23%) of vitamin B_{12} deficiency in free-living elderly people.[74,78,79] This may be due to undetected pernicious anemia, or more likely a condition of gastric acid hyposecretion, gastric atrophy. The prevalence of gastric atrophy increases with advancing age, and it exists in approximately 24% of persons aged 60 to 69 years, 32% of persons aged 70 to 79 years, and more than 37% of persons aged older than 80 years, predicted by low pepsinogen I levels.[80]

Gastric atrophy may interfere with vitamin B_{12} bioavailability because there is less secretion of acid and pepsin. This leads to impaired digestion of cobalamin (vitamin B_{12}) from food sources as well as to the binding of cobalamin to bacteria that are usually killed in the more acid environment of a normal stomach. Although there is a normal output of intrinsic factor, not enough vitamin B_{12} is released from its food carriers to be absorbed in adequate amounts.

For patients who have atrophic gastritis, providing supplemental intrinsic factor will not correct the malabsorption; however, giving acid or acid plus pepsin with supplemental vitamin B_{12} reverses the malabsorption.[81] Another study demonstrated that a course of tetracycline therapy aimed at killing the bacteria that binds the vitamin B_{12} will correct abnormal absorption of the vitamin.[82]

Vitamin B_{12} deficiency is a concern in elderly people because it has been associated with impaired cognitive function, dementia and neuropsychiatric disorders. These symptoms are associated with normal serum vitamin B_{12} levels, normal Schilling tests, and the absence of anemia or macrocytosis but with elevated serum homocysteine or methylmalonate levels.[83] Vitamin B_{12} deficiency frequently manifests itself in nonspecific symptoms; one case report describes oral epithelial dysplasia associated with vitamin B_{12} deficiency that responded to vitamin therapy.[84] It is important to be aware that a vitamin B_{12} deficiency is a possible cause of vague complaints of lethargy, malaise, and forgetfulness.

Vitamin C

Vitamin C has been a controversial nutrient for many years. Although there is no evidence that vitamin C absorption or use is impaired in elderly persons, vitamin C intake has been associated with a reduced risk for cancer, cataracts, and coronary heart disease and an increased life expectancy.[78] Vitamin C has been identified as the most potent antioxidant in the blood and may, therefore, be effective in protecting against stress-related and degenerative diseases.[74,85] Some investigators have suggested that 140 mg/day is necessary to saturate tissues with ascorbic acid (vitamin C) and recommend that maintaining tissues at full saturation may be desirable.[86]

In epidemiologic studies, vitamin assessments in elderly people, particularly among sedentary, homebound, institutionalized, and chronically ill elderly, have shown significant vitamin C deficiency, using plasma ascorbic acid levels as the marker. In the Dutch Nutrition Surveillance Study, vitamin C status was examined in both free-living and institutionalized elderly women. The investigators found that vitamin C status is most closely associated with daily dietary intake and that food preparation practices were a significant factor in the losses of vitamin C in food.[87]

Among the fat-soluble vitamins, there tends to be less risk of deficiency because of the ability to store these nutrients in liver and adipose tissue. There are risks, however, that are associated with some of these vitamins, particularly vitamins A and D.

Vitamin A

In older people, there are greater vitamin A storage pools, an age-related delay in clearance of retinyl esters, and elevated levels of unbound circulating plasma vitamin A. These factors suggest that there is a lower margin of safety in vitamin A intake requirements.[74] Although population surveys often indicate an inadequate dietary intake of vitamin A, liver levels of vitamin A do not drop with age.[78] There is evidence that this finding may be attributed to the decreased clearance of blood vitamin A levels, particularly retinyl esters, which are indicators of toxicity.[88] Vitamin A requirements may actually be lower in older adults, but more extensive longitudinal studies are needed.

Vitamin A has been associated with the possible prevention of some types of cancer. Studies on the roles of retinol, preformed vitamin A, and β-carotene are somewhat controversial.[89,90] Thus far, there are no observed toxic side effects from ingestion of high levels of carotenoids in either young or old subjects.[78]

Vitamin D

Vitamin D is one of the nutrients for which elderly women may be at risk for deficiency. Older adults maintain lower levels of active vitamin D (1,25-dihydroxyvitamin D) than do younger adults because of a lower dietary consumption and a decrease in sunlight exposure.[78] Vitamin D is unique in that the body has the ability to synthesize its biologically active form, but advancing age is associated with a decreased capacity to produce 7-dehydrocholesterol (provitamin D_3) in the skin and to convert 25-hydroxyvitamin D to the active 1,25-dihydroxyvitamin D.[78]

The various roles of vitamin D in the body make it a very important dietary component. The best known function of vitamin D is to retain bone and to facilitate calcium absorption and use.[91] A recently elucidated role of vitamin D is that it acts as a modulator of mononuclear phagocyte and lymphocyte biology; clinically it regulates host immune defenses.[92] Curiously, depressed immune function has been noted in elderly people, and this observation raises questions regarding the relationship between dietary vitamin D intake and immune responsiveness in the elderly.

The RDA for vitamin D for older adults is 200 IU. Despite one study in which the average vitamin D intake was approximately 380 IU/day, it is apparent that many elderly people require supplementation to maintain serum calcitriol levels.[93] Dietary vitamin D intake is often inadequate[94–96] and, therefore, contributes to the risk of vitamin deficiency, which contributes to reduced bone mass in elderly women.[94] Offering vitamin D supplementation to elderly women has a beneficial effect on maintaining bone density[97,98] and should be considered in at-risk populations.

Other Vitamins

Other vitamins that are often associated with potential problems in elderly people are folic acid and vitamins E and K. Folic acid at the level of the RDA will barely meet the needs of most healthy elderly. For older adults who have folate malabsorption related to gastric atrophy, folic acid requirements may be slightly higher than presently identified to provide an adequate margin for those who have absorption problems.

There is no RDA for vitamin E but rather an "allowance" based on usual U.S. intake levels.[78] Vitamin E deficiencies are very rare and are not generally considered a risk in elderly people. There is some speculation that high dietary or supplemental intakes of vitamin E are associated with reduced risks for atherogenesis, cataracts, and ischemic heart disease. The protection vitamin E offers when it quenches free radicals has been associated with a decrease in age-related conditions in which the etiology may be cellular damage.[78] Vitamin K status may be at risk in elderly individuals who are on sulfa drugs, antibiotics, and anticoagulant therapies.

MINERALS

Establishing mineral requirements in humans is very difficult despite their essentiality to the maintenance of life. For example, no RDAs have ever been established for sodium and potassium although they are indispensable in the diet. These two major minerals may be affected by various chronic diseases and their treatments, but they are rarely deficient in the diets of elderly people. Concern for these nutrients arises when older patients are receiving drug therapy that affects fluid and electrolyte balance; where these conditions exist, it is important to monitor sodium and potassium status.[99]

There are, however, requirements established for other minerals, including calcium, phosphorus, and magnesium.[99,100] Calcium remains the most controversial of all the minerals because of the crucial role it has in the maintenance of bone.

Calcium

The present RDA for calcium is 800 mg/day for women aged 51+. There have been many discussions over whether this recommendation should be raised to 1000 mg, 1200 mg, or 1500 mg/day for this group. Because of the high incidence of osteoporosis in postmenopausal women, this nutrient is of great importance. There is a direct relationship between dietary calcium intake and bone mineral density in postmenopausal women.[101,102] Adequate ingestion of calcium is very important all through the life cycle, but in young women who are still building bone density and in older women who are at risk of losing bone density rapidly, it is crucial.

Recently, the National Institutes of Health held a Consensus Development Conference on Optimal Calcium Intake (June 1994). The recommendation for calcium intake for postmenopausal women who are on estrogen replacement therapy is for 1000 mg/day, and for postmenopausal women who are not receiving estrogen therapy, it is 1500 mg/day.[103] This level of calcium intake in older women not receiving estrogen may limit bone mass loss but it is not as effective as hormone replacement therapy in maintaining bone density.

There are, however, other factors in addition to dietary calcium intake that must be present to preserve bone density in older women.[103] Adequate intake of vitamin D is also necessary to enhance the absorption and use of calcium. A third factor is weight-bearing exercise.[104] Many older women are at high risk for developing osteoporosis because these three factors are frequently deficient in their diet and life style. Weight and body mass index also have an impact on bone density. For example, women who are heavier have a slower rate of bone loss than leaner women.[105,106] Bone health in women is complex, and many other factors contribute to the maintenance of a healthy skeleton.[107] Certainly, prevention of osteoporosis through early nutrition intervention efforts targeted to girls and young women is essential for optimum bone health.

Phosphorus

Phosphorus requirements are usually established as a one-to-one ratio with calcium. Presently, the RDA for phosphorus in women older than age 50 is 800 mg/day to maintain balance with calcium requirements; if calcium requirements are increased, then phosphorus requirements will also have to be increased. Phosphorus deficiency occurs infrequently but may be due to an inadequate intake of calcium-rich and/or protein-rich food, or an excessive use of phosphate-binding antacids.[99]

Magnesium

Magnesium requirements in older women are approximately 280 mg/day. In healthy women, this is an adequate level to maintain magnesium nutriture. However, in any person who has a problem with gastrointestinal malabsorption or excessive gastrointestinal losses, chronic alcoholism, renal dysfunction, or protein-calorie malnutrition, magnesium deficiency becomes a concern. Magnesium deficiency is treatable; it is, however, difficult to recognize.[99] Symptoms are primarily neuromuscular, including Trousseau and Chvostek signs, muscle spasms, personality changes, anorexia, nausea, and vomiting. These signs and symptoms are often ascribed to other etiologies than nutritional deficit, and it is a condition not commonly recognized by most physicians who do not have training in nutrition.

TRACE MINERALS

Although many trace minerals are essential, most are required in such small amounts that there have been no RDAs identified. Rather, there are quantities that have been described as an Estimated Safe and Adequate Daily Dietary Intake (ESADDI). These trace minerals are associated with excesses and deficiencies in very rare and unusual circumstances and do not require dietary evaluation because in a nutritionally adequate diet these nutrients should be present in adequate amounts. When patients are given enteral and parenteral solutions for extended periods of time, the trace minerals (iodine, copper, selenium, chromium, boron, manganese) must be supplemented and status monitored.[108]

In contrast, iron and zinc do have RDAs and must be evaluated in assessing dietary adequacy. Both of these minerals are important in elderly women.

Iron

Iron is an important nutrient for women of all ages. The recommendation for dietary iron decreases in postmenopausal women due to the cessation of menstrual blood loss. In older women the RDA for iron decreases to 10 mg/day from 15 mg/day. Older people tend to have higher tissue iron stores so the requirement for iron to replace or maintain these stores is diminished.[109]

Anemia is one of the most common hematologic findings in older people; however, it appears to be independent of iron nutriture. When iron-deficiency anemia occurs in older people, it is usually associated with gastrointestinal blood losses. It is important to first diagnose the iron deficiency and identify the etiology before treatment can be initiated. Elderly people respond appropriately to oral iron salt therapy, but it should only be used when the cause of the anemia is clearly established.[109]

Zinc

Zinc is an essential nutrient that has captured considerable attention in recent years. Data on the prevalence of zinc deficiency in elderly people is highly variable, which makes it difficult to generalize about zinc status in this population. Of greatest interest regarding older adults is the role that zinc has in taste sensitivity, wound healing, and immune function. It is known that taste sensitivity decreases with advancing age[110]; this loss of taste has been linked to the fact that zinc deficiency is associated with hypogeusia.[111] However, zinc supplementation will only improve taste acuity in zinc-deficient individuals. In the nutriture of elderly people, zinc has been associated with many different problems. Zinc status is affected by dietary intake; meats, fish, and poultry are good sources of absorbable zinc, whereas vegetable sources are not absorbed as well. Many medications used widely by elderly people also have an effect on zinc status: diuretics, laxatives, and antacids.[108]

Zinc plays an important role in wound healing, but supplementation with zinc in individuals who are not zinc-deficient does not improve the quality or rate of wound healing.[108] Zinc has also been linked to cellular immunity. In zinc-deficient persons, zinc supplementation does improve immune responsiveness,[112] and recommendations have been made to provide small amounts of supplemental zinc to ensure proper immune functioning in elderly people.[108] It is wise to monitor any mineral supplementation carefully because of the hazards associated with aggressive supplementation, and zinc is no different.[113] The unique characteristics and issues related to nutritional needs of elderly women are summarized in Exhibit 10-3.

Exhibit 10-3 Nutrition Needs of Elderly Women: Unique Characteristics and Issues

Energy	• RDA based on extrapolated data from young adults. • Needs decrease with age, but no recommendations available for young versus elderly.
Fat	• Needs do not change. • Restriction of intake to prevent development of chronic diseases has been questioned.
Carbohydrates	• Needs do not change. • Dietary intake is reduced. • Incorporation of high-fiber foods rather than fiber additives needs to be encouraged.
Protein	• Protein-energy malnutrition has been reported. • RDA is inadequate to maintain nitrogen balance. • Rich sources are often voluntarily excluded.
Fluids	• Great risk of dehydration.
Vitamin B_6	• Deficiency has been observed using biochemical indices. • RDA may be too low. • Consumption of fruits and vegetables needs to be encouraged.
Vitamin B_{12}	• Deficiency is prevalent (23%) based on biomedical indices. • RDA needs to be increased to compensate for abnormal absorption.
Vitamin C	• Deficiency has been observed using biochemical indices. • An intake of 140 mg/day may be needed to keep tissues fully saturated. • Food preparation practices contribute to losses.
Vitamin A	• Lower margin of safety in requirements as compared to younger adults.
Vitamin D	• Risk of deficiency is increased. • Decreased dietary consumption. • Decreased sunlight exposure.
Folic Acid	• RDA needs to be increased to compensate for malabsorption in some individuals.
Calcium	• RDA is low.
Iron	• Needs are decreased. • Anemia is common but is independent of iron nutriture.
Zinc	• Generalizations about status are difficult to make due to variability in the data.

FUTURE RESEARCH NEEDS

There is a great need for continuing research on the nutrient needs of elderly people, particularly women. Much of what is presently known about the nutrient needs of adults is derived from cross-sectional studies that include individuals of all ages. Research that examines the need for specific nutrients for maintenance of health in the elderly is essential for developing therapies that reduce the risk of chronic diseases as well as enhancing recovery from acute illnesses. Because of the increasing number of elderly in the U.S., concerted efforts need to be made to understand the nutritional needs of elderly people.

Meeting the nutritional needs of elderly women is challenging because their energy requirements drop while their macronutrient requirements and most of their micronutrient requirements do not change or increase. The planning and implementation of a low calorie, nutrient-dense diet suitable for elderly women that also meets contemporary dietary recommendations requires knowledge about appropriate food choices. Nutrition education programs would benefit elderly women and persons responsible for their care.

References

1. American Geriatrics Society Task Force on Older Women's Health. *Older Women's Health.* Washington, DC; 1993.

2. Gilford DM, ed. *The Aging Population in the Twenty-First Century: Statistics for Health Policy.* Washington, DC: National Academy Press; 1988.

3. Chernoff R, ed. Demographics of aging. In: Chernoff R, ed. *Geriatric Nutrition: The Health Professional's Handbook.* Gaithersburg, Md: Aspen Publishers; 1991:1–10.

4. Smith DW. Is greater female longevity a general finding among animals? *Biol Rev Cambridge Philos Soc.* 1989;64(1):1–12.

5. Johansson S. Longevity in women. *Cardiovasc Clin.* 1989;19(3):3–16.

6. Hazzard WR. Why do women live longer than men? Biological differences that influence longevity. *Postgrad Med.* 1989;85(5):271–278.

7. Pegels CC. *Health Care and the Older Citizen.* Gaithersburg, Md: Aspen Publishers; 1988.

8. Heidrich SM. The relationship between physical health and psychological well-being in elderly women: a developmental approach. *Res Nurs Health.* 1993;16:123–130.

9. Alexander BB, Rubinstein RL, Goodman M, et al. A path not taken: a cultural analysis of regrets and childlessness in the lives of older women. *Gerontologist.* 1992;32(5):618–626.

10. Rubinstein RL, Alexander BB, Goodman M, et al. Key relationships of never married, childless older women: a cultural analysis. *Gerontol Soc Sci.* 1991;46(5):S270–277.

11. Roughan PA. Mental health and psychiatric disorders in older women. *Clin Geriat Med.* 1993; 9(1):173–190.

12. Goldstein MZ, Perkins CA. Mental health and aging women. *Clin Geriat Med.* 1993;9(1):191–196.

13. Löwik MRH, Schneijder P, Hulshof KFAM, et al. Institutionalized elderly women have lower food intake than do those living more independently (Dutch Nutrition Surveillance System). *J Am Coll Nutr.* 1992;11(4):432–440.

14. Löwik MRH, van den Berg H, Schrijver J, et al. Marginal nutritional status among institutionalized elderly women as compared to those living more independently (Dutch Nutrition Surveillance System). *J Am Coll Nutr.* 1992;11(6):673–681.

15. Carter WJ. Macronutrients requirements for elderly persons. In: Chernoff R, ed. *Geriatric Nutrition: The Health Professional's Handbook.* Gaithersburg, Md: Aspen Publishers; 1991:11–24.

16. Shepard JW. Interrelationships of exercise and nutrition in the elderly. In: Armbrecht HJ, Prendergast J, Coe R, eds. *Nutritional Intervention in the Aging Process.* New York, NY: Springer-Verlag; 1984.

17. Reilly JJ, Lord A, Bunker WW, et al. Energy balance in healthy elderly women. *Br J Nutr.* 1993;69:21–27.

18. Morley JE, Glick Z. Endocrine aspects of nutrition and aging. In: Chernoff R, ed. *Geriatric Nutrition: The Health Professional's Handbook.* Gaithersburg, Md: Aspen Publishers; 1991:311–335.

19. Voorrips LE, Tineke M-CVA, Deurenberg P, et al. Energy expenditure at rest and during standardized activities: a comparison between elderly and middle-aged women. *Am J Clin Nutr.* 1993;58:15–20.

20. Niskanen L, Piirainen M, Koljonen M, et al. Resting energy expenditure in relation to energy intake in patients with Alzheimer's disease, multi-infarct dementia and in control women. *Age Aging.* 1993;22:132–137.

21. Arciero PJ, Goran MI, Gardner AM, et al. A practical equation to predict resting metabolic rate in older females. *J Am Geriatr Soc.* 1993;41:389–395.

22. Butterworth DE, Nieman DC, Perkins R, et al. Exercise training and nutrient intake in elderly women. *J Am Diet Assoc.* 1993;93:653–657.

23. Voorrips LE, van Staveren WA, Hautvast JGAV. Are physically active elderly women in a better nutritional condition than their sedentary peers? *Eur J Clin Nutr.* 1991;45:545–552.

24. Fiatarone MA, O'Neill EF, Doyle N, et al. The Boston FICSIT study: the effects of resistance training and nutritional supplementation on physical frailty in the oldest old. *J Am Geriatr Soc.* 1993;41:333–337.

25. Antonini FM, Vannucci A. Exercise and nutrition in the elderly. In: Labus L, Pernigotti I, Ferrario F, eds. *Sedentary Life and Nutrition.* New York, NY: Raven Press; 1990:89–94.

26. Kohrt WM, Obert KA, Holloszy JO. Exercise training improves fat distribution patterns in 60- to 70-year-old men and women. *J Gerontol Med Sci.* 1992;47(4):M99–M105.

27. Owens JF, Matthews KA, Wing RR, et al. Can physical activity mitigate the effects of aging in middle-aged women? *Circulation.* 1992;85:1265–1270.

28. Rutherford OM, Jones DA. The relationship of muscle and bone loss and activity levels with age in women. *Age Ageing.* 1992;21:286–293.

29. Ideno KT, Kubena KS. Nutrition, physical activity, and blood pressure in the elderly. *J Nutr Elderly.* 1990;9(2):3–15.

30. Evans WJ. Exercise, nutrition and aging. *J Nutr.* 1992;122:796–801.

31. Shangold MM. Exercise in the menopausal woman. *Obstet Gynecol.* 1990;75(suppl 4):53S–58S;81S–83S.

32. Lee C. Factors related to the adoption of exercise among older women. *J Behav Med.* 1993;16(3):323–334.

33. Siguel EN, Schaefer EJ. Aging and nutritional requirements of essential fatty acids. In: Beare-Rogers J, ed. *Dietary Fat Requirements in Health and Disease.* Champaign, Ill: American Oil Chemists Society; 1988:163–189.

34. Sorenson A, Chapman N, Sundwall D. Health promotion and disease prevention in the elderly. In: Chernoff R, ed. *Geriatric Nutrition: The Health Professional's Handbook.* Gaithersburg, Md: Aspen Publishers;1991:449–483.

35. American Heart Association. *Dietary Guidelines for Healthy American Adults: A Statement for Physicians and Health Professionals by the Nutrition Committee.* Dallas, Tx: American Heart Association; 1986.

36. Garry PJ, Hunt WC, Koehler KM, et al. Longitudinal study of dietary intakes and plasma lipids in healthy elderly men and women. *Am J Clin Nutr.* 1992;55:682–688.

37. Löwik MRH, Wedel M, Kok FJ, et al. Nutrition and serum cholesterol levels among elderly men and women (Dutch Nutrition Surveillance System). *J Gerontol Med Sci.* 1991;46(1):M23–M28.

38. Kaiser FE. Cholesterol, heart disease, and the older adult. *Clin Appl Nutr.* 1992;2(1):35–43.

39. Harris T, Cook EF, Kannel WB, et al. Proportional hazards analysis of risk factors for coronary heart disease in individuals aged 65 or older. *J Am Geriatr Soc.* 1988;36:1023–1028.

40. Benfante R, Reed D. Is elevated serum cholesterol level a risk factor for coronary heart disease in the elderly? *JAMA.* 1990;263:393–396.

41. Pariza MW. Diet, cancer, and food safety. In: Shils ME, Olson JA, Shike M, eds. *Modern Nutrition in Health and Disease.* 8th ed. Philadelphia, Pa: Lea & Febiger; 1994:1545–1558.

42. Crighton IL, Dowsett M, Hunter M, et al. The effect of a low-fat diet on hormone levels in healthy pre- and postmenopausal women: relevance for breast cancer. *Eur J Cancer* 1992;28A(12):2024–2027.

43. Lissner L, Kroon U-B, Björntrop P, et al. Adipose tissue fatty acids and dietary fat sources in relation to endometrial cancer: a retrospective study of cases in remission, and population-based controls. *Acta Obstet Gynecol Scand.* 1993;72:481–487.

44. Vinik AI, Jenkins DJA. Dietary fiber in the management of diabetes. *Diabetes Care.* 1988;11:160–173.

45. Schneeman BO, Tietyen J. Dietary fiber. In: Shils ME, Olson JA, Shike M, eds. *Modern Nutrition in Health and Disease.* 8th ed. Philadelphia, Pa: Lea & Febiger; 1994:89–100.

46. Snustad D, Lee V, Abraham I, et al. Dietary fiber in hospitalized geriatric patients: too soft a solution for too hard a problem? *J Nutr Elderly.* 1991;10(2):49–63.

47. Wolfsen CR, Barker JC, Mitteness LS. Constipation in the daily lives of frail elderly people. *Arch Fam Med.* 1993;2:853–858.

48. Cashman MD. The aging gut. In: Chernoff R, ed. *Geriatric Nutrition: The Health Professional's Handbook.* Gaithersburg, Md: Aspen Publishers; 1991:183–227.

49. Hermann JR, Hanson CF, Kopel BH. Fiber intake of older adults: relationship to mineral intakes. *J Nutr Elderly.* 1992;11(4):21–32.

50. Timmons KH, DuFord S. Quick and easy steps to a high fiber diet for the elderly. *JNE.* 1991;23:250G.

51. Steinmetz KA, Potter JD. Food-group consumption and colon cancer in the Adelaide case-control study. I. Vegetable and fruit. *Int J Cancer.* 1993;53:711–719.

52. Munro HN, Young VR. Protein metabolism in the elderly. *Postgrad Med.* 1978;63(3):143–152.

53. Uauy R, Winterer JC, Bilmazes C, et al. The changing pattern of whole body protein metabolism in aging humans. *J Gerontol.* 1978;33:663–671.

54. Crim MC, Munro HN. Proteins and amino acids. In: Shils ME, Olson JA, Shike M, eds. *Modern Nutrition in Health and Disease.* 8th ed. Philadelphia, Pa: Lea & Febiger; 1994:3–35.

55. Gersovitz M, Motil K, Munro HN, et al. Human protein requirements: assessment of the adequacy of the current recommended allowance for dietary protein in elderly men and women. *Am J Clin Nutr.* 1982;35:6–14.

56. Bienia R, Ratcliff S, Barbour GS, et al. Malnutrition in the hospitalized geriatric patient. *J Am Geriatr Soc.* 1982;30:433–436.

57. Linn BS. Outcomes of older and younger malnourished and well-nourished patients one year after hospitalization. *Am J Clin Nutr.* 1984;39:66–73.

58. Sullivan DH, Patch GA, Walls RC, et al. Impact of nutritional status on morbidity or mortality in a select population of geriatric patients. *Am J Clin Nutr.* 1990;51:749–758.

59. Sullivan DH, Walls RC, Lipschitz DA. Protein-energy undernutrition and the risk of mortality within 1 yr of hospital discharge in a select population of geriatric rehabilitation patients. *Am J Clin Nutr.* 1991;53:599–605.

60. Volkert D, Kruse W, Oster P, et al. Malnutrition in geriatric patients: diagnostic and prognostic significance of nutritional parameters. *Ann Nutr Metab.* 1992;36:97–112.

61. Rudman D, Mattson DE, Feller AG, et al. Fasting plasma amino acids in elderly men. *Am J Clin Nutr.* 1989;49:559–566.

62. Caballero B, Gleason RE, Wurtman RJ. Plasma amino acid concentrations in healthy elderly men and women. *Am J Clin Nutr.* 1991;53:1249–1252.

63. Mitchell CO, Chernoff R. Nutritional assessment of the elderly. In: Chernoff R, ed. *Geriatric Nutrition: The Health Professional's Handbook.* Gaithersburg, Md: Aspen Publishers; 1991:363–396.

64. Schoeller DA. Changes in total body water with age. *Am J Clin Nutr.* 1989;50:1176–1181.

65. Reiff TR. Water loss in aging and its clinical significance. *Geriatrics.* 1987;42(6):53–62.

66. Rowe J, Shack N, Defronzo R. The influence of age on the renal response to water deprivation in man. *Nephron.* 1976;17:270–278.

67. Rolls B, Wood R, Rolls E, et al. Thirst following water deprivation in humans. *Am J Physiol.* 1980;239:R476–R482.

68. Phillips P, Rolls BJ, Ladingham DM, et al. Reduced thirst after water deprivation in healthy elderly men. *N Engl J Med.* 1984;311:753–759.

69. Leaf A. Dehydration in the elderly. *N Engl J Med.* 1984;311:791–792.

70. Rolls BJ, Phillips PA. Aging and disturbances in thirst and fluid balance. *Nutr Rev.* 1990;48:137–143.

71. Editorial. Thirst and osmoregulation in the elderly. *Lancet.* 1984;2(8410):1017–1018.

72. Chernoff R. Thirst and fluid requirements in the elderly. *Nutr Rev.* 1994;52:S3–S5.

73. USDA Human Nutrition Information Service. *Food Facts for Older Adults.* Washington, DC: 1993. U.S. Government Printing Office; Home and Garden Bulletin no. 251.

74. Russell RM. Micronutrient requirements of the elderly. *Nutr Rev.* 1992;50(12):463–466.

75. Ribaya-Mercado JD, Russell RM, Sahyoun N, et al. Vitamin B_6 requirements of elderly men and women. *J Nutr.* 1991;121:1062–1074.

76. Meydani S, Ribaya-Mercado JD, Russell RM, et al. Vitamin B_6 deficiency impairs interleukin-2 production and lymphocyte proliferation in elderly adults. *Am J Clin Nutr.* 1991;53:1275–1280.

77. Manore MM, Vaughan LA, Lehman WR. Contribution of various food groups to dietary vitamin B_6 intake in free-living, low-income elderly persons. *J Am Diet Assoc.* 1990;90(6):830–834.

78. Blumberg JB. Changing nutrient requirements in older adults. *Nutr Today.* 1992;Sept/Oct:15–20.

79. Pedrosa MC, Russell RM. Folate and vitamin B_{12} absorption in atrophic gastritis. In: Holt PR, Russell RM, eds. *Chronic Gastritis and Hypochlorhydria in the Elderly.* Boca Raton, Fla: CRC Press; 1993:157–169.

80. Krasinski SD, Russell RM, Samloff M, et al. Fundic atrophic gastritis in an elderly population. *J Am Geriatr Soc.* 1986;34:800.

81. King CE, Leibach J, Toskes PP. Clinically significant vitamin B_{12} deficiency secondary to malabsorption of protein-bound vitamin B_{12}. *Dig Dis Sci.* 1979;24:397–402.

82. Suter PM, Golner BB, Goldin BR. Reversal of protein-bound vitamin B_{12} malabsorption with antibiotics in atrophic gastritis. *Gastroenterology.* 1991;101:1039–1045.

83. Lindenbaum J, Healton EB, Savage DG, et al. Neuropsychiatric disorders caused by cobalamin deficiency in the absence of anemia or macrocytosis. *N Engl J Med.* 1988;318:1720–1728.

84. Theaker JM, Porter SR, Fleming KA. Oral epithelial dysplasia in vitamin B_{12} deficiency. *Oral Surg Oral Med Oral Pathol.* 1989;67:81–83.

85. Balz F, Stocker R, Ames BN. Antioxidant defenses and lipid peroxidation in human blood plasma. *Proc Natl Acad Sci.* 1988;85:9748–9752.

86. Jacob RA, Skala JH, Omaye ST. Biochemical indices of human vitamin C status. *Am J Clin Nutr.* 1987;46:818–826.

87. Löwik MRH, Hulshof KFAM, Schneijder P, et al. Vitamin C status in elderly women: a comparison between women living in a nursing home and women living independently. *J Am Diet Assoc.* 1993;93:167–172.

88. Krasinski SD, Cohn JS, Schaefer EJ, et al. Postprandial plasma retinyl ester response is greater in older subjects compared with younger subjects. *J Clin Invest.* 1990;85:883–892.

89. Slater TF, Block G. Antioxidant vitamins and beta carotene in disease prevention. *Am J Clin Nutr.* 1991;53:189S–396S.

90. The Alpha-Tocopherol, Beta Carotene Cancer Prevention Study Group: The effect of vitamin E and beta carotene on the incidence of lung cancer and other changes in male smokers. *N Engl J Med.* 1994;330:1029–1035.

91. Anderson JJB. The role of nutrition in the functioning of skeletal tissue. *Nutr Rev.* 1992;50(12):388–394.

92. Yoder MC, Manolagas SC. Vitamin D and its role in immune function. *Clin Appl Nutr.* 1991;1(1):35–44.

93. O'Dowd KJ, Clemens TL, Kelsey JL, et al. Exogenous calciferol (vitamin D) and vitamin D endocrine status among elderly nursing home residents in the New York City area. *J Am Geriatr Soc.* 1993;41:414–421.

94. Villareal DT, Civitelli R, Chines A, et al. Subclinical vitamin D deficiency in postmenopausal women with low vertebral bone mass. *J Clin Endocrinol Metab.* 1991;72(3):628–634.

95. Webb AR, Pilbeam C, Hanafin N, et al. An evaluation of the relative contributions of exposure to sunlight and of diet to the circulating concentrations of 25-hydroxyvitamin D in an elderly nursing home population in Boston. *Am J Clin Nutr.* 1990;51:1075–1081.

96. Gloth FM, Tobin JD, Sherman SS, et al. Is the recommended daily allowance for vitamin D too low for the homebound elderly? *J Am Geriatrics Soc.* 1991;39:137–141.

97. Dawson-Hughes B, Dallal GE, Krall EA, et al. Effect of vitamin D supplementation on wintertime and overall bone loss in healthy postmenopausal women. *Ann Intern Med.* 1991;115(7):505–512.

98. Chapuy MC, Arlot ME, Duboeuf F, et al. Vitamin D3 and calcium to prevent hip fractures in elderly women. *N Engl J Med.* 1992;327:1637–1642.

99. Lindeman RD, Beck AA. Mineral requirements. In: Chernoff R, ed. *Geriatric Nutrition: The Health Professional's Handbook.* Gaithersburg, Md: Aspen Publishers;1991:53–76.

100. Freeland-Graves JH, Bales CW. Dietary recommendations of minerals for the elderly. *Curr Top Nutr Dis.* 1989;21:3–14.

101. Andon MB, Smith KT, Bracker M, et al. Spinal bone density and calcium intake in healthy postmenopausal women. *Am J Clin Nutr.* 1991;54:927–929.

102. Hasling C, Søndergaard K, Charles P, et al. Calcium metabolism in postmenopausal osteoporotic women is determined by dietary calcium and coffee intake. *J Nutr.* 1992;122:1119–1126.

103. National Institutes of Health Consensus Development Conference statement. *Optimal Calcium Intake.* June 6–8, 1994.

104. Nelson ME, Fisher EC, Dilamnian FA, et al. A 1-yr walking program and increased dietary calcium in postmenopausal women: effects on bone. *Am J Clin Nutr.* 1991;53:1304–1311.

105. Felson DT, Zhang Y, Hannan MT, et al. Effects of weight and body mass index on bone mineral density in men and women: the Framingham Study. *J Bone Miner Res.* 1993;8(5):567–573.

106. Tremollieres FA, Pouilles J-M, Ribot C. Vertebral postmenopausal bone loss is reduced in overweight women: a longitudinal study in 155 early postmenopausal women. *J Clin Endocrinol Metab.* 1993;77:683–686.

107. Heaney RP. Nutritional factors in elderly subjects: methodological and contextual problems. *Am J Clin Nutr.* 1989;50:1182–1189.

108. Fosmire GJ. Trace metal requirements. In: Chernoff R, ed. *Geriatric Nutrition: The Health Professional's Handbook.* Gaithersburg, Md: Aspen Publishers; 1991:77–105.

109. Lipschitz DA. Impact of nutrition on the age-related declines in hematopoiesis. In: Chernoff R, ed. *Geriatric Nutrition: The Health Professional's Handbook.* Gaithersburg, Md: Aspen Publishers; 1991:271–287.

110. Schiffman SS. Perception of taste and smell in elderly persons. *Crit Rev Food Sci Nutr.* 1993;33(1):17–26.

111. Henkin RI, Patten BM, Re PK, et al. Syndrome of acute zinc loss. *Arch Neurol.* 1975;32:745–751.

112. Wagner PA, Jernigan JA, Bailey LB, et al. Zinc nutriture and cell-mediated immunity in the aged. *Int J Vitam Nutr Res.* 1983;53:94–101.

113. Fosmire GJ. Possible hazards associated with zinc supplementation. *Nutr Today.* 1989;May/June:15–18.

Part II

Preventive Nutrition Throughout the Life Cycle

11

Preventive Nutrition in Adolescent Girls

Linda Van Horn and Annie O. Wong

If optimal nutritional practices were attained, all babies would be breast-fed; all children, regardless of ethnic background or socioeconomic status, would consume an adequate diet; and all adolescents would adopt health-promoting, nutritious dietary habits that would carry them through adulthood with minimal risk for chronic disease. Nutritional intake would come from a variety of foods from all food groups, in moderate portions, balanced with adequate activity to maintain ideal body weight. Girls, in particular, would have a realistic perception of their bodies and the confidence to consume calories adequate for normal growth and development. Of course, dietary fat intake would be less than 30% of total calories. Fruits and vegetables would be consumed in abundance. Foods would be prepared without excessive sodium, caffeine, or alcohol. Children would learn to cook, not just to reheat. They would read and understand labels. They would be informed and discriminating consumers. They would have access to lower-fat, high-fiber foods at school, popular fast-food restaurants, cafeterias, and sporting events. Finally, children would develop an appreciation for variety in their food choices and a willingness to experiment with different cuisines, and all this would be shared on a social level without fear of ostracism from peers.

Is this vision pure fantasy or are there glimpses of hope for the future? How far removed from these objectives are we? What guidelines and recommendations exist to facilitate progress? How effective are they? What else should be done for adolescent girls to improve their overall health and future risk for disease? Why bother during adolescence when girls are experiencing so many physical and emotional changes and are generally at low risk for morbidity or mortality from chronic disease?

The primary diseases that cause death and disability in women include cardiovascular disease, breast and colon cancer, osteoporosis, diabetes, and obesity. Each of these is considered preventable, or at least modifiable, through dietary and life-style changes. None of these diseases is acute in onset, progression, or treatment. Months and even years of dietary behavior, often evident during adolescence, contribute to the gradual development of risk factors for each disease. The longer these behaviors have been implemented, the more refractory they may be to change. Fifty years of a high-fat, high-salt, low-fiber eating pattern is likely to be more difficult to change than 13 or 14 years of such a pattern. Levels of motivation and dietary adherence may be greater in older populations as they confront their own mortality, but there are no data to compare the efficacy and feasibility of initiating a risk reduction program across two different age groups of women. Despite evidence, for example, of atherosclerotic regression in men who followed an aggressive program of very low-fat diet and exercise, the benefits of primary prevention and avoiding progression of atherosclerosis are clearly superior.

Adolescence is a period of involuntary and perhaps, unwanted, rapid physical growth. The psychological and emotional maturity needed to comprehend and accept the body's changing form may or may not accompany these changes. Adolescents increasingly assume responsibility for their own behavior but may not base decisions on accurate information or sound judgment. Parents, teachers, and other authority figures become secondary in importance and credibility is given to fashion, media, and most significantly, peers. Can prevention efforts succeed under such tumultuous conditions?

TARGETS FOR PREVENTION

The *Healthy People 2000: National Health Promotion and Disease Prevention Objectives* of the U.S. Department of Health and Human Services identify three broad goals for public health.[1] The goals are to increase the span of healthy life for Americans, reduce health disparities among Americans, and achieve access to preventive services for all Americans. Of the 298 specific objectives that were identified in 22 separate priority areas, several are devoted to nutrition, and some of those involve adolescents. *Healthy Children 2000* provides national health promotion and disease prevention objectives related to mothers, infants, children, and adolescents.[2] Objectives related to adolescent nutrition are summarized in Exhibit 11-1. Detailed discussion of those objectives related to prevention of specific chronic disease follows.

Also, at least three of The *Healthy People 2000* objectives can be applied to adolescents. These relate to reading and using the new food labels to help make wise food choices and include:

2.13 Increase to at least 85% the proportion of people aged 18 and older who use food labels to make nutritious food selections.

There are no data documenting the proportion of children or adolescents who read food labels. With the advent of the Nutrition Labeling and Education Act

Exhibit 11-1 Healthy Children 2000: Nutrition Objectives

---

1. Reduce overweight to a prevalence of no more than 20% among people aged 20 and older and no more than 15% among adolescents aged 12 through 19. (Baseline: 26% for people aged 20 through 74 in 1976 to 1980, 24% for men and 27% for women; 15% for adolescents aged 12 through 19 in 1976 to 1980.)

2. Reduce growth retardation among low-income children aged 5 and younger to less than 10%. (Baseline: Up to 16% among low-income children in 1988, depending on age and race/ethnicity.)

3. Reduce dietary fat intake to an average of 30% of calories or less and average saturated fat intake to less than 10% of calories among people aged 2 and older. (Baseline: 36% of calories from total fat and 13% from saturated fat for people aged 20 through 74 in 1976 to 1980; 36% and 13% for women aged 19 through 50 in 1985.)

4. Increase to at least 50% the proportion of overweight people aged 12 and older who have adopted sound dietary practices combined with regular physical activity to attain an appropriate body weight. (Baseline: 30% of overweight women and 25% of overweight men for people aged 18 and older in 1985.)

5. Increase calcium intake so at least 50% of youth aged 12 through 24 and 50% of pregnant and lactating women consume three or more servings daily of foods rich in calcium, and at least 50% of people aged 25 and older consume two or more servings daily. (Baseline: 7% of women and 14% of men aged 19 through 24 and 24% of pregnant and lactating women consumed three or more servings, and 15% of women and 23% of men aged 25 through 50 consumed two or more servings in 1985 to 1986.)

6. Reduce iron deficiency to less than 3% among children aged 1 through 4 and among women of childbearing age. (Baseline: 9% for children aged 1 through 2, 4% for children aged 3 through 4, and 5% for women aged 20 through 44 in 1976 to 1980.)

7. Increase to at least 75% of the proportion of mothers who breast-feed their babies in the early postpartum period and to at least 50% the proportion who continue breast-feeding until their babies are 5 to 6 months old. (Baseline: 54% of discharge from birth site and 21% at 5 to 6 months in 1988.)

8. Increase to at least 75% the proportion of parents and caregivers who use feeding practices that prevent baby bottle tooth decay. (Baseline data available in 1991.)

9. Increase to at least 90% the proportion of restaurants and institutional food service operations that offer identifiable low-fat, low-calorie food choices, consistent with the Dietary Guidelines for Americans. (Baseline: About 70% of fast-food and family restaurant chains with 350 or more units had at least one low-fat, low-calorie item on their menu in 1989.)

10. Increase to at least 90% the proportion of school lunch and breakfast services and child care food services with menus that are consistent with the nutrition principles in the Dietary Guidelines for Americans.

11. Increase to at least 75% the proportion of the nation's schools that provide nutrition education from preschool through 12th grade, preferably as part of quality school health education.

12. Increase to at least 75% the proportion of primary care providers who provide nutrition assessment and counseling and/or referral to qualified nutritionists or dietitians. (Baseline: Physicians provided diet counseling for an estimated 40 to 50% of patients in 1988.)

Source: Reprinted from *Healthy Children 2000: National Health Promotion and Disease Prevention Objectives Related to Mothers, Infants, Children, Adolescents, and Youth*, US Department of Health and Human Services, DHHS Pub No HRSA M, 1991.

(NLEA) of 1993, the format and standardization of food labels has been simplified and label reading should be encouraged among literate children as well as adults. The National Adolescent Study Health Survey published in 1987 reported that only 27% of students in 8th through 10th grades had received any previous instruction on interpreting food labels.[3]

> **2.14** Achieve useful and informative nutrition labeling for virtually all processed foods and at least 40% of fresh meats, poultry, fish, fruits, vegetables, baked goods, and ready-to-eat-carry-away foods. Standardized labeling is now in place, but the level of effectiveness has not been evaluated among children or adults.

> **2.15** Increase to at least 5000 brand name items the availability of processed food products that are reduced in fat and saturated fat. The food industry has readily responded to this request, but data to evaluate the impact of these modified products on the nutritional status of children are not yet available.

CARDIOVASCULAR DISEASE

Risk Factors

There is growing evidence that atherogenesis begins in childhood.[4,5] The primary risk factors for coronary heart disease (CHD) are high blood cholesterol and low-density lipoprotein cholesterol (LDL-C), hypertension, and smoking. Clinical trials continue to demonstrate that life-style intervention aimed at reducing these risk factors results in decreased morbidity and mortality from cardiovascular disease (CVD).[6,7] Despite dramatic reductions that have occurred over the past three decades, CVD remains the leading cause of death and disability in this country in both men and women.

Blood Cholesterol

The Expert Panel on Blood Cholesterol Levels in Children and Adolescents (NCEP Pediatric Panel)[8] summarized the significance of cholesterol levels in children and adolescents as follows:

> Children and adolescents in the United States have higher blood cholesterol levels and higher dietary intakes of saturated fatty acids (SFA) and cholesterol than their counterparts in many other countries.

Autopsy studies demonstrate that early coronary atherosclerosis or precursors of atherosclerosis often begin in childhood and adolescence.

High blood total cholesterol, LDL-C and VLDL-C and low HDL-C levels are correlated with the extent of early atherosclerotic lesions in adolescents and young adults.

Children and adolescents with elevated blood cholesterol, particularly LDL-C levels, frequently come from families in which there is a high incidence of CHD among adult members.

High blood cholesterol aggregates in families as a result of both shared environments and genetic factors.

Children and adolescents with high cholesterol levels are more likely than the general population to have high levels as adults.

Consequently, the NCEP Pediatric Panel, like its predecessor, the Population-Based Panel,[9] recommended that all children older than 2 years follow a Step I Diet to prevent and/or treat high blood cholesterol levels. This approach was targeted at reducing the population mean total and LDL-C levels for children and adolescents. Also, the report advocated an individualized approach to identify and treat those children who are at greatest risk of developing high blood cholesterol as adults, thereby increasing their risk of CHD. The panel recommended selective screening of blood cholesterol in the pediatric population within the context of usual health care, based on family history or other risk factors (Table 11-1). These cutpoints are neither gender- nor age-specific. The Lipid Research Clinics (LRC) Prevalence Study published in 1980[10] reported the mean total, LDL-C, and HDL-C levels for girls aged 10 to 14 years were 164 mg/dL, 100 mg/dL, and 54 mg/dL, respectively. More recent data from NHANES III are forthcoming.

Table 11-1 Classification of Total and LDL-C Levels in Children and Adolescents from Families with Hypercholesterolemia or Premature Cardiovascular Disease

Category	Total Cholesterol (mg/dL)	LDL-Cholesterol (mg/dL)
Acceptable	<170	<110
Borderline	170–199	110–129
High	≥200	≥130

Source: Reprinted from *Report of the Expert Panel on Blood Cholesterol Levels in Children and Adolescents,* National Heart Lung and Blood Institute, US Department of Health and Human Services, DHHS Pub No 91-2732, September 1991.

Several studies have measured lipid levels in children longitudinally to determine whether the rank order of blood cholesterol is preserved over time. In the Muscatine study of children (aged 5 to 18 years at baseline) who were remeasured at 20 to 30 years of age, tracking of blood cholesterol was observed.[11] Of those who were observed to have cholesterol levels greater than the 90th percentile at a younger age, 43% remained above the 90th percentile at the older age, 62% were above the 75th percentile, and 81% were greater than the 50th percentile. Furthermore, individuals whose total cholesterol levels declined over time had made healthy life-style changes during youth. Gidding[12] summarized results from several studies that had tracked cholesterol levels from childhood to early adulthood (Table 11-2). Despite diverse racial and geographic populations, the results were similar. Individuals at the upper percentile had a 40 to 50% chance of remaining there 15 to 20 years in the future. Thus, blood cholesterol levels do track, although not as well as height and weight. Hence, not all children with elevated blood cholesterol become adults with elevated cholesterol. However, those at the highest percentiles are most likely to remain higher than the population mean.

Regardless of age or gender, dietary intervention to reduce elevated blood cholesterol levels is warranted.[8] As stated in Healthy Children 2000 Objective **2.5,** all people older than age 2 should reduce dietary fat intake to an average of 30% of calories or less and saturated fat intake to an average of less than 10% of calories.

Diet

In the National Health and Nutrition Examination Survey (NHANES) II, adolescent girls aged 11 to 17 years consumed an average of 36 to 38% of calories

---

Table 11-2 Tracking of Children's Cholesterol Levels into Adulthood

Study Site	Correlation Coefficient Early to Current[a]	Predictors of Elevated Cholesterol Levels as an Adult
Muscatine, IA	.49–.72	Elevated childhood cholesterol levels most important; obesity; smoking; oral contraceptive use; positive family history
Bogalusa, LA	.38–.66	Elevated childhood cholesterol levels most important; obesity
Beaver County, PA	.38–.51	Elevated childhood cholesterol levels most important; smoking; oral contraceptive use; failure to make dietary changes to lower fat content

[a]Coefficients vary by gender, age at first examination, and race.
Source: Adapted with permission from *American Journal of Diseases of Children* (1993;147:386–392), Copyright © 1993, Publications Medicales International.

from fat.[13] Black girls reported consuming slightly more total fat, SFA, and cholesterol than white girls. Furthermore, 59% and 58% of black and white female adolescents, respectively, reported consuming more than 125% of the recommended intake of 10% of total calories from SFA. Results from the LRC Prevalence Study indicated that black girls, aged 10 to 14 years, consumed more energy from meat, fish, poultry, and eggs than white girls ($p<0.05$).[14] Another smaller study found that only 17% of Texan adolescents consumed diets that contained less than 30% of calories from fat.[15] Newer data from NHANES III indicate some improvements in certain groups (Table 11-3). Total fat intake in white adolescent girls was down to 33 to 34% of calories. SFA was 13% and 12% for black and white girls, respectively. Average cholesterol intakes of all groups was below recommended levels.

Dietary Recommendations

Step I Diet

The Pediatric Panel recommended that the Step I Diet be adopted by all healthy children older than age 2 . The pattern of nutrient intake is the same as that recommended for adults:

- SFA: less than 10% of total calories per day
- total fat: an average of no more than 30% of total calories per day
- dietary cholesterol: less than 300 mg/day

Table 11-3 Mean Dietary Intakes of Selected Macronutrients by Age and Race Group for U.S. Female Girls 12 to 19 Years of Age, NHANES III

	Age Groups			
	12–15 Years		16–19 Years	
	Black	White	Black	White
Energy intake (kcal)	2079 (91)[a]	1783 (58)	2107 (83)	1885 (74)
Total fat (% kcal)	38 (1.0)	33 (0.9)	36 (0.8)	34 (0.7)
Saturated fat (% kcal)	13 (0.4)	12 (0.4)	13 (0.4)	12 (0.4)
Monounsaturated fat (% kcal)	14 (0.4)	12 (0.4)	13 (0.3)	13 (0.4)
Polyunsaturated fat (% kcal)	8 (0.5)	6 (0.3)	7 (0.4)	7 (0.3)
Cholesterol (mg)	275 (27.4)	181 (12.3)	232 (17.1)	204 (14.4)
Total carbohydrate (% kcal)	49 (1.1)	56 (1.2)	51 (0.9)	53 (1.2)
Protein (% kcal)	14 (0.5)	13 (0.4)	14 (0.4)	14 (0.4)

[a]Standard error of the mean.
Source: Reprinted from *Energy and Macronutrient Intakes of Persons Ages 2 Months and Over in the United States: Third National Health and Nutrition Examination Survey,* Phase I, 1988–1991, by McDowell MA, Briefel RR, Alaimo K, et al, advance data from Vital Health Statistics no 255, National Center for Health Statistics, 1994.

Also, nutrient adequacy should be achieved by eating a wide variety of foods, and energy intake should be sufficient to support optimal growth and development. A Step I Diet for adolescents is shown in Table 11-4. Girls must pay close attention to an adequate intake of calcium, iron, and zinc when consumption of animal products is reduced. Use of low-fat dairy products and lean meats can satisfy these nutrient requirements. Exhibit 11-2 illustrates sample menus with a fast food lunch for girls aged 11 to 14 years old.

Rationale

Epidemiologic evidence indicates that premenopausal women are at reduced risk of cardiovascular morbidity and mortality compared with men. The incidence of cardiovascular disease in women is highest after age 50. Why, then, should an adolescent girl be concerned about following a low-fat, low-cholesterol, high-fiber diet? At least three reasons emerge:

- because it offers nutritional benefits beyond those related to lipid lowering
- because it is consistent with weight management
- because it introduces an eating pattern that is encouraged for life and adherence tends to improve the longer the eating pattern is followed

What are the potential risks or concerns with adopting such an eating pattern early in life? It has been argued that American children are generally healthier than most other children in the world; why interfere? What evidence is there that changing from the typical American diet to a lower fat intake is feasible, efficacious, and safe in growing children?

Interventions

One study that will help answer these questions is the Dietary Intervention Study in Children (DISC).[17] DISC is a multicenter, prospective study involving more than 600 girls and boys (between 8 and 10 years old at baseline) with moderately elevated LDL-C levels. Children were randomized to a modified Step I Diet (28% calories from total fat, and less than 75 mg dietary cholesterol per 1000 calories) that was designed to meet the nutritional requirements for growing children. Intensive and long-term maintenance intervention involved children and their families participating in group and individual sessions. Nutrition education combined with emphasis on achieving self-efficacy characterize the DISC intervention provided for both parents and children.[17] Follow-up is expected to be maintained for a minimum of 7 years, throughout adolescence, until the age of 18 years. The primary outcome measure of efficacy in DISC is

Table 11-4 Step I Diets for Adolescents

	Age (yr)						
	Child			11–14		15–18	
	2–3	4–6	7–10	Male	Female	Male	Female
Food Group							
Meat, poultry, and fish (oz)	2	5	6	6	6	6	6
Eggs (per week)[a]	3	3	3	3	3	3	3
Dairy products (servings)	3	3	4	4	4	4	4
Fats and oils (servings)	4	5	5	7	5	10	5
Breads and cereals (servings)[b]	5	6	7	9	8	12	8
Vegetables (servings)	3	3	3	4	3	4	3
Fruits (servings)	2	3	3	3	3	5	3
Sweets and modified fat desserts (servings)	1	2	2	4	3	4	3
Nutrients							
Recommended dietary allowance for energy (cal)	1300	1800	2000	2500	2200	3000	2200
Actual energy (cal)	1317	1786	2025	2522	2221	3011	2221
Fat (g)	46	62	70	86	73	103	73
(% cal)	(30)	(31)	(31)	(30)	(29)	(30)	(29)
Carbohydrate	177	230	255	338	294	418	294
(% cal)	(52)	(50)	(49)	(52)	(52)	(54)	(52)
Protein (g)	59	87	104	114	109	125	109
(% cal)	(18)	(19)	(20)	(18)	(19)	(16)	(19)
Fatty acids and cholesterol							
Saturated fatty acids (g)	15	20	23	26	24	29	24
(% cal)	(10)	(10)	(10)	(9)	(9)	(9)	(9)
Monounsaturated fatty acids (g)	16	23	25	31	26	37	26
(% cal)	(11)	(11)	(11)	(11)	(11)	(11)	(11)

[a]Nutrient analysis is for three eggs per week; with four eggs per week, the average dietary cholesterol increases by 30 mg/day.
[b]The breads and cereals food group includes bread, cereal, pasta, rice, starchy vegetables, and dry beans and peas.
Source: Reprinted from *Report of the Expert Panel on Blood Cholesterol Levels in Children and Adolescents,* National Heart Lung and Blood Institute, US Department of Health and Human Services, DHHS Pub No 91-2732, September 1991.

Exhibit 11-2 Sample Menus for Girls Aged 11 to 14 Years with Fast-Food Lunch

Typical	Step I Diet	Step II Diet
Breakfast at home	**Breakfast at home**	**Breakfast at home**
Orange juice (1 cup)	Orange juice (1 cup)	Orange juice (1 cup)
Presweetened cereal (1 cup)	Corn flakes (3/4 cup)	Corn flakes (3/4 cup)
Whole milk (1 cup)	1% milk (1 cup)	Skim milk (1 cup)
		English muffin (1/2)
		Margarine[c] (1 tsp)
Fast-food lunch	**Fast-food lunch**	**Sandwich shop**
Cheeseburger	Hamburger (1/4 lb)	Tuna sandwich
French fries (1 regular order)	French fries (1 regular order)	Bread (2 slices)
Catsup (3 packets)	Lettuce, tomato, onion, catsup	Tuna, water pack (3 oz)
Cola drink (1 small)	Animal crackers (1/2 box)	Tomato, celery, relish
	Cola drink (1 medium)	Mayonnaise (4 tsp)
		Pretzels (3/4-oz bag)
		Oatmeal cookies, homemade[c] (4)
		Cola drink (1 medium)
Snack at home	**Snack at home**	**Snack at home**
Ginger snaps (2 medium)	Multigrain low-fat crackers (4)	Multigrain low-fat crackers (4)
Club soda (1 can)	Low-fat cheese (3/4 oz)	Low-fat cheese (3/4 oz)
	Club soda (1 can)	Club soda (1 can)
Dinner at home	**Dinner at home**	**Dinner at home**
Fried chicken breast, breaded and fried in shortening, skin eaten	Broiled chicken breast, no skin (3 oz)	Broiled chicken breast, no skin (3 oz)
Boiled potato[a] (1)	Boiled potato[b] (1)	Boiled potato[c] (1)
Broccoli spears[a] (1/2 cup)	Broccoli spears[b] (4)	Broccoli spears[c] (4)
Roll (1 small)	Tomato (4 slices)	Tomato (4 slices)
Margarine[b] (1 tsp)	Bread (1 slice)	Bread (1 slice)
Iced tea (1 cup)	Strawberries (1/2 cup)	Margarine[c] (2 tsp)
	Nonfat yogurt (1 container)	Strawberries (1/2 cup)
	Water	Nonfat yogurt (1 container)
		Water
Snack at home	**Snack at home**	**Snack at home**
American cheese (3/4 oz)	Cupcake, commercial (1)	Cupcake, homemade (1)
Crackers (4)	1% milk (1 cup)	Skim milk (1 cup)
Fruit drink (1/2 cup)		
Calories: 2219	**Calories:** 2240	**Calories:** 2248
Fat, % cal: 35	**Fat, % cal:** 29	**Fat, % cal:** 27
SFA, % cal: 15	**SFA, % cal:** 10	**SFA, % cal:** 6
Cholesterol, mg: 264	**Cholesterol, mg:** 188	**Cholesterol, mg:** 159

[a]Seasoned with butter.
[b]Stick margarine used in food preparation.
[c]Tub margarine used in food preparation.
Source: Reprinted from Report of the Expert Panel on Blood Cholesterol Levels in Children and Adolescents, National Heart Lung and Blood Institute, US Department of Health and Human Services, DHHS Pub No 91-2732, September 1991.

change in LDL-C between the two groups. Safety is assessed by comparing linear growth and serum ferritin levels. Secondary safety outcome measures include serum zinc, folate, retinol and albumin levels, ratio of LDL-C to HDL-C, sexual maturation, cognitive development, and child behavior.[17] After 36 months, the mean net LDL-C difference between the two groups was −3.3 mg/dL

(p = 0.02).[18] There were no differences observed in height or other safety parameters between groups.

Although DISC is a clinical trial of efficacy in children with elevated LDL-C, another study, the Child and Adolescent Trial of Cardiovascular Health (CATCH) is a school-based study of diet, exercise, and educational intervention to reduce CVD risk in healthy 8- to 10-year-old children from 96 schools in California, Minnesota, Texas, and Louisiana.[19,20] Outcome measures include blood lipids lipoproteins, anthropometrics, self-reported dietary intake and activity expenditure data, and various psychosocial parameters.[20] The CATCH Eat Smart School Nutrition Program successfully implemented changes in menu planning, food purchasing, recipe modification, food preparation, food production, and food merchandising[21] (Exhibit 11-3). Preliminary results from CATCH illustrate the feasibility of implementing school-based health intervention efforts. The effects on biologic variables are forthcoming.

The "Know Your Body" Program, sponsored by the American Health Foundation, has been implemented among elementary school children since the 1980s.[22] Favorable results were reported from a school-based educational intervention in more than 3,300 children in 37 New York schools.[23] Teacher-delivered education on diet, physical activity, and cigarette smoking was provided to children in the fourth through eighth grades. Significant reductions in total cholesterol were reported after 5 years of intervention and favorable trends in dietary intake and health knowledge were observed, but other targeted risk factors were not significantly altered. The net change in plasma total cholesterol levels was 5.1% in the Westchester County schools and –2.9% in the Bronx area schools.

The Children's Health Project is also a study of preadolescent children with elevated blood cholesterol levels who are randomly assigned to either a parent-child autotutorial intervention (PCAT) or usual care.[24] Unlike DISC or CATCH, this study involves recruitment within a primary care setting, and the intervention is self-directed because it uses tape-recorded dietary education with corresponding written materials. Intervention is directed at both the randomized child and his or her family. Preliminary results reported increases in knowledge scores as well as significant reductions in LDL-C in the PCAT group versus usual care.[24,25]

HYPERTENSION

Hypertension is another major risk factor for cardiovascular mortality in adults. Epidemiologic evidence demonstrates that blood pressure levels in adults are correlated with blood pressure and body size in childhood.[26] As with hyperlipidemia, the prevalence of high blood pressure is low during childhood and adolescence, but higher levels appear to track well into the third and fourth decades of life, as is shown in Table 11-5.[27] Primary prevention of hypertension in child-

Exhibit 11-3 CATCH Eat Smart Modifications

Menu Planning	Food Preparation	Food Purchasing
Choose lower-fat and lower-sodium commodities for reimbursable meals.	Whip butter.	Identify specifications for new items for bid.
Stay within federal guidelines.	Defat ground meat.	Change from canned to fresh or frozen foods.
Offer one seafood and poultry item each week.	Skin chicken.	Check prices of new food items to see if it is within budget.
Increase the use of poultry products in the place of ground beef and wieners.	Oven-bake French fries.	Encourage vendors to bid on products in small quantities.
Increase the use of part-skim mozzarella cheese.	No salt or oil in rice and spaghetti.	Taste test new products.
Increase the use of fresh fruits and vegetables.	Bake, broil, steam instead of fry.	Purchase part-skim mozzarella cheese if not offered in commodities.
Choose lower-fat and lower-sodium recipes.	Use vegetable spray on baking pans instead of butter or shortening.	Use certain commodities (ground turkey, chicken) in place of ground beef.
	Use egg whites instead of butter on top of bread for browning.	Purchase lower-fat ham.
		Purchase lower-fat mayonnaise.
		Purchase lower-fat hamburger patties.
		Purchase different foods for the CATCH schools in a district.
		Increase the purchases of skim milk, low-fat milks ($1^1/2$% to $^1/2$% fat) and nonfat dried milk.

Food Production	Recipe Modification	Food Merchandising
Follow the recipe exactly.	Defat ground meat.	Use posters-Hearty Heart Characters in cafeteria.
Use proper serving utensils.	Reduce salt.	Feature posters on serving line indicating Eat Smart food items.
Keep a notebook of all Eat Smart recipes.	Reduce fat.	Each day post menus in cafeteria with heart next to Eat Smart food items.
Measure all ingredients.	Replace beef wieners with turkey wieners.	Offer gifts such as book markers.
Use the same recipe each time a menu item is prepared.	Replace smoked sausage with turkey sausage.	Place Hearty Heart centerpieces on tables-flower vases.
	Use vegetable oil instead of shortening.	Make Eat Smart announcements on PA.
	Use part-skim mozzarella cheese instead of American cheese.	
	Use fresh potatoes instead of canned potatoes.	
	Use fresh or frozen vegetables instead of canned vegetables.	
	Skin chicken.	
	Write down ingredients and amounts for each recipe.	
	Use wheat flour instead of white flour.	
	Whip butter.	
	Make an oilless roux.	
	Skim broths and gravies.	

Source: Reprinted with permission from *School Food Service Research Review* (1992;16[2]:114–121), Copyright © 1992, American School Food Service Association.

Table 11-5 Correlations of Adult Diastolic Blood Pressure with Childhood Measure[a]

			Childhood			
Childhood Age (yr) and Sex	*Systolic Blood Pressure (mm Hg)*	*Diastolic Blood Pressure (mm Hg)*	*Height (cm)*	*Wt (kg)*	*Quetelet Index*	*Change in Quetelet Index*
Adults 20–25						
7–8						
F	0.28	0.57	0.10[b]	−0.4[b]	−0.03[b]	0.15[b]
M	0.06[b]	−0.01[b]	0.12[b]	0.25[b]	0.27	0.21[b]
9–10						
F	0.13	0.23	0.18	0.18	0.13	0.15
M	0.07[b]	0.13	−0.02[b]	−0.06[b]	−0.05[b]	0.12
11–12						
F	0.26	0.17	0.20	0.22	0.17	0.19
M	0.15	0.15	0.12	0.10	0.05[b]	0.24
13–14						
F	0.13	0.21	0.16	0.15	0.10	0.22
M	0.10[b]	0.20	0.09	0.08[b]	0.05[b]	0.20
15–16						
F	0.08	0.22	0.13	0.09[b]	0.04[b]	0.18
M	0.11	0.26	0.10[b]	0.10[b]	0.04[b]	0.21
17–18						
F	0.15	0.30	0.08[b]	0.05[b]	0.01[b]	0.14
M	0.24	0.26	0.08[b]	0.11[b]	0.10[b]	0.21
Adults 26–30						
13–14						
F	0.34[b]	0.31	0.11[b]	0.37	0.34	0.14[b]
M	0.12	0.26	0.09[b]	0.12[b]	0.14[b]	0.20
15–16						
F	0.25	0.29	−0.03[b]	0.20	0.23	0.20
M	0.11	0.21	0.11[b]	0.19	0.17	0.27
17–18						
F	0.17	0.27	0.04[b]	0.08[b]	0.09[b]	0.22
M	0.12[b]	0.24	−0.11[b]	0.08[b]	0.15	0.27

[a] $p < .05$
[b] $p < .01$

Source: Data from *Pediatrics* (1989;84:633–641), American Academy of Pediatrics, 1989.

hood has been recommended as the optimal approach to treatment.[28] Classification of hypertension by age is presented in Table 11-6.

Sodium and Blood Pressure

The *Healthy People 2000* Objective 2.9 states that 40% of adults decrease salt and sodium intake so that 65% of home meal preparers prepare foods without adding salt, at least 80% of people avoid using salt at the table, and at least 40% regularly purchase foods modified or lower in sodium.[1]

In 1988, the INTERSALT Cooperative Research Group reported findings from cross-cultural comparisons of urinary sodium and blood pressure in adults from 52 centers worldwide.[31] Increase in blood pressure with age was significantly related to sodium intake. Presently, there are no biologic markers to determine exactly who is susceptible to sodium-induced high blood pressure. And, in children, there are no definitive data regarding the sodium-blood pressure relationship. Because there are no known health benefits of a high sodium intake, the potential risks for increased blood pressure with age provide a rationale for reducing salt intake for any age level.

Weight loss, sodium reduction, increased potassium intake, and alcohol reduction offer potentially effective, nonpharmacologic approaches to blood pressure

Table 11-6 Classification of Hypertension by Age

	Significant Hypertension (mm Hg)	Severe Hypertension (mm Hg)
10–12 yr		
Systolic blood pressure	126–133	≥134
Diastolic blood pressure	82–89	≥90
13–15 yr		
Systolic blood pressure	136–143	≥144
Diastolic blood pressure	86–91	≥92
16–18 yr		
Systolic blood pressure	142–149	≥150
Diastolic blood pressure	92–97	≥98

	Stage 1 (mild)	Stage 2 (moderate)	Stage 3 (severe)	Stage 4 (very severe)
19+ yr (Adults)				
Systolic blood pressure	140–159	160–179	180–209	≥210

Note: The Fifth Report of the Joint National Committee on Detection, Evaluation and Treatment of High Blood Pressure (JNCV) classified hypertension by age based on data from the National Health and Nutrition Examination Survey (NHANES III).
Source: Data from Guidelines for Adolescent Nutrition by I Alton and M Story, US Department of Health and Human Services, 1993, and from *Archives of Internal Medicine* (1993;153:154–183), American Medical Association, 1993.

reduction.[30,32,33] Clinical trials have shown that dietary sodium restriction reduces blood pressure in some normotensive and hypertensive adults. Most of these studies have employed short-term interventions, leaving unanswered the question of long-term efficacy of sodium restriction for hypertension control.

Pediatric intervention studies involving sodium reduction and/or potassium supplementation are limited and have mixed results in normotensive children and adolescents.[34-36] It has been suggested that below a certain threshold level, reduction in sodium intake will not reduce a low blood pressure farther. In adolescents with high blood pressure, Sinaiko et al[37] reported significant reductions in blood pressure in girls by decreasing the sodium/potassium ratio over a 3-year period. Differences in blood pressure response were reported between boys and girls, and the authors concluded that different sensitivities to these changes may exist between boys and girls.

Nutritionally, the biologic requirement for sodium is far less than 1 g/day.[38] The average sodium intake is estimated to be at least five times that amount. There is no method for detecting sodium-sensitive hypertension, and long-term studies of sodium restriction have suffered from poor dietary adherence. Another study of adolescent blood pressure comparing Seventh-Day Adventists (SDA) with non-SDA adolescents failed to show significant differences in mean blood pressure levels between the two groups, despite marked differences in diet and life style.[39] Boys older than age 12 years had higher trends in mean systolic blood pressure than younger boys or girls at any age. Also, black children of both sexes had slightly higher blood pressure levels at all ages, suggesting greater risk in this ethnic group even during childhood.[40] Primary prevention efforts to maintain low blood pressure long term must include moderate sodium and increased potassium intake, as well as weight control.[41]

The Task Force on Blood Pressure Control in Children[42] recommends limiting sodium intake in children to 4 to 6 g of salt (1.5 to 2.5 g sodium) per day if the child is hypertensive. Increased dietary potassium intake is also recommended, but no limits have been established.

Prevention of Obesity

Healthy People 2000 Objective 2.3 states: reduce overweight to a prevalence of no more than 20% among people aged 20 and older and no more than 15% among adolescents aged 12 through 19. For definitions of adolescent overweight, see Table 11-7. These values represent the age- and gender-specific 85th percentile values of the 1976 to 1980 NHANES II, corrected for sample variation.

Obesity is a major public health problem that is a risk factor for increased blood pressure, blood cholesterol, fasting blood glucose, and a myriad of psychological and emotional problems even in youth.[43-45] There is concern that the

Table 11-7 Recommended Cutoff Values for Body Mass Index (BMI)

Age (yr)	At Risk of Overweight		Overweight	
	Male	Female	Male	Female
10	20	20	23	23
11	20	21	24	25
12	21	22	25	26
13	22	23	26	27
14	23	24	27	28
15	24	24	28	29
16	24	25	29	29
17	25	25	29	30
18	26	26	30	30
19	26	26	30	30
20–24	27	26	30	30

BMI = kg/m^2
Source: Adapted with permission from *American Journal of Clinical Nutrition* (1994;59:307–316), Copyright © 1994, American Society for Clinical Nutrition.

prevalence of obesity is increasing in both adults and children by comparing results of NHANES I and II. A prevalence of 21.9% obesity and 9% superobesity, defined as triceps skinfolds greater than the 95th and 98th percentiles, respectively, was reported among 12- to 17-year-old children in NHANES II, more than double the levels reported in NHANES I. Studies have estimated that 14% of infants, 40% of obese 7-year-olds, and 70% of obese 10- to 13-year-olds will become obese adults.[46] Thus, obesity in adolescence is more likely to persist into adulthood than obesity in younger children. Black women have twice the prevalence of obesity as white women.[47] Adolescence has been suggested as a critical period for intervention in black teenage girls.[48] Very few studies have systematically investigated primary prevention of obesity in the young.

In adults, obesity intervention has been generally unsuccessful, with less than 10% maintaining weight loss over time.[49] More than $30 billion is spent per year by Americans trying to lose weight, often without medical supervision, with potential complications from unrecognized and untreated side effects of inadequate nutritional practices.[50] Because attempts at weight loss among adults are notoriously unsuccessful, primary prevention of obesity in childhood and adolescence remains the goal.[49]

Obesity Intervention

By combining behavioral, dietary, and exercise change, Epstein et al[51,52] reported successful reduction of body weight and accompanying decreases in blood pressure and blood cholesterol levels in children. These changes remained

10 years later. Modest success has also been reported by the Shapedown Program that involves group intervention in 11- to 13-year-old children who participate in a camp-type experience to learn new life-style behaviors.[53] Change in aerobic fitness, more than dietary change, was a strong predictor of long-term weight loss.[54]

Other studies among obese adolescents have shown mixed results. Penna et al[54] studied 80 obese adolescents who were placed in one of four treatments for 4 weeks: increased-fiber diet and exercise, increased-fiber diet and no exercise, low-fiber diet and increased exercise, or low-fiber diet and no exercise. Significant effects of exercise on weight and an interaction between fiber and exercise was found in girls, but not boys. No long-term data were reported.

Although obesity is more prevalent in minorities than in the white population, few studies have addressed this problem. Wadden et al[55] conducted a 16-week behavioral weight control program with 36 obese black girls (aged 14 years). Girls were randomized to child alone, child and mother together, and child and mother in separate but concurrent sessions. At 16 weeks, average weight loss was 0.7 kg, 8.2 kg, and 1.4 kg, respectively. At 6 months, 54% of all girls were below their baseline weight, but only 11% showed a reduction in body mass index (BMI) greater than 5%. Weight loss was significantly related to mother's attendance.

Physical activity is a crucial factor in prevention and treatment of obesity. Studies among children of obese parents have shown that less energy per kg body weight is expended than among normal-weight children of normal-weight parents. Encouraging regular, daily, aerobic exercise balanced with lower dietary fat intake is the strategy most often recommended for prevention.[56] Based on a physical activity questionnaire, adolescent girls in Pittsburgh reported significantly less physical activity than boys, and a negative association was found between activity and age in these girls.[57] Studies are needed to further identify risk factors and effective interventions for improving long-term adherence to active life styles in children into adulthood.

Overall, obesity is the most prevalent of the CVD risk factors in adolescent girls. The greatest potential for successful primary prevention is similar to that recommended for intervention—dietary fat restriction, behavioral skill development, and regular exercise as part of life-style change.[50,51]

CANCER

Cancer is the second leading cause of death among adults in the United States. This disease is characterized by uncontrolled growth of cells that can occur in any part of the body at any age. During the past few decades, considerable progress has been made in the understanding of cancer etiology and pathophysiology. Attempts to delineate specific causes, methods of detection, prevention, and cure continue to evolve. There is growing evidence that diet plays a role in cancer prevention and could reduce cancer incidence.[58–60] Most damaging to women's health are cancers of the lung, breast, and colon. Breast cancer incidence rate among women is about 107 per 100,000, and it is estimated that approximately one of every nine women will develop breast cancer by age 85.[61] Possible links between pubertal development, diet, and later risk of breast cancer have been suggested.[60]

Risk Factors

Diet-related cancers are not common among children and adolescents. Migrant studies suggest that many cancers develop due to long-term habitual exposure to an unfavorable dietary pattern.[62] There is evidence that even early in life, one or more risk factors associated with the development of cancer may be present.

Dietary practices and exercise routines can be modified at any stage of life. It has been estimated that two-thirds of cancer cases are associated with two lifestyle practices: 35% with the typical American diet, and 30% with tobacco use.[60] Based on the evidence collected from international studies, an estimated 10 to 70% of all cancer mortality in the United States is related to diet.[63] In women, 57% of cancer incidence is related to diet.[64]

Dietary Patterns Potentially Related to Risk

Exposure to environmental influences on cancer risk begins in childhood. The current diet of American children is not consistent with dietary recommendations for reducing cancer risk. NHANES III revealed that female adolescents eat an average of 34% calories from total fat and 53% of calories from carbohydrates.[16] The problem may not only be lack of knowledge but rather an unwillingness or inability to change behavior. According to the National Adolescent Student Health Survey conducted in 1987, 62.6% of all girls did not know that eating too little fiber may cause colon cancer; only 13.9% knew that baked beans contain more fiber than baked potatoes; 38.1% ate fried food at least four times a week; only 25.3% who eat chicken removed the skin; and 43.8% of girls ate three or more snacks per day and of those, 60% were high-fat, low-fiber foods such as chips or candy.[65] Fruit and vegetable intakes have also been associated with lower risks of some cancers.[66] The number of female high school students who reported consuming five or more daily servings of fruits and vegetables was only 10%.[67]

Rationale for Early Intervention

Increased awareness, understanding, and acceptance of dietary recommendations for reducing cancer risk have been reported among adults as a result of successful education efforts in the past decade.[58] Adolescents have received relatively little attention in this area.[68,69] There is conceptual agreement that children and youth should be provided nutrition education in school, but federal funding is limited to the Nutrition Education and Training Program (NET) initiated in 1978. The intent of NET is to "teach children, through a positive daily lunchroom experience and appropriate classroom reinforcement, the value of a nutritionally balanced diet; and to develop curricula and materials to train teachers and school food-service personnel to carry out this task." The funding for this program was cut from the original $26 million in 1978 to $20 million in 1980, to $15 million in 1981, and to $5 million in 1982.[68] Currently, nutrition education is not part of school health education in every American school.[1] Many of the nutrition curricula that are used offer technical information on essential nutrition concepts without the practical skills to effectively implement them. Although knowledge is not the only criterion, it is a necessary factor for healthy life-style behavior.

In *Fighting Cancer in America: Achieving the Year 2000 Goal,* the National Cancer Advisory Board included a specific recommendation directed at the nation's schools.[69] The board recommends that America's schools be encouraged to participate actively in cancer prevention and early detection programs. Specifically for teenagers, the board recommended a combination of motivational programs and innovative curricula for cancer prevention and detection. Curriculum content should be developed to encourage and guide school food services to provide foods and beverages that are consistent with the nutritional guidelines of the National Cancer Institute, the American Cancer Society, the National Heart, Lung and Blood Institute, and the U.S. Surgeon General.

Cancer Prevention Efforts

There is promising evidence that school-based intervention is feasible in improving young people's diets. One of the largest school-based cancer prevention intervention programs is the "Know Your Body" curriculum, targeted at reducing cigarette smoking and modifying behaviors in the areas of diet and physical activity.[70] Beginning from the fourth grade and continuing through the ninth grade, the intervention group received 2 hours per week of learning and activities while the control group received the standard curriculum. A diet reduced in total and saturated fat, and high in complex carbohydrate and fiber was recommended, and students were taught to identify foods based on their fat, carbohydrate, and fiber contents. Results indicated that students in the intervention group consumed significantly less total fat and saturated fat and more total carbohydrate than the control group. This program was successful in modifying students' knowledge, attitudes, and behavior.

A pilot program supported by the American Cancer Society and Boy Scouts of America helped Boy Scouts to increase their understanding of risk factors associated with cancer, to evaluate family meal plans using a cancer prevention score sheet, and to prepare meals using diet and cancer prevention guidelines.[71] Results indicated that Boy Scouts were able to retain learned materials about diet and cancer.

The school is an obvious setting for implementing health education programs that can reach more than 46 million students each year.[72] Because children are already divided into appropriate grade levels, it is feasible to deliver information and skills appropriate to the students' cognitive development.

The American Cancer Society and the National Cancer Institute have developed a curriculum entitled "Changing the Course." This program delivers knowledge, as well as skills in evaluating personal intake patterns, decision making, goal setting, and self-evaluation. A manual for school food service personnel is provided to address menu planning, food purchasing, and food preparation strategies. This program has been successfully pilot tested, and it is anticipated that it will be implemented nationwide at the community level within the next decade.[72]

OSTEOPOROSIS

Osteoporosis is a universal multifactorial disorder characterized by asymptomatic reduction of the mineral and protein components of bones.[73] The remaining bones become thinner and porous, although the bone composition remains unaltered and normal. When reduction of bone mass reaches the level below that necessary for adequate support of the body, the bone will become brittle and vulnerable to fractures. Chronic pain, decreased mobility, and increased risk of fracture-related complications or death are common. Factors associated with increased risk of developing osteoporosis have been identified, but the fundamental pathogenesis remains unclear. Primary prevention offers the best strategy for effective control.

Osteoporosis is responsible for at least 1.5 million fractures of the hip, wrist, and vertebrae in the United States each year. Of these, 500,000 postmenopausal women experience their first vertebral fracture, often resulting in chronic disability and permanent reduction of the quality of life in these women. The health care cost associated with the acute care and rehabilitation of fracture patients is approximately $10 billion per year.[74]

Risk Factors

Reduced calcium intakes contribute to osteoporosis development. Thus, a *Healthy People 2000* objective states: increase calcium intake so at least 50% of youth aged 12 through 24 consume three or more servings of calcium-rich foods daily. When these objectives were written, 7% of women aged 19 through 24 consumed three or more servings daily. Data from NHANES III report the mean intakes of calcium for women aged 12 to 15 and 16 to 19 years were 796 mg and 822 mg, respectively.[16] This is far below the 1989 Recommended Dietary Allowance (RDA) of 1200 mg/day for people aged 12 to 24, and thus is a risk factor for many young women.

Aside from significant trauma, decreased skeletal mass is the most important risk factor for bone fracture. Genetic and ethnic factors potentially account for 50 to 70% of the contribution to bone mass up to about 20 years of age; the remainder is probably determined by dietary and other life-style factors.[75] Factors associated with damaging effects on bone mass are alcohol intake, smoking, caffeine consumption, inactivity, and a low calcium/phosphorus ratio in the diet. Optimal development of bone mass and bone density during adolescence may be the most effective preventive strategy against osteoporotic fracture later in life.[76] Calcium intake plays a critical role in the development of bone during growth, and physical activity has an independent positive effect on bone mass development during adolescence.[77] Optimizing bone mass during growth and deterring the rate of bone loss in the early postmenopausal years are considered the optimal preventive strategies.[76,77]

Bone Mass Development

The acquisition of bone mass is a result of the interactions among genetic factors, the amount of mechanical loading such as physical exercise, and the hormonal and nutritional environment.[77] The rate of bone growth and bone modeling varies greatly with different developmental stages. Bones are in rapid growth from birth until about age 21. Experts in this field now believe that the critical period for maximum bone mass formation occurs during growth spurt, which is between 10 and 21 years of age. Girls experience their growth spurt about 2 years earlier than boys. During this stage, the longitudinal bone growth occurs. In girls, maximum velocity of growth in height is reached at approximately 12 years of age and the cessation of linear growth occurs at about 16 years of age.[77]

Bone mass is increased by mechanical loading and decreased by disuse. Close to 60% of the weight of mature bone is mineral, mainly in the form of calcium phosphate.[78] This mineral cannot be manufactured intrinsically, it must be obtained from the diet. The need for calcium is highest from 10 to 20 years of age. During longitudinal bone growth, the skeleton retains up to 350 mg calcium per day and results in approximately 37% accumulation of the total skeletal mass.

Because urinary calcium loss increases with age until it reaches its maximum by the cessation of puberty, calcium intake is one of the main determinants of calcium balance. During the age when bone growth occurs, individuals need to ingest sufficient calcium to ensure that they absorb more calcium from their intestines than they excrete and thus achieve positive balance. It is important that young individuals maintain a positive balance to support this process. Adequate consumption of dietary calcium as well as regular weight-bearing exercise during growth is thought to be important in achieving genetically programmed peak bone mass, because the greater the mass attained before age-related loss, the less likely bone loss will reach the level at which a fracture will occur.

The 1989 RDA for calcium for adolescents is 1200 mg/day.[38] At this amount, adolescents retain about 350 mg of calcium per day. A dietary intake of calcium approaching RDA values appears to be adequate to allow acceptable peak bone mass in women. Anderson and Metz[76] compared data from several cross-sectional studies of late adolescent and young adult women to quantify contributions of dietary calcium and physical activity to radial bone development. They concluded that a moderate intake of calcium approaching or exceeding the age-specific RDA, in addition to adequate physical activity, permits the attainment of optimal bone mass in American white women. The influences of dietary calcium and physical activity on optimal bone development appear to be independent but complementary of each other.

Dietary Patterns and Bone Mass

The current dietary practices of typical American teenagers place them at increased risk of osteoporosis.[79] According to national nutrition surveys, teenagers and young adults consume high-phosphorus, low-calcium diets.[76] Calcium intake falls below the RDA as early as 12 years of age whereas phosphorus intake exceeds the RDA.[78] Data collected from the NFCS in 1987-88 indicated that 40% of teenage girls did not drink any milk over the 3-day period and that 90% of all teenagers did not include any dark green vegetables in their diet.[80] Dairy products have typically provided about 75%[75] of dietary calcium in U.S. diets, but as the number of nondairy calcium-fortified foods increase, dietary adequacy may also improve.[38] Questions of bioavailability need further consideration. Because calcium is concentrated primarily in one food group and phosphorus is widely distributed in foods, especially popular foods such as soft drinks, it is clear that adolescents need education to make appropriate food choices.

Alcohol use is also prevalent among teenagers, especially between 18 to 24 years of age. More than 65% of young people from this age group reported using alcohol during the previous month. In a 1987 national survey, 28% of 8th graders and 38% of 10th graders reported occasions of heavy drinking.[65]

Rationale for Prevention

Based on the available data, adolescents appear to be at risk for future development of osteoporosis. The relatively high prevalence of alcohol intake and smoking contributes to risk even though these two risk factors are relatively weak. More significant is the proportion of adolescent girls and young women who consume less than the RDA for calcium intake and do not participate in daily physical activity beneficial to bone development.[76,77]

Two approaches offer potential prevention of osteoporosis.[78] One is to reduce the rate of bone loss after menopause. The second and preferred approach is to increase peak bone mass at skeletal maturity.[78] The prevention of osteoporosis in adolescents emphasizes the importance of a balanced diet, with adequate energy, protein, and calcium, and physical activity. Girls should be encouraged to meet the RDA for calcium of 1200 mg/day and to participate in weight-bearing exercises on a regular basis.

ROLE OF THE FEDERAL GOVERNMENT IN ADOLESCENT HEALTH

The federal government has a direct role in influencing the health of adolescents through funding various federal departments. They conduct research, develop policies, design and implement programs, and provide services designed to serve adolescents specifically or adolescents as part of the general adult or child population. For example, the 1987 National Adolescent Student Health Survey was administered by the Centers for Disease Control and Prevention.[3] School-based nutrition education projects and smoking cessation interventions are sponsored by the National Cancer Institute within the National Institute of Health[79]; and the school breakfast and school lunch programs are provided by U.S. Department of Agriculture's Food and Nutrition Services.[80] A more detailed description of the roles of various federal agencies in providing adolescent care is in the report of the Office of Technology Assessment (OTA) on adolescent health.[79]

Some federal agencies set aside specific funds to serve adolescents, depending on the agency's priorities. Federal agency long- and short-term priorities are established by the U.S. Congress. If Congress emphasized the need to improve adolescent health, federal agencies could potentially secure additional funding for such purposes. Currently, the government heavily supports programs and projects on acquired immunodeficiency syndrome and human immunodeficiency virus infection, as well as use of illicit drugs. This leaves little or no resources for other adolescent health problems.

The federal government also has an indirect role in influencing the health of adolescents. It provides block grants to state and local agencies, and these groups often determine their own priorities. Whether grant awards assist adolescents in positive ways depends on where adolescent health issues stand among all local priorities.

Recommendations for Adolescent Health

The OTA committee reviewed adolescents' nutritional and fitness problems and identified specific preventive strategies. These include the following:

- **Support federal data collection and research.**
  1. *Data collection:* survey schools and communities to determine the availability of facilities for a range of physical education and the competence of adults supervising physical education. Support the routine collection of data on adolescents' nutritional status with oversamplings of disabled, minority, and poor adolescents in population-based surveys.
  2. *Research:* support research on the effects of adolescents' nutrition and fitness choices on their current and future health. Support research on the nutritional and fitness preferences of adolescents to help target educational and other preventive interventions. Support research on the relationships between nutritional needs and varying levels of physical activity.
- **Foster changes in adolescents' environments.**
  1. Support the provision of healthy nutritional choices to adolescents in schools and the community (e.g., in fast-food outlets).
  2. Support efforts to improve access to fitness activities for adolescents with special health care needs (e.g., the chronically ill and disabled), overweight, and poor adolescents.
  3. Support the education of physical education teachers, coaches, trainers, and others about adolescent-specific factors that could influence adolescents' physical abilities.

Future Directions

Adolescent diets are similar to those of adults living in the United States and are not currently consistent with recommendations for chronic disease prevention.[13,79,81] The Committee on Diet and Health concluded that a diet of less than 30% calories from fat, saturated fat limited to 10% of calories, and cholesterol limited to 300 mg/day is safe for children older than 2.[82] In a new era of standardized food labeling, all consumers including adolescents should be encouraged to become informed and discriminating shoppers. Nutrition education including label reading, shopping and food preparation skills, and knowing how to be selective in restaurants is essential to this process. Beginning education early in life could lower the cost of educating adults and the cost of treating diet and lifestyle-related diseases in the future.

Dwyer[83] addressed the concerns of adolescent nutrition to meet the year 2000 objectives and beyond. She advocated that special attention be paid to adolescents with certain sociodemographic characteristics and/or special physiologic conditions that place them at higher nutritional risk. For example, adolescents who live in poor families especially in rural areas of the Southeast, Appalachia, and parts of the Southwest often lack access to nutrition-related health services. Members of ethnic minorities, including African-Americans, Hispanics, Native Americans, Asian-Americans, and Pacific Islanders, are often at nutritional risk as well. Dr. Dwyer offered the following recommendations: [83]

Improving Adolescent Nutrition

- Improve the nutrition component of health services for adolescents, including pregnant adolescents and those with special health care needs (i.e., chronic illness).
- Ensure quality nutrition education programs for school-aged children and adolescents, including children with special health care needs.
- Strengthen and improve food services for children and adolescents.
- Improve the nutrition knowledge base and skills of food service providers, educators, parents, and other caregivers.
- Expand the research base in adolescent nutrition.

CONCLUSION

Prevention of chronic diseases could have a major impact on future society through improved quality of life, reduced health care costs, and increased work productivity.[83] This is a long-term endeavor that will challenge the progression of chronic diseases throughout a lifetime. It requires consistent monitoring and evaluation as time goes by. Diet is a significant contributor to the complex interactions of genetic and environmental factors that influence health and disease. Without the societal commitment to dedicate the necessary resources to achieve the health goals, many adolescents will grow into high-risk adults. Primary prevention efforts in this age group have been shown to be efficacious and feasible. Establishing good nutrition habits can be the best investment for improving public health.

References

1. U.S. Department of Health and Human Services. *Healthy People 2000: National Health Promotion and Disease Prevention Objectives.* Washington, DC: U.S. Government Printing Office; 1990. DHHS (PHS) Publication no. 91-50213.

2. U.S. Department of Health and Human Services. *Healthy Children 2000: National Health Promotion and Disease Prevention Objectives Related to Mothers, Infants, Children, Adolescents, and Youth.* Washington, DC: U.S. Department of Health and Human Services, Public Health Services, Health Resources and Services Administration, Maternal and Child Health Bureau; 1991.

3. American School Health Association for the Advancement of Health Education Society for Public Health Education Inc. *The National Adolescent Student Health Survey: A Report on the Health of America's Youth.* Oakland, Calif: Third Party Publishing Co.; 1989.

4. Stary HC. Evolution and progression of atherosclerotic lesions in coronary arteries of children and young adults. *Arteriosclerosis.* 1989;9:I–31.

5. Roche A, Wilson M, Gidding S, Siervogel R. Lipids, growth, and development. *Metabolism.* 1993;42:36–44.

6. LaRosa J, Hunninghake D, Bush D. The cholesterol facts: a summary of the evidence relating dietary fats, serum cholesterol and coronary heart disease. A joint statement by the American Heart Association and the National Heart Lung and Blood Institute. *Circulation.* 1990;81:1721–1733.

7. Brown G, Albess J, Fisher L. Regression of coronary artery disease as a result of intensive lipid–lowering therapy in men with high levels of apolipoprotein B. *N Engl J Med.* 1990;323:1289–1298.

8. National Heart Lung and Blood Institute. *Report of the Expert Panel on Blood Cholesterol Levels in Children and Adolescents.* Washington, DC: U.S. Department of Health and Human Services; 1991. DHHS Publication no. 91-2732.

9. National Cholesterol Education Program. Report of the Expert Panel on Population Strategies for a Blood Cholesterol Reduction. *Circulation.* 1991;83:2132–2154.

10. National Heart Lung and Blood Institute. *The Lipid Research Clinics Population Studies Data Book: The Prevalence Study.* Bethesda, Md: U.S. Dept. of Health and Human Services; 1980. National Institutes of Health Publication no. 80-1527.

11. Lauer R, Lee J, Clarke WR. Factors affecting the relationship between childhood and adult cholesterol levels: the Muscatine study. *Pediatrics.* 1988;82:309–318.

12. Gidding S. The rationale for lowering serum cholesterol levels in American children. *Am J Dis Child.* 1993;147:386–392.

13. Kimm SY, Gergen P, Malloy M, Dresser C, Carroll M. Dietary patterns of U.S. children: implications for disease prevention. *Prev Med.* 1990;19:432–442.

14. Prewitt TE, Haynes SG, Graves K, Haines PS, Tyroler HA. Nutrient intake, lipids, and lipoprotein cholesterols in black and white children: the Lipid Research Clinics Prevalence Study. *Prev Med.* 1988;17:247–262.

15. McPherson RS, Nichaman MZ, Kohl HW, Reed DB, LaBarthe DR. Intake and food sources of dietary fat among school children in the Woodlands, Texas. *Pediatrics.* 1990;86:520–526.

16. McDowell MA, Briefel RR, Alaimo K, et al. *Energy and Macronutrient Intakes of Persons Ages 2 Months and Over in the United States: Third National Health and Nutrition Examination Survey, Phase I, 1988–91.* Hyattsville, Md: National Center for Health Statistics; 1994. Advance data from Vital and Health Statistics no. 255.

17. DISC Collaborative Research Group. Dietary Intervention Study in Children (DISC) with elevated low-density-lipoprotein cholesterol. Design and baseline characteristics. *Ann Epidemiol.* 1993;3:393–402.

18. DISC Collaborative Research Group. Dietary Intervention Study in Children (DISC) with elevated low-density-lipoprotein cholesterol—36 month results. *JAMA.* 1995;273:1429–1435.

19. Perry C, Stone E, Parcel G, et al. School-based health promotion: the child and adolescent trial for cardiovascular health (CATCH). *J School Health.* 1990;60:406–413.

20. Belcher J, Ellison RC, Shepard EN, et al. Lipid and lipoprotein distributions in children by ethnic group gender and geographic location. *Prev Med.* 1993;22:143–151.

21. Nicklas T, Reed D, Rupp J, et al. Reducing total fat, saturated fatty acids, and sodium: the CATCH Eat Smart School Nutrition Program. *School Food Serv.* 1992;16:114–121.

22. Walter HJ, Hofman A, Connelly PA, Barrett L, Kost K. Primary prevention of chronic disease in childhood: changes in risk factors after one year of intervention. *Am J Epidemiol.* 1985;122:772–781.

23. Walter H, Hofman A, Vaughn R, Wynder E. Modification of risk factors for coronary heart disease. Five year results of a school-based intervention trial. *N Engl J Med.* 1988;318:1093–1100.

24. Shannon B, Tershakovec A, Achterberg C, Martel J, McKenzie J, Mitchell D. Cholesterol education for at-risk children (abstract). Presented at American Heart Association 66th Scientific Sessions, Atlanta; November 1993.

25. Shannon B, Greene G, Stallings V, et al. A dietary education program for hypercholesterolemic children and their parents. *J Am Diet Assoc.* 1991;91:208–212.

26. Daniels S. Primary hypertension in childhood and adolescence. *Pediatr Ann.* 1992;21:224–235.

27. Lauer RM, Clarke WR. Childhood risk factors for high adult blood pressure: the Muscatine study. *Pediatrics.* 1989;84:633–641.

28. Joint National Committee on Detection Evaluation and Treatment of High Blood Pressure. The Fifth Report of the Joint National Committee on Detection, Evaluation and Treatment of High Blood Pressure (JNC-V). *Arch Intern Med.* 1993;153:154–183.

29. Alton I, Story M. *Guidelines for Adolescent Nutrition.* U.S. Department of Health and Human Services, Washington, DC: Public Health Service, Region V; September 1993.

30. Stamler J. Blood pressure and high blood pressure: aspects of risk. *Hypertension.* 1991;18(suppl I):I–97–I–107.

31. INTERSALT Cooperative Research Group. Intersalt: an international study of electrolyte excretion and blood pressure: results for 24 hour urinary sodium and potassium excretion. *BMJ.* 1988;297:319.

32. Law MR, Frost CD, Wald NJ. By how much does dietary salt reduction lower blood pressure? III. Analyses of data from trials of salt reduction. *BMJ.* 1991;302:819–824.

33. Cutler J, Fotlman D, Elliott P, Such I. An overview of randomized trials of sodium reduction and blood pressure. *Hypertension.* 1991;17(suppl I):I–27–I–33.

34. Miller J, Weinberg M, Daugherty S, Fineberg N, Christian J, Grim C. Blood pressure response to dietary sodium restriction in healthy normotensive children. *Am J Clin Nutr.* 1988;47:113–119.

35. Howe P, Cobrac L, Smith R. Lack of effect of short term changes in sodium intake on blood pressure in adolescent school children. *J Hypertens.* 1991;9:181–186.

36. Ellison R, Copper A, Stephenson W, et al. Effects on blood pressure of a decrease in sodium use in institutional food preparation: the Exeter-Andover Project. *J Clin Epidemiol.* 1989;42:201–208.

37. Sinaiko A, Gomez-Marin O, Prineas R. Effect of low-sodium diet or potassium supplementation on adolescent blood pressure. *Hypertension.* 1993;21:989–994.

38. National Research Council. *Recommended Dietary Allowances.* 10th ed. Washington, DC: National Academy Press; 1989.

39. Harris R, Phillips R, Williams P, Kuzma J, Traser G. The Child-Adolescent Blood Pressure Study: distribution of blood pressure levels in Seventh-Day Adventist (SDA) and Non-SDA children. *Am J Public Health.* 1981;71:1342–1349.

40. Voors AW, Foster T, Fredrichs R. Studies of blood pressure in children ages 5–14 in a total biracial community: the Bogalusa Heart Study. *Circulation.* 1976;54:319–327.

41. Kaplan N. Dietary aspects of the treatment of hypertension. *Annu Rev Public Health.* 1986;7:503–519.

42. Task Force on Blood Pressure Control in Children. American Academy of Pediatrics. Report of the Second Task Force on Blood Pressure Control in Children—1987. *Pediatrics.* 1987;79:1.

43. Krasnegor NA, Grave GD, Kretchmer N, eds. *Childhood Obesity: A Biobehavioral Perspective.* NJ: The Telford Press; 1988.

44. Van Itallie TB. Health implications of overweight and obesity in the United States. *Ann Intern Med.* 1985;103:983–988.

45. Pipes P. Prevention of chronic disease with dietary intervention in childhood. In: Pipes P, Trahms C, eds. *Nutrition in Infancy and Childhood.* 5th ed. Chicago, Ill: Mosby; 1993:288–308.

46. Garn SM, LaVelle M. Two-decade follow-up of fatness in early childhood. *Am J Dis Child.* 1985;139:181–185.

47. Kuczmarski RJ, Flegal KM, Campbell SM, Johnson CL. Increasing prevalence of overweight among US adults. The National Health and Nutrition Examination Surveys, 1960 to 1991. *JAMA.* 1994;272:205–211.

48. Melnyk MG, Weinstein E. Preventing obesity in black women by targeting adolescents: a literature review. *J Am Diet Assoc.* 1994;94:536–540.

49. National Institutes of Health. Consensus development panel on the health implications of obesity. *Ann Intern Med.* 1985;103:1073–1077.

50. Bray GA. Complications of obesity. *Ann Int Med.* 1985;103:1052–1062.

51. Epstein LH, Valoski A, Koeske R, Wing RR. Family-based behavioral weight control in obese young children. *J Am Diet Assoc.* 1986;86(4):481–484.

52. Epstein LH, Valoski A, Wing RR, McCurley J. Ten-year follow-up of behavioral, family-based treatment for obese children. *JAMA.* 1990;264(19):2519–2523.

53. Mellin L, Slinkard L, Irwin C. Adolescent obesity intervention validation of the shapedown program. *J Am Diet Assoc.* 1988;87:333–338.

54. Penna M, Bacallao J, Barta L, Amador M, Johnston FE. Fiber and exercise in the treatment of obese adolescents. *J Adol Hlth Ctr.* 1989;10:30–34.

55. Wadden TA, Stunkard AJ, Rich L, Rubin CJ, Swiedel G, McKenney S. Obesity in black adolescent girls: a controlled clinical trial of treatment by diet, behavior modification, and parental support. *Pediatrics.* 1990;85:345–352.

56. Sallis J, Patterson T, Buono M, Atkins C, Nader R. Aggregation of physical activity habits in Mexican-American and Anglo families. *J Behavioral Med.* 1988;11:31–41.

57. Aaron D, Kriska A, Dearwater S, et al. The epidemiology of leisure physical activity in an adolescent population. *Med Sci Sports Exer.* 1993;25:847–853.

58. Greenwald P. NCI Cancer prevention and control research. *Prev Med.* 1993;22:624–660.

59. Reddy BS. Dietary fat, calories, and fiber in colon cancer. *Prev Med.* 1993;22:738–749.

60. Bal DG, Foerster SB. Dietary strategies for cancer prevention. *Cancer.* 1993;72:1005–1010.

61. American Cancer Society Cancer Facts and Figures—1993.

62. Winick M. The role of early nutrition in subsequent development and optimal future health. *Bull NY Acad Med.* 1989;65:1020–1025.

63. Doll R, Peto R. The causes of cancer: quantitative estimates of avoidable risks of cancer in the US today. *JNCI.* 1981;66:1191–1308.

64. Wynder EL, Gori GB. Contribution of the environment to cancer incidence: an epidemiologic exercise. *JNCI.* 1977;5–32.

65. Portnoy B, Christenson GM. Cancer knowledge and related practices: results from the National Adolescent Student Health Survey. *J School Health.* 1989;59:218–223.

66. Block G, Patterson B, Subar A. Fruit, vegetables, and cancer prevention: a review of the epidemiologic evidence. *Nutr Cancer.* 1993;18:1–19.

67. Participation in school physical education and selected dietary patterns among high school students—United States, 1991. *MMWR.* 1992;41(33):597–607.

68. Olson CM. Childhood nutrition education in health promotion and disease prevention. *Bull NY Acad Med.* 1989;65:1143–1153.

69. Korn D. Fighting cancer in America: achieving the year 2000 goal. *J School Health.* 1989;59:224.

70. Walter HJ, Waughan RD, Wynder EL. Primary prevention of cancer among children: changes in cigarette smoking and diet after six years of intervention. *JNCI.* 1989;81:995–999.

71. Iammarino NK, Weinberg AD. Cancer prevention in the schools. *J School Health.* 1985;55:86–95.

72. Mettlin C. Dietary cancer prevention in children. *Cancer.* 1993;71(10 suppl):3367–3369.

73. Greenfield GB. *Radiology of Bone Diseases.* 5th ed. Philadelphia: JB Lippincott Company;1990.

74. Warlaw GM. Putting osteoporosis in perspective. *J Am Diet Assoc.* 1993;93:1000–1006.

75. Raper N. Nutrient Content of the US Food Supply. *Food Review.* 1991;July-September:17.

76. Anderson JJB, Metz JA. Contributions of dietary calcium and physical activity to primary prevention of osteoporosis in females. *J Am Coll Nutr.* 1993;12:378–383.

77. Matkovic V, Dekanic D, Kostial K. Calcium, Teenagers, and Osteoporosis. In: *Osteoporosis: Current Concepts. Report of the Seventh Ross Conference on Medical Research.* Ross Laboratories; Columbus;1987.

78. Chest CH. Theoretical overview: bone development, peak bone mass, bone loss, fracture risk. *Am J Med.* 1991;91(suppl 5B): 2S–4S.

79. U.S. Congress Office of Technology Assessment. *Adolescent Health, Vol III: Crosscutting Issues in the Delivery of Health and Related Services.* OTA-H-466. Washington, DC: Government Printing Office; 1991.

80. Williams CL, Wynder EL. A Child Health Report Card: 1992. *Prev Med.* 1993;22:604–628.

81. U.S. Congress Office of Technology Assessment. *Adolescent Health, II: Background and the Effectiveness of Selected Prevention and Treatment Services.* Washington, DC: U.S. Government Printing Office; 1991. OTA-H-466.

82. Committee on Diet and Health, Food and Nutrition Board, National Research Council. *Diet and Health: Implications for Reducing Chronic Disease Risk*. Washington, DC: National Academy Press; 1989.

83. Dwyer JT. Great expectations: overview of adolescent nutrition for the year 2000 and beyond. In: Nussbaum M, Dwyer JT, eds. *State of the Art Reviews: Adolescent Nutrition and Eating Disorders*. 1992;3:377–390.

12

ಎ

Obesity

Sachiko T. St. Jeor, Lori J. Silverstein, and Stanley R. Shane

Obesity is the most common nutritional disorder in the United States. It is a serious, prevalent, and refractory public health problem,[1] imposing an economic burden of almost $40 billion, or 5.5% of the costs of illness.[2] The prevalence of obesity has significantly increased, such that we are moving farther away from the 1991 health-promotion, disease-prevention goal as described in *Healthy People 2000* to "reduce overweight to a prevalence of no more than 20 percent among people aged 20 and older."[3] Indeed, according to the most recent report released from the 1988 to 1991 National Health and Nutrition Examination Survey (NHANES) III, phase 1, one-third (33.3%) of all American adults (35% women; 31% men) are overweight.[4] The adult population has undergone an alarming 8% increase in the prevalence of overweight, from a baseline of 26% (27% for women and 24% for men, aged 20 through 74), as reported from NHANES II a decade earlier in 1976 to 1980 (Figure 12-1). This is particularly important in contrast with the small 2% increase over the previous two decades, from 24.3% as reported from National Health Examination Survey (NHES)1 (1960 to 1962) and 25% from NHANES I (1971 to 1974).

Although obesity is independent of ethnicity, minority populations have a higher prevalence. Poverty and lower educational attainment increase susceptibility to obesity and its progression.[5] Nearly one-half of non-Hispanic black women (48.6%) and Mexican-American women (46.7%) are overweight as compared with the non-Hispanic white women (32.9%). Further, the prevalence is notably increased in younger Mexican-American women compared with non-Hispanic white and black women; the highest prevalence of overweight being 40 to 49 years for Mexican-American women, 50 to 59 years for non-Hispanic white women, and 60 to 69 years for non-Hispanic black women, as shown in Figure 12-2.[4] Obesity has also been increasing at a greater rate among black girls and

This work was supported by grant no. HL34589 from the National Heart, Lung and Blood Institute of the National Institutes of Health.

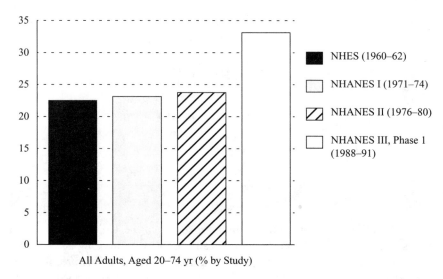

Figure 12-1 Prevalence of Overweight Is Steadily Increasing.   *Source:* Data from *Journal of the American Medical Association* (1994;272:205–211*),* American Medical Association, 1994.

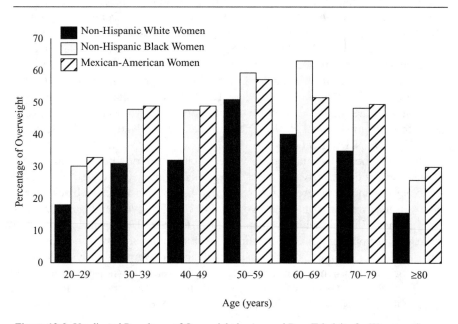

Figure 12-2 Unadjusted Prevalence of Overweight by Age and Race/Ethnicity for Women.   *Source:* Reprinted from *Journal of the American Medical Association* (1994;272:205–211), American Medical Association, 1994.

adolescents (aged 6 to 17) than among non-Hispanic whites,[6] and the limited success of non-Hispanic black American women at weight loss highlights the need for culturally specific programs. Thus, if obesity prevention and treatment interventions are to be effectively implemented and maintained, special attention must be given to the diversity in the way various "obesities" develop; the way obesities are differentially affected by age, gender, ethnicity, and socioeconomic factors; and the way obesities are individually expressed with regard to body fat distribution, weight patterns, and other related disease risk factors.

OBESITY INCREASES MORBIDITY AND MORTALITY

Obesity has been considered an independent risk factor for cardiovascular disease,[7] contributing directly to the leading cause of death among American women.[8] Also, obesity has been recognized for its indirect contributions toward increasing morbidity and mortality through the enhancement of other diseases and/or their risk factors, such as insulin resistance, diabetes, hypertension, dyslipidemia, gallstones and cholecystitis, respiratory dysfunction, and osteoarthritis.[9] In most cases, the effects of being overweight also increase with its severity and duration, which, in turn, are usually related to age and hormonal status, especially in women.[10]

The optimal weight for health is currently under debate,[11] but data from several large population studies indicate that mortality increases as weight increases.[12] Exhibit 12-1 summarizes increases in risk associated with obesity. A body mass index (BMI or weight [kg]/height^2 [m]) of greater than 35 is associated with a twofold increase in total mortality.[13] In women, the risk of obesity has been predominantly expressed through its associations with increased morbidity and mortality from coronary heart disease, diabetes, and cancer. Data from the Nurses' Health Study implicated overweight in more than 40% of all heart disease cases in U.S. women, and the risk notably doubled with weight gains of more than 20 lb in adulthood.[14] This may be partially due to increased plasma cholesterol associated with increased relative weight and increased triglycerides and/or hyperinsulinemia enhancing the production of very low-density lipoprotein in the liver,

Exhibit 12-1 Obesity Increases Morbidity and Mortality

- BMI > 35 is associated with 2 times total average mortality
- Overweight is associated with 40% of heart disease in women
- Overweight is associated with 3 times the risk for hypertension
- Weight gain of 20 lb doubles the risk of cardiovascular disease
- Diabetes occurs at 3 times the rate in obese women
- Overweight associated with 1.55 times average mortality for some cancers in women

as observed with weight gains.[9,15] Furthermore, the increased prevalence of hypertension among the obese has been well documented. The relative risk for hypertension for overweight adults was found to be three times that of nonoverweight adults, with the risk in younger adults (aged 20 to 45 years) 5.6 times greater than that of older adults (aged 45 to 75).[13] Similarly, diabetes occurs at three times the rate in obese as compared with nonobese women,[13] particularly in relationship to those with abdominal or central fat distribution patterns.[16] The Cancer Prevention Study I confirmed increased mortality risk for women 40% or more overweight, with relative risks of 2.07 for coronary heart disease, 7.90 for diabetes, and 1.55 for cancer of all sites (specifically, 5.42 for endometrial, 4.65 uterine, 3.58 gallbladder, 2.39 cervical, 1.63 ovarian, and 1.53 breast cancers, respectively).[17] Importantly, the risk for increased mortality from breast cancer in postmenopausal women has been associated with the degree and duration of the obese state.[18]

Weight cycling, also known as "yo-yo dieting," has been a concern for researchers and individuals involved in obesity treatment, as it applies psychological and physiologic stress on dieters. The degree of concern was great enough to stimulate preparation of a special communication from the National Task Force on the Prevention and Treatment of Obesity,[19] which concluded that weight cycling does not significantly alter metabolism and that data on long-term health effects are lacking. Although some observational studies show increased mortality in weight cyclers, many studies demonstrate no effect on cardiovascular risk factors and diabetes risk. At this point in time, the task force concluded that the health risks of obesity outweigh the possible hazards of weight loss attempts among the obese.

It is clear that obese individuals are at increased risk for health complications and suffer from increased rates of morbidity and mortality from the leading causes of death. However, due to the chronic nature and current limitations in treatment, obesity is too often overlooked or not treated at all. Complex psychological, behavioral, and environmental factors set the stage for dieting failures and further exacerbate the disease process.

DIETING CONCERNS AND PRACTICES

Psychological and sociocultural pressures may cause, promote, or lead to an intense preoccupation with weight and body image in women throughout their lives. Thus, it is no surprise that dieting concerns and practices occur across all age and weight categories with a willingness to try almost any weight loss strategy.[20] Approximately 60% of young girls between grades 1 and 6 develop distorted body images and overestimate their weight, and 70% diet between the ages of 14 and 21 years.[21] The 1990 self-administered Youth Risk Behavior Survey of 11,467 high school students reported that 44% of girls (15% of boys) were trying to lose weight and that an additional 26% of girls (15% of boys) were trying to keep from gaining weight by exercising, skipping meals, taking diet pills, and vomiting.[22] Among 60,681 adults in the Behavioral Risk Factor Surveillance System, a random digit dial survey, 38% of women (24% of men) were trying to lose weight, with another 28% of both women and men trying to maintain their weight.[22] Furthermore, according to the 1990 National Health Interview Survey (NHIS), 52% of women (36.7% of men) considered themselves to be overweight and were trying to lose weight by eating less and/or increasing their physical activity.[23] Of concern are reports that the dieting population includes as many as one in three who need not restrict their calories (i.e., those individuals who are underweight [8.9% women versus 4.5% men] and average weight [20% women versus 10.2% men]).[24]

Self-reported dieting behaviors in women differed significantly from those of men in the RENO Diet Heart Study, comprised of 508 normal weight and obese men and women. As outlined in Table 12-1, weight programs (i.e., Weight Watchers, TOPS, and Overeaters Anonymous) were most likely to have been used by obese females relative to all other groups (mean lifetime frequency of 1.8 times). Being both female and overweight were also associated with subjects' use of diet pills/products (mean lifetime frequency of 4.5 times) and with total diet methods used (mean lifetime frequency of 21.3 times). Fad diets were used more often by females of both weight groups than by males. Generally, it appeared that normal-weight males were far less likely to engage in dieting (mean lifetime frequency of 2.6 times) than were normal-weight females, obese females, or obese males. Interestingly, obese males and normal-weight females were equally likely to diet

Table 12-1 Mean Lifetime Frequency of Diet Method Use by Gender and Weight Group

Diet Method	Females		Males	
	Normal Weight	Obese	Normal Weight	Obese
Weight programs[a]	0.4	1.8	0.1	0.2
Diet pills/products[b]	2.7	4.5	0.2	1.2
Psychological treatments	0.6	1.0	0.4	1.1
Fasting	0.9	2.4	0.5	0.8
"Fad" diets[c]	2.3	3.3	0.3	1.4
Exercise programs	0.5	8.1	1.0	2.4
Total diet methods[b]	7.5	21.3	2.6	7.1

[a]Gender differences, weight group differences, and gender × weight group interaction ($p < .05$).
[b]Gender differences and weight group differences ($p < .05$).
[c]Gender differences ($p < .05$).
No superscript denotes no significant effect.
Source: Data from Horm J and Anderson K, Who in America is Trying to Lose Weight?, *Annals of Internal Medicine* (1993;119:672–676), American College of Physicians, 1993.

(by total diet methods), and exercise programs were the most common diet method used by obese as well as normal-weight males (mean lifetime frequency of 2.4 and 1.0 times, respectively).[25] Most weight loss attempts are self-directed. In a survey consisting of 20,000 readers of *Consumer Reports,* of those losing and maintaining the loss of a significant amount of weight (mean=34 lb), 72% had done so on their own, 20% participated in commercial programs, 3% used diet pills, and 5% enrolled in hospital- or university-based programs.[26] Moreover, a population survey conducted among working men and women found that 75% of women (47% of men) had dieted, but only 31% of women (6% of men) had enrolled in an organized weight loss program.[27]

Behavior modification includes both eating and exercise behaviors and is an essential part of any weight reduction program. Specific behaviors are targeted for change after a systematic evaluation of associated antecedents and conse-quences.[28] Foreyt and Goodrick[28] identified the five major behavior modification treatment components as self-monitoring (recording), stimulus control (restrict-ing environmental factors), contingency management (rewards), changing behav-ioral parameters (altering topology), and cognitive-behavior modification (thinking patterns) as outlined in Table 12-2. Of the behavioral strategies report-edly used by the RENO Diet heart participants as part of any past weight loss plan, stimulus control was the highest in all groups, especially in obese females (Table 12-3). Physical activity was higher in normal-weight males and females as compared with their obese counterparts, and more women used cognitive restruc-turing and nutrition education. More normal-weight women controlled their eat-ing behaviors. In comparison, more obese women used self-monitoring as means

Table 12-2 Behavior Treatment Components

Component	Description	Examples
Self-monitoring	Recording of target behaviors and factors associated with behaviors	Food and exercise records, moods, and environment associated with overeating
Stimulus control	Restricting environmental factors associated with inappropriate behaviors	Keep away from high-fat foods; eat at specific times and places; set aside time and place for exercise
Contingency management	Rewarding appropriate behaviors	Give prizes for achieving exercise goals
Changing behavior parameters	Directly altering target behavior topology	Slow down eating; self-regulate exercise
Cognitive-behavior modification	Changing thinking patterns related to target behaviors	Counter social pressure to be thin to reduce temptation to diet

Source: Reprinted with permission from Foreyt, JP, and Goodrick, GK, Evidence for Success of Behavior Modification in Weight Loss and Control, *Annals of Internal Medicine* (1993;119:699), Copy-right © 1993, American College of Physicians.

Table 12-3 Self-Reported Behavioral Strategies Used[a]

Specific Behavior	Total Possible Points	Total Sample	Women		Men	
			Normal Weight	Obese	Normal Weight	Obese
Stimulus control[b]	42	22.1	23.6	26.0	19.5	19.2
Eating behavior[c]	18	6.2	6.7	6.3	6.2	5.7
Reward[c]	12	1.3	1.3	2.1	0.9	0.6
Self-monitoring[b]	9	0.4	0.5	0.9	0.2	0.1
Nutrition education[d]	12	3.3	4.0	3.8	2.8	2.7
Physical activity[e]	18	5.6	6.0	5.3	6.1	5.0
Cognitive restructuring[b]	15	5.2	5.5	5.5	4.8	4.9

[a]Behavioral strategies were derived from a questionnaire administered to subjects at baseline. Questions were answered on a 0 (never) to 3 (always) frequency scale with regard to how often that particular strategy was part of the subject's weight loss plans. Those responses were summed for each type of strategy, to yield composite scores. The scale scores and its selection were based on a review of behavioral strategies for weight loss (Stunkard and Berthold, *Am J Clin Nutr.* 41(4):821–823, 1985).
[b]Gender effect, weight effect, and gender X weight group interaction ($p < .05$).
[c]Gender and weight group effects ($p < .05$).
[d]Gender effect only ($p < .05$).
[e]Weight group effect only ($p < .05$).
Source: Data from Horn J and Anderson K, Who in America is Trying to Lose Weight?, *Annals of Internal Medicine* (1993;119:672–676), American College of Physicians, 1993.

for weight control.[25] It is clear that a better understanding of motivational factors, dieting behaviors, choices of programs, and methods with improved outcomes are drastically needed to meet the challenges of obesity treatment and prevention, especially in women.

WEIGHT LOSS PRACTICES AND RESULTS

The 1990s have been labeled by Brownell[26] as the "antidieting decade" because it represents a time when critical attention is being cast on the limitations of treatment as well as the high costs and serious consequences of dieting. The diet industry is being challenged. For example, the New York Department of Consumer Protection has developed regulations governing the services of diet centers, designed to improve disclosure of the health risks and overall costs of their weight loss programs.[29] Further, regulation of obesity management through an accrediting agency has been proposed to ensure patient safety,[30] and new challenges are evident for health care professionals to responsibly increase their involvement and effectiveness.

The limitations of professional treatment programs have been painfully recognized, attesting to the fact that on the average (1) weight losses do not exceed approximately 0.4 to 0.5 kg/wk; (2) only 8.5 kg are lost in behavioral programs lasting 15 to 20 weeks; (3) one-third of the weight lost is regained in 1 year after treatment; and (4) most will regain all the weight lost within 5 years.[31] Because traditional methods appear to be limited in the amount and maintenance of weight losses, other options such as very low-calorie diets (VLCDs) consisting of 400 to 800 kcal/day and resulting in an average weight loss of 20 kg over 12 weeks (but also regain of weight within 5 years) have been recommended for the moderately to severely overweight (BMI of 30 or more) who have failed to lose weight by more conventional methods.[32]

Recent studies suggest that drugs may have a role in long-term obesity treatment. Weintraub[33] demonstrated that fenfluramine (a centrally acting serotonin agonist) and phentermine (a centrally active adrenergic-stimulating agent) produced and maintained moderate weight losses for 3.5 years in some subjects.[34] Further, studies using placebo versus active drugs (appetite suppressants that act on noradrenergic and dopaminergic receptors to produce satiety) produced net weight losses of 2 to 20 kg compared with placebo with maintenance up to 36 months and weight regain after terminating drug treatment.[35] Thus, it has been speculated that specific biochemical defects may be responsible for treatment-resistant subtypes of obesity and that different drugs may correct these defects.[34] An NIH Workshop on Pharmacologic Treatment of Obesity recently concluded that the long-term results of fenfluramine alone and in combination with phentermine are promising in reducing body weight over an extended period of time.[36] The potential use for these and other drugs in obesity treatment was recognized, and further research was encouraged. Drugs should be considered as only one component of a weight control program, and their long-term use should involve other members of the health care team, particularly because individuals respond differently to drugs and healthy life styles and eating habits must be maintained.

Surgical interventions produce weight losses that are almost never achieved with behavioral or medical therapy and are considered for patients whose BMI exceeds 40 or is between 35 and 40 with accompanying, high-risk, comorbid conditions.[37] Jejunoileal bypass surgery has been replaced by two procedures that are presented in Figure 12-3.[38] These are vertical banded gastroplasty (a small pouch constructed with a restricted outlet along the lesser curvature of the stomach) and Roux-en-Y gastric bypass (proximal gastric pouch whose outlet is a Y-shaped limb of small bowel of varying lengths).[37] With these surgical interventions, maximum weight losses are achieved between 18 and 24 months postoperatively and weight loss maintained at 5 years or longer is from 48 to 74% with gastric bypass and from 50 to 60% with vertical banded gastroplasty.[39] The mechanism of weight loss with vertical banded gastroplasty appears to be the mechanical barrier to food intake. Although it is easier to perform than gastric bypass with fewer perioperative complications, it is also associated with lesser long-term weight loss. Weight loss with gastric bypass surgery is associated with dumping

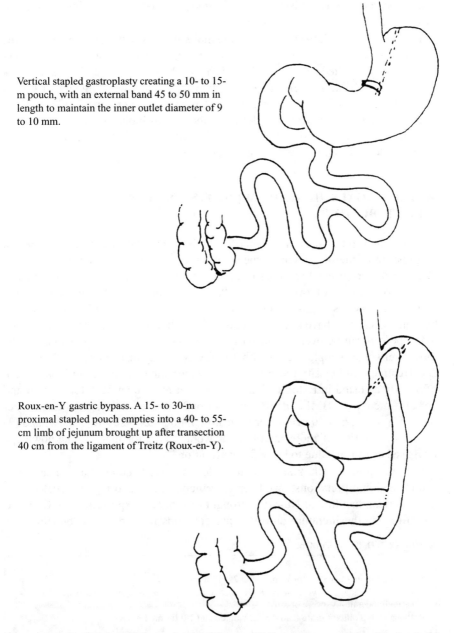

Vertical stapled gastroplasty creating a 10- to 15-m pouch, with an external band 45 to 50 mm in length to maintain the inner outlet diameter of 9 to 10 mm.

Roux-en-Y gastric bypass. A 15- to 30-m proximal stapled pouch empties into a 40- to 55-cm limb of jejunum brought up after transection 40 cm from the ligament of Treitz (Roux-en-Y).

Figure 12-3 Vertical Stapled Gastroplasty and Roux-en-Y Gastric Bypass. *Source:* Reprinted with permission from *American Journal of Clinical Nutrition* (1992;55[2]:553S), Copyright © 1992, American Society for Clinical Nutrition.

syndrome and a rapid transit of nutrients into the small intestine, but the mechanism of action is still largely unknown.[34,39]

The complexity of obesity has become more obvious with the realization of the limitations of treatment. Also, the increasing prevalence of obesity and unsuccessful, self-directed dieting efforts further challenge professionals to look toward a revitalization of efforts. Reasonable and healthy weight goals for weight loss and maintenance along with an understanding of prevention of weight gain at critical periods, efforts to better delineate the role of biobehavioral, psychological, and physiologic attributes, and individualization of treatment will help us focus needed efforts to improve our effectiveness.

WEIGHT GOALS, HEALTHY WEIGHTS, AND FAT DISTRIBUTION

New weight guidelines are needed not only to prevent obesity but to prevent progression of the obese state, especially with regard to fat accumulation in the abdominal area (truncal or upper body fat) and viscera (intra-abdominal cavity). Current definitions of overweight as "an excess amount of body weight that includes all tissues—muscle, bone, and fat—as well as water" and obesity as "having excess fat" have been established.[40] Furthermore, it has been recognized that a person can be overweight but not obese (such as a body builder), but the most overweight people are also obese. The National Task Force on Prevention and Treatment of Obesity recently set forth recommendations for the assessment of obesity as listed in Exhibit 12-2: (1) body fat more than 30% for women and 25% for men; (2) a BMI at age 35 or older of 27 or greater, at age 34 or younger of 25 or greater, and 30 or greater indicating moderate-to-severe obesity; and (3) waist-to-hip ratios of more than 0.8 for women (1.0 for men) to acknowledge increased health risk due to body fat distribution.[40]

With recognition that many weight guidelines have been used and their applications and interpretations have been extremely limited and highly debated,[41–47] the American Institute of Nutrition brought together an Expert Steering Committee to review the literature and hear presentations relevant to establishing new

Exhibit 12-2 Definitions of Obesity

- Body fat more than 30% for women and 25% for men
- BMI of 27+ at age 35 yr or older; BMI of 25 at age 34 yr or younger; and a BMI >30 indicating moderate-to-severe obesity
- Waist-to-hip ratio of more than 0.8 for women and 1.0 for men

Source: Information from National Task Force on Prevention of Obesity, *Journal of the American Medical Association* (1994;272:1196–1202), American Medical Association, 1994.

weight guidelines. The committee summarized its deliberations, emphasizing the following points[11]:

1) weight guidelines should be directed at healthy, nonpregnant adults age 21 and over, and serve primarily for the *prevention* of obesity and obesity-related complications;

2) due to the increasing prevalence of overweight among children and adolescents, complexities created by growth and development, frequency of eating disorders, and potential for psychosocial harm because of labeling, the task of creating further guidelines requires additional effort (i.e., the creation of an additional committee closely coordinated with the American Academy of Pediatrics);

3) a separate document should be created for health practitioners to provide guidelines for the management of overweight among individuals whose weight falls outside the recommended guidelines;

4) guidelines should be in the form of weight-for-height tables or figures and should be accompanied by the statement that they should not be used as a basis for discrimination in any form and should not be used as a basis for obesity treatment; furthermore, in the absence of validation of the effectiveness, a simplified three-part approach consisting of weight-for-height, waist-to-hip, and treatment for medical conditions was recommended.

5) evidence was insufficient to justify separate tables for categories of age, gender, or ethnicity, although there is a clear need for additional data;

6) no more than 10 (or possibly 15) pounds should be gained after age 21; any unexplained weight loss of more than 10 pounds requires medical attention; waistline measurement should not increase more than approximately 2–3 inches after age 21;

    a) the preferred format was a table for ages 21 and older, using a single BMI criterion of 18–25 kg/m^2 for both sexes (although this needs further consideration) with a notation that most people will be healthier toward the lower end of the range and guidance about limiting weight gain;

    b) considered a format that depicts a range of lowest risk (or optimal) weight with additional ranges indicating gradations of risk

Table 12-4 Body Weight in Pounds According to Height and Body Mass Index[a]

Body Mass Index (kg/m^2)

Height (in.)	19.0	20.0	21.0	22.0	23.0	24.0	25.0	26.0	27.0	28.0	29.0	30.0	35.0	40.0
							Body Weight (lb)							
58.0	90.7	95.5	100.3	105.0	109.8	114.6	119.4	124.1	128.9	133.7	138.5	143.2	167.1	191.0
59.0	93.9	98.8	103.8	108.7	113.6	118.6	123.5	128.5	133.4	138.3	143.3	148.2	172.9	197.6
60.0	97.1	102.2	107.3	112.4	117.5	122.6	127.7	132.9	138.0	143.1	148.2	153.3	178.8	204.4
61.0	100.3	105.6	110.9	116.2	121.5	126.8	132.0	137.3	142.6	147.9	153.2	158.4	184.8	211.3
62.0	103.7	109.1	114.6	120.0	125.5	130.9	136.4	141.9	147.3	152.8	158.2	163.7	191.0	218.2
63.0	107.0	112.7	118.3	123.9	129.6	135.2	140.8	146.5	152.1	157.7	163.4	169.0	197.2	225.3
64.0	110.5	116.3	122.1	127.9	133.7	139.5	145.3	151.2	157.0	162.8	168.6	174.4	203.5	232.5
65.0	113.9	119.9	125.9	131.9	137.9	143.9	149.9	155.9	161.9	167.9	173.9	179.9	209.9	239.9
66.0	117.5	123.7	129.8	136.0	142.2	148.4	154.6	160.8	166.9	173.1	179.3	185.5	216.4	247.3
67.0	121.1	127.4	133.8	140.2	146.5	152.9	159.3	165.7	172.0	178.4	184.8	191.1	223.0	254.9
68.0	124.7	131.3	137.8	144.4	151.0	157.5	164.1	170.6	177.2	183.8	190.3	196.9	229.7	262.5
69.0	128.4	135.2	141.9	148.7	155.4	162.2	168.9	175.7	182.5	189.2	196.0	202.7	236.5	270.3
70.0	132.1	139.1	146.1	153.0	160.0	166.9	173.9	180.8	187.8	194.7	201.7	208.6	243.4	278.2
71.0	135.9	143.1	150.3	157.4	164.6	171.7	178.9	186.0	193.2	200.3	207.5	214.6	250.4	286.2
72.0	139.8	147.2	154.5	161.9	169.2	176.6	183.9	191.3	198.7	206.0	213.4	220.7	257.5	294.3
73.0	143.7	151.3	158.8	166.4	174.0	181.5	189.1	196.7	204.2	211.8	219.3	226.9	264.7	302.5
74.0	147.7	155.4	163.2	171.0	178.8	186.5	194.3	202.1	209.9	217.6	225.4	233.2	272.0	310.9
75.0	151.7	159.7	167.7	175.6	183.6	191.6	199.6	207.6	215.6	223.5	231.5	239.5	279.4	319.4
76.0	155.8	164.0	172.2	180.4	188.6	196.8	205.0	213.2	221.4	229.5	237.7	245.9	286.9	327.9

[a]Each entry gives the body weight in pounds (lb) for a person of a given height and body mass index.

(e.g., BMI 18–23 = lowest risk, 24–25 = mild risk, 26–29 = medium risk, 30+ = high risk)

7) the acknowledgment that a BMI of less than 16 may be an indication of an eating disorder or underlying illness and individuals should obtain evaluation, education, and counseling or treatment, particularly with weight loss of more than 5% of body weight or 10 pounds.

8) for individuals whose weight falls outside the range, the cited BMI ranges may neither be attainable nor practical; for these individuals, avoidance of further weight gain should be the first objective with recognition that even modest weight reductions, such as 10 pounds, can be beneficial;

9) methods of weight control should emphasize physical activity, include aerobic exercise coupled with modest, sustainable caloric restraint, using food choices within the overall USDA/HHS Dietary Guidelines for Americans; cigarette smoking should not be used to control weight.

Emphasis on the distribution and composition of fat in relation to total body weight and disease risk, anticipated weight gains with age, and notable differences between gender and ethnic groups necessitates the need for new weight guidelines.

A risk classification system that compares waist to hip ratio (WHR) effects within the context of BMI was recently developed by Bray.[48] In this system, the degree of risk was classified in five stages (very low to very high). For example, in the optimal BMI range from 20 to less than 25, the respective WHR cutoffs for very low, low and moderate risks are less than 0.70, 0.70 to 0.85, and greater than 0.85 for women and less than 0.85, 0.85 to 1.0, and greater than 1.0 for men, respectively. The naturally higher WHRs for men, which indicate greater abdominal fat, partially explain their increased health risks for various diseases. A further recommendation includes no weight gain after the age of 20 years for men and only a small (if any) weight gain in women (equivalent to 0.5 BMI/decade or 2 BMI units, or approximately 10 to 15 lb depending on height) from ages 25 to 65 years. This more sensitive index, which combines BMI and WHR, shows promise in refining assessment and prognostic efforts and places further emphasis on the prevention of undesirable weight gain with age.

Table 12-4 lists the BMI in pounds according to height in inches.[48] The optimal BMI range is from 20 to 25, with a BMI of 22 associated with the lowest mortality. Overweight classifications traditionally used by the National Center for Health Statistics in their surveys[4] and many research studies are weight at the

85th percentile or BMI of 27.3 or greater for women (27.8 for men), 120% or greater ideal body weight (midpoint of the 1959 or 1983 Metropolitan Life Insurance height for weight tables), and obesity indices of BMI of 32.3 or greater for women (31.1 for men) for classification at the 95th percentile as severely overweight.[49,50] Others have recommended a more practical and easy-to-use breakdown of BMIs with the normal range as 20 to 25, overweight as 25 to 30, severe overweight as 30 or greater, and massive overweight as 40 or greater.[51]

Although the WHR is currently the most practical surrogate measure of abdominal or visceral fat, there is still argument regarding its overall use, particularly related to change.[52,53] Some argue that it is a stronger independent risk factor than BMI.[54] In a sample of 41,837 women aged 55 to 69 years, the WHR was more incremental and positively associated with mortality than was BMI; a 15-cm (6 in.) increase in waist size in a woman with a 100-cm (40 in.) hip was associated with a 60% greater relative risk of mortality.[55]

The accumulation and distribution of fat has been related to four separate factors: genetics (25% of human variability); age (weight gains that begin in middle age and increase thereafter); gender differences (women tend to distribute fat around the thighs and men around the abdomen); and life-style factors (positive energy balance, physical inactivity, stress, smoking, alcohol, and dietary fat).[56,57] Sex steroids directly influence fat accumulation and regulation. In women, the accumulation of fat in the femoral region is influenced primarily by estrone (E_1), which activates lipoprotein lipase activity (the rate-limiting step for the uptake of fat into the cell as opposed to lipolysis for lipid mobilization) and influences the development of fat cells.[57] By contrast, women who tend to deposit fat in the abdominal region and exhibit central obesity similar to that of men have a higher level of androgens and free testosterone.[56,58]

The specific recommendations for a healthy weight goal and/or realistic weight loss goal remains a challenge for all involved in weight management efforts. Weight history including the highest adult body weight, lowest adult body weight, usual weight, weight gains and losses during critical times (e.g., pregnancy), and desired weight should always be assessed when setting realistic and achievable weight goals. To increase effectiveness in weight management, smaller and more achievable weight losses (10 lb) that can be maintained should be more commonly recommended with incremental staging of smaller additive weight losses and a focus on weight maintenance when weight loss is no longer being achieved.

EATING BEHAVIORS AND FOOD PATTERNS

Weight fluctuations (gains and losses) are common in women and are not always related to eating and/or dieting or unique to women who are obese. A study of 87 women not associated with a weight loss program indicated that the obese subjects experienced the greatest weight changes, but dietary, attitudinal, behavioral, psychological, and energy balance (intake and expenditure) factors associated with obesity were not necessarily correlated with weight changes.[59] Other studies of eating patterns have demonstrated that neither microbehavior (mouthfuls, chews, drinks, and pauses) nor macrobehaviors (type and amount of food consumed and total eating and drinking time) were significantly different between obese and nonobese individuals.[60]

The overall diet composition and eating frequency are newer areas that are receiving attention, especially with regard to gender differences, adiposity, effect on energy balance, and potential effects on overall health.[10] A nibbling diet providing 17 snacks was associated with lower serum total cholesterol, low-density lipoprotein cholesterol, apolipoprotein B, and serum insulin levels as compared with a traditional three-meal diet.[61] Similarly, modest increases in reported meal frequency (4 or more meals a day versus 1 to 2 meals a day) without increases in caloric intake were related to reduced cholesterol concentrations in a sample of 2034 white men and women aged 50 to 89 years in Rancho Bernardo, California.[62] The overall diet composition in relation to macronutrient balance may also have differential effects on body weight and adiposity. When a high-carbohydrate (60% kcal) and a high-fat diet (60% kcal) were fed in a randomized, crossover design to eight subjects on a clinical research ward, nutrient oxidation rates of both fat and carbohydrate changed in response to changes in intake, and with longer periods, significant difference in total body energy and body composition could be favorably elicited by a high-carbohydrate diet.[63] Similarly, decreases in adiposity and weight were observed in 303 women enrolled in a low-fat dietary intervention trial and randomly assigned to either the low-fat (21% kcal as fat) or control (37.3% kcal as fat) diet.[64] However, Leibel et al[65] demonstrated that a very high-fat (70%) and a very low-fat (0%) diet did not significantly alter energy need over an 8-week period. Obesity may be caused by a positive fat balance, and because fat intake does not stimulate fat oxidation, it is plausible that the obese state is promoted by the effects of a high-fat diet on the maintenance and/or increase of fat stores[66] but the effects on energy balance are equivocal. The greatest effect of the high-fat diet is believed to be during the period after weight loss, when energy requirements are reduced and rate of fat oxidation may be low, because negative energy balance is the strongest determinant of the amount and rate of weight loss during the weight reduction phase.[67]

Table 12-5 presents data from 7-day food records from the RENO Diet Heart Study, in which the number of eating incidents (classified as defined meals, start of eating 30 minutes apart and/or eating at a different location), although not significantly different, were higher in the obese subjects as compared with the normal-weight subjects. Total calories per day were significantly higher in obese women (lower in obese men), whereas the percentage of kilocalories from fat was

Table 12-5 Eating Incidents and Dietary Intake Measures

	Females			Males		
	All	Normal Weight	Obese	All	Normal Weight	Obese
Mean no. of eating incidents per day[a]	5.6±1.5	5.4±1.6	5.7±1.6	5.7±1.6	5.5±1.3	6.0±1.8
Total calories[b]	1888±457	1869±414	1909±499	2643±719	2780±727	2508±687
Total fat (g)[c]	78±25	74±23	83±27	108±37	110±38	107±36
Percentage of calories from fat[d]	37±6	35±6	38±6	36±6	35±6	37±6
Saturated fat (g)[e]	28±10	27±10	30±11	39±15	39±16	38±14
Cholesterol (mg)[f]	260±91	246±95	274±84	378±152	371±162	385±143

[a]No significant (ns) differences by gender or weight group.
[b]Gender differences ($p < .001$); weight group differences ($p < .05$); gender × weight group interactions ($p < .01$).
[c]Gender differences ($p < .001$); weight group differences ($p < .001$); gender × weight group interactions ($p < .05$).
[d]Gender differences (ns); weight group differences ($p < .001$); gender × weight group interactions (ns).
[e]Gender differences ($p < .001$); weight group differences (ns); gender × weight group interactions ($p < .05$).
[f]Gender differences ($p < .001$); weight group differences ($p < .06$); gender × weight group interactions (ns).
Source: Data from Leibel RL, Hirsch J, Appel BE, Checani GC, Energy Intake Required to Maintain Body Weight is Not Affected by Wide Variation in Diet Composition, *American Journal of Clinical Nutrition.* (1992;55:350–355), American Society for Clinical Nutrition, 1992.

significantly higher in the obese women (and obese men) as compared with normal-weight women (and men), respectively.[68] These data stimulate interest in the role of fat in weight gain and eating patterns, with specific regard for increased energy intake and increased eating incidents in obese women.

CRITICAL PERIODS FOR WEIGHT GAIN IN WOMEN

Women tend to outlive men by 5 to 9 years, with their average life expectancy now approximately 80 years in 15 countries.[69] Although this generally indicates that women have a lower mortality rate than men in all age groups, it is hypothesized that this gender difference will decline in time. The most probable reason for this decline is their propensity toward weight gain (for whatever reason) and increasing overweight moving women into higher risk categories over time. Also, special problems with osteoporosis, eating disorders, and menstrual irregularities affect and are affected by body weight throughout life.[8]

The Fetal and Infant Nutrition and Susceptibility to Obesity workshop sponsored by the Food and Nutrition Board of the National Research Council in 1978[70] concluded that correlations between weight, weight gain, or skinfold measurements at birth or the first year with comparable measures at ages 7 to 16 years are low (r=.25), and evidence was not convincing at that time to associate the obese child with the obese adult. However, Dietz[71] later suggested that three critical periods for the development of obesity were gestation and early infancy, ages 5 and 7 years, and adolescence. During early uterine growth, it was hypothesized that nutrition may affect the differentiation of hypothalamic centers responsible for the control of food intake (appetite regulation), and during the third trimester and postnatal period, nutrition may influence adipose tissue cellularity and protect or promote later obesity. During the first year of life, BMI increases and then subsequently decreases. The second increase in BMI or "adiposity rebound" occurs beginning at approximately 5 years of age, and this period has also been hypothesized to be a vulnerable period for increased fatness. Although not clearly established, the hypothesis that children who rebound earlier (before 5.5 years of age), compared with average (6.0 to 6.5 years) or late (after 7 years), grow fatter for a longer period of time. Last, during adolescence, girls have a greater risk than boys for both the onset and persistence of obesity, with 30% of all obese adult women (compared with 10% obese adult males) being obese early in adolescence. Only 20% of obese females returned to normal weight over a 10-year period compared to 70% of obese males. Interestingly, men tend to suffer more from the consequences of obesity present during childhood than women, most likely because of their central fat distribution pattern enhanced by their androgen production.

The age of puberty is an important time when body fat and total body weight are critically important to hormonal expressions. Frisch and McArthur[72] found that a minimum weight for height, representing a critical level of fat as the percentage of body weight, was related to the onset of menarche. This weight was equivalent in composition to approximately 17% body fat. As the population gets heavier, it is notably significant that the average age of puberty has dropped to 12.8 years, with the mean weight at menarche of 105 lb (47.8 kg) with approximately 22% body fat as compared with 100 years ago when menarche was reached at age 15 or 16 years.[72,73] Although girls are usually less fat at the onset of menarche, the average weight gain of 4.5 kg to age 18 years is represented by mean body fat at age 16 years of approximately 27% and at age 18 years at approximately 28%. It has been hypothesized that a minimum level of stored body fat as energy is necessary to be used for ovulation and menstrual cycling. Thus, weight changes associated with cessation and restoration of menstrual cycles were reported to be in the 10 to 15% of body weight range. Further, the minimal weight for height necessary for the restoration and maintenance of menses of women aged 16 years and older was equivalent to 22% body fat. It is not surprising to note the delayed menarche and amenorrhea common in ballet dancers,[74] highly trained athletes,[75] and those with anorexia nervosa.[76] The incidence of irregularities in the menstrual cycle increased during times of increased training when the fat in relation to the lean mass decreased with weight loss but similarly returned to normal with weight gains of approximately 2.3 kg. Female fat tissues are a significant extragonadal source of estrogen and may affect hormonal feedback mechanisms controlling ovulation and the menstrual cycle. Other factors have been postulated, however, to affect these abnormalities and include decreased estrogen production, increased energy expenditure (physical activity and training), leanness (lean/fat ratio), temperature changes, and stress or related psychological factors.

An important study involving 16,000 white females by Garn et al[77] related the timing of menarche to subsequent weight and fatness in adulthood (ages 20 to 35 years). These studies classified women according to their age at menarche as early (at age of 11 years or younger), intermediate (12 to 13 years), or late (age 14 years or older) maturers. In all age groups, the early maturers were slightly shorter by approximately 1 cm and weighed approximately 4 kg more than the late maturers (3.8 kg in the 20 to 24 age group to 5.7 kg in the 30 to 35 age group) with the differences in weight attributable to body fatness. It was concluded that a difference of 3 years at the age of menarche (11 years or less) was associated with a difference of about 4 to 5 kg (8.8 to 11 lb) in weight by age 30, or 30% more in relative fatness. Further, it was estimated that more than 26% of the early maturers were obese by the age of 30 as compared with only 15% of the intermediate and 15% of the late maturers. Thus, the findings that menarcheal age is inversely related to fatness levels in older women make room for new research. It is not to say that we should attempt to delay menarche or limit exercise but, conversely, to mediate and encourage activity to avoid excessive weight gains and fat deposition during these critical periods. A more thorough understanding of the etiologic mechanisms, biologic susceptibilities, and behavioral expressions are needed to help us develop effective counseling and educational strategies at this important age. Further, the importance of good eating and exercise habits, weight stability in lieu of chronic dieting, and earlier intervention to prevent anticipated weight (fat) gain will not only help in the prevention of obesity but also in reducing the future risk of the obesity-related diseases (especially breast cancer) in women.

The predictive value of BMIs in childhood (ages 1 to 18 years) were studied with regard to their relationships to BMI as an adult (age 35 years). Figure 12-4 presents Pearson correlation coefficients for BMI at ages 1 to 18 years and BMI at age 35 as constructed by Guo et al.[78] For females, the correlation increased from years 1 to 18, with the exceptions from 1 to 3 and from 10 to 13 years; for males, the correlations increased from 1 to 4 years, remained stable from 4 to 9 years, and then increased. The correlations were higher for females, reaching 0.7 (0.6 for males) at age 18 years. Childhood obesity has increased over the past two decades, with estimates from four population surveys indicating that 27.1% of 6- to 11-year-olds and 21.9% of 12- to 18-year-olds are obese and the likelihood being higher in adolescent girls than boys (25.5 versus 18.3%).[79] Most preadolescent obese children (10 to 13 years old) (70%) remain obese as adults. Although the development and maintenance of obesity occurs more frequently in adulthood, childhood (21%) and adolescent (25%) obesities are important problems and contribute to treatment-resistant subtypes as adults.[80–82] Furthermore, obesity aggregates in families, with genetic heritability accounting for approximately

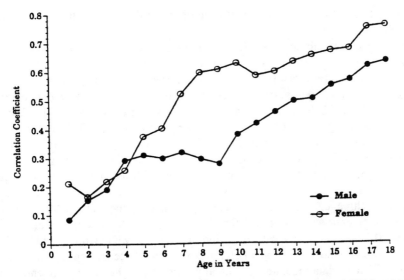

Figure 12-4 Correlation Coefficients between Body Mass Index at Age 35 and Childhood Body Mass Index from 1 to 18. *Source:* Reprinted with permission from Guo SS, Roche AF, Chumlea WC, Gardner JD, and Siervogel RM, The Predictive Value of Childhood Body Mass Index Values for Overweight at Age 35, *American Journal of Clinical Nutrition* (1994;59:810–819), Copyright © 1994, American Society for Clinical Nutrition.

25% of the age-gender-adjusted phenotypic variance of fat mass or percentage body fat.[83] Familial resemblance is also influenced by shared life styles, environments, and sociocultural systems. For example, in black females, where the origin of obesity begins in adolescence, cultural attitudes may be more accepting of overweight, and successful intervention should begin early and use existing support systems.[7] Thus, early intervention for obesity prevention over treatment is of paramount importance.[84] The Centers for Disease Control and Prevention emphasizes that young adults in their early 20s, especially young women who are already overweight, should be targeted for obesity prevention.[85]

Major weight gain, defined as at least a 20% increase in body weight or approximately 14 kg (range, 8.8 to 21.0 kg), was two times higher in women than in men studied in the 10-year follow-up study of NHANES I.[86] This weight gain was greatest in women (8.4%) as compared with men (3.9%), ages 25 to 35 years, and peaked in both sexes between the ages 35 and 44 years, after which it declined in men and continued to rise in women until age 55 years. From ages 25 through 54 years, women gained an average of 7.3 kg (16.1 lb), or approximately 1.6 times the men's average of 4.5 kg (9.9 lb).[86,87] This is a critical period during which intervention and prevention efforts would be better rewarded, and more practical, smaller, achievable weight losses should be emphasized. Also, weight maintenance strategies for the prevention of predictable future weight gain should be promoted.

Pregnancy contributes to the higher prevalence of obesity among women. In a study of 41,184 postmenopausal women reporting lifetime parity and weight at ages 18, 30, 40, and 50, BMI increased with age, and parity was only weakly associated with weight gain and overweight. Women gained an average of 11.05 kg (0.35 kg/yr) between ages 18 and 50 years. Parity was associated with an increase in body weight (0.55 kg per live birth), with women with lifetime parity of one or two live births having a lower BMI and lower proportion of overweight than either nulliparous women or those with 3 or more lifetime births.[88] However, it has been noted that on the average, women with average gestational weight gains (25 to 35 lb) retain about 1 kg (2.2 lb) above and beyond their expected increase with age.[89] Studies specifically investigating the relationships of weight gain and retention 10 to 18 months after delivery in the national Maternal and Infant Health Survey showed a retention of 1.6 lb for white women and 7.2 lb for black women who gained the amount of total weight recommended during pregnancy.[90] These data indicate the critical period of weight gain and retention during pregnancy can increase susceptibilities toward future obesity and that interventions should be sensitive toward and target susceptible populations, such as black women, and times when small weight gains can be avoided, controlled, or more rapidly reduced.

The danger of the "chronic dieting syndrome" is common among women,[91] and as years progress, the need to normalize eating patterns becomes more important to sustain health and prevent further weight gains. Much of the weight accumulation is subtle and builds over time such that obesity treatment is not a priority, especially in middle-aged women. However, attention to these women (aged 35 to 50 years) has recently been emphasized due to their increased risk for cardiovascular disease, which is largely associated with progressive weight gains and increasing prevalence of obesity. The Nurses Health study of 115,886 women aged 30 to 35 years related 70% of coronary events attributable to excess weight in women of the highest weight category (BMI of 29 or greater) but even mild-to-moderate obesity increased the risk of coronary disease.[14,92] Thus, the challenge is to educate and counsel these women toward healthier diets and eating patterns, especially because they are also more frequently the ones who are responsible for the nutritional health of their families.

Weight gain is common at the time of menopause, but the contributing factors have not yet been clearly delineated. Although changes in hormonal status and their effects are notable, their direct effects on weight gain are poorly understood. Wing et al[93] studied the prospective weight change in 485 middle-aged women over a 3-year span and noted that they gained an average of 2.25 ± 4.19 kg, with 20% gaining 4.5 kg or more and 3% losing 4.5 kg or more. There were no significant differences between the women who remained premenopausal and those who had a natural menopause (+2.07 versus +1.35 kg), and they concluded that weight gain was due more to other factors than menopause per se. There are many behavioral and psychological factors that are changing with age, and long-term positive and negative effects seem to cumulate around the "mid-life crisis." Hormonal changes may affect these expressions and their subtle effects are often blamed as causal rather than contributory. This is important in view that many of the factors are modifiable and good targets for intervention, particularly with regard to weight management.

As noted earlier, weight decreases in non-Hispanic white women after age 59 and in non-Hispanic black women after age 69 years.[4] The current definition of overweight has been questioned with regard to its applicability to the 55- to 74-year-old age group who have no evidence of obesity-related risk factors or who are at risk for a significant increase in mortality due to weight.[94] Rather the issue regarding the relationship of low weight (BMI 22 or less) to mortality (relative risk, 1.3 to 1.6 except for women aged 55 to 64 years) in this age group was thought to be more dramatic than those related to overweight per se. These findings suggest that sensitivity to weight management issues across the spectrum from low to high BMI needs further attention, especially in this elderly population.

TREATMENT RECOMMENDATIONS AND CHALLENGES

Obesity in women is a life-long concern that has challenged professionals. However, due to the current limitations of treatment, increasing prevalence, and significant associations with morbidity and mortality, the field needs revitalization. Further, understanding how common and predictable life stages and life-cycle events affect weight and how individual differences (socioeconomics, ethnicity, genetics, etc.) come into play will be an important new beginning. Such recommendations as those outlined in Figure 12-5 by Brownell and Wadden[95] in matching individuals with treatment is another needed step that will improve our effectiveness. Further, guidelines including the three components of diet, physical activity, and behavior modification are essential,[96] and more specific recommendations as outlined by the Michigan Task Force in Exhibit 12-3[97,98] help move forward the basic considerations of what should and can be done responsibly. Table 12-6 summarizes current treatment recommendations outlined in the 1995 National Academy of Science publication *Weighing the Options*.[99] This report also emphasizes important questions to be addressed by both the consumer and programs to improve outcomes.

Because negative psychological attributes have been associated with weight fluctuations (gains/losses) and weight maintenance has been associated with well-being, eating self-efficacy, and lower stress,[100] these areas require further attention with regard to their role in smaller weight changes as they occur. An immense

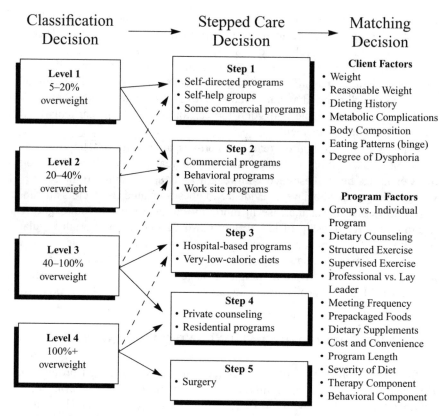

A conceptual scheme showing the three-stage process in selecting a treatment for an individual. The first step, the classification decision, divides individuals according to percentage overweight into four levels. These levels dictate which of the five steps would be reasonable in the second stage, the stepped care decision. This indicates that the least intensive, costly, and risky approach will be used from among alternative treatments. The third stage, the matching decision, is used to make the final selection of a program and is based on a combination of client and program variables. The dashed lines with arrows between the classification and stepped care stages show the lowest level of treatment that may be beneficial, but more intensive treatment is usually necessary for people at the specified weight level.

Figure 12-5 Conceptual Scheme for Matching Individuals with Treatments. *Source:* Reprinted with permission from Brownell KD and Wadden TA, The Heterogeneity of Obesity: Fitting Treatments to Individuals, *Behavior Therapy* (1991;162), Copyright © 1991, Association for the Advancement of Behavior Therapy.

challenge remains for health professionals in the area of weight management to (1) increase the understanding of the complexities and multiple interactions in the development of the "obesities"; (2) to develop more effective, long-term strategies targeted toward specific behavioral expressions and individual differences; and (3)

Exhibit 12-3 Recommendations for Adult Weight Loss Program

	Task Force Recommendation
Screening	The client should be screened to verify that there are no medical or psychological conditions that would make weight loss inappropriate. The client's level of health risk should be identified: low-risk, moderate-risk, or high-risk.
Level of care	The weight loss program should provide the level of care appropriate to the client's level of health risk: levels of care 1, 2, or 3.
Individualized treatment plans	Factors contributing to the client's weight status should be identified. These factors serve as the basis of each client's individualized weight loss plan, which includes the weight goal and plans for nutrition, exercise, behavioral change, medical monitoring or supervision, and health supervision.
Staffing	Weight loss service providers should be trained and supervised adequately for the level of health risk of clients receiving care.
Full disclosure	The client should give informed consent, having been informed of potential physical and psychological risks from weight loss and regain, likely long-term success of the program, full cost of the program, and credentials of the weight loss care providers.
Reasonable weight goal	The weight goal for the client should be based on personal and family weight history, *not* exclusively on height and weight charts.
Rate of weight loss	The advertised and actual rate of weight loss, after the first 2 weeks, should not exceed an average of 2 lb/wk.
Calories per day	The daily calorie level should be adjusted so that each client can achieve but not exceed the recommended rate of weight loss. The daily caloric intake should not be lower than 1,000 calories at level 1, 800 calories at level 2, and 600 calories at level 3. If the daily caloric level is below 800 calories, additional safeguards should be in place.
Diet composition	Protein: between 0.8 and 1.5 g of protein per kilogram of goal body weight, but no more than 100 g of protein per day. Fat: 10–30% of calories as fat Carbohydrate: at least 100 g/day for level 1; at least 50 g/day for level 2.
Nutritional adequacy	Fluid: at least 1 quart of water daily. The food plan should allow the client to obtain 100% of the client's recommended dietary allowances (RDA). If nutrition supplements are used, nutrient levels should not greatly exceed 100% of the RDA.
Nutrition education	Nutrition education encouraging permanent healthful eating patterns should be incorporated into the weight loss program.

continues

Exhibit 12-3 Recommendations for Adult Weight Loss Program (continued)

	Task Force Recommendation
Formula products	The food plan should consist of a variety of foods available from the conventional food supply. Formula products are not recommended for the treatment of moderate obesity and should not be used at low-calorie formulations without specialized medical supervision.
Exercise component	The weight loss program includes an exercise component that is safe and appropriate for the individual client. The client is screened for conditions that would make medical clearance before exercise appropriate. The client is instructed to recognize and deal with potentially dangerous physical responses to exercise. The client works toward 30–60 minutes of continuous exercise five to seven times per week, with gradual increases in intensity and duration.
Psychological component	Behavior modification techniques appropriate for the specific client should be taught.
Appetite suppressants	Appetite suppressant drugs are not recommended and should not take the place of changes in diet, exercise, and behavior.
Weight maintenance	A maintenance phase is included in the treatment program.

Health Care Levels

Level 1: low-risk clients have no known health problems that, in the judgment of the personal physician, require direct medical monitoring during weight loss. It is the responsibility of weight loss care providers to exclude moderate-risk or high-risk clients, unless they have specific clearance from their own physician. Providers should preferably be health professionals but could be specially trained lay leaders. The essential components of nutrition, exercise, and behavior change should be approved by appropriate health professionals.

Level 2: moderate-risk clients have medical conditions that could be complicated by weight loss or the treatment program. Medical monitoring is essential; a health care team is recommended.

Level 3: high-risk clients have severe, life-threatening conditions necessitating direct medical supervision during weight loss. Care is best provided in a hospital in-patient setting or an outpatient clinic staffed by an interdisciplinary team specializing in the treatment of obesity.

Evaluation of health status, rather than weight, should be the key factor in deciding level of care. Admitting high-risk clients to programs while failing to provide necessary health services is irresponsible and dangerous.

Weight loss is not appropriate for clients who are pregnant, suffer from anorexia or bulimia or psychological problems that may be aggravated by a weight loss program, are of normal weight or below, or who have low motivation or unrealistic expectations.

Source: Reprinted with permission from *Obesity and Health* (1991;2[5]:28–29), Copyright © 1991, Health Living Institute.

Table 12-6 Approaches to Treatment*

Strategy	Description	Assessment
1. Balanced deficit diets	1,200+ kcal/day usually nutritionally adequate. Average weight loss 0.25 kg/week for every −500 kcal/day deficit.	Require little supervision for healthy individuals without underlying medical conditions. Group support and monitoring by a health care professional have been shown to yield better results.
2. Low-calorie diets	800 to 1,200 kcal/day; use regular foods, specially formulated or fortified products and/or prepackaged foods; may require vitamin/mineral supplementation. Average weight loss of 0.5 to 1.5 kg/week (8.5 kg over 20 weeks): most regain weight lost in 5 years.	Safe but need physician approval and supervision by a health care provider (especially for patients with comorbid conditions).
3. Very low-calorie diets	< 800 kcal/day-modified fast; replace usual food with supplements; based in hospitals or clinics; supply 45–100 g HBV protein (0.8 to 1.5 mg/kg% IBM). 100 g CHO minimum fat for EFA and RDAs of vitamins, minerals, and electrolytes. Average weight loss of 20 kg over 12 weeks. Most regain weight lost in 5 years.	Medically supervised and administered by a multi-disciplinary team. BMI > 30 (moderate to severe obesity) who have failed at other Rx; may also be appropriate for BMI 27 to 30 who have comorbid conditions. Usually prescribed for 12 to 16 weeks; improvements noted in glycemic control, BP, and cholesterol in approximately 3 weeks.
4. Pharmacotherapy (used in conjunction with caloric restriction, behavior modification, and increased activity/exercise)	Current recommendations include *phentarmine*, a cate-cholaminergic agent (15 mg Ionamin) for appetite and *fenfluramine*, a serotonin agonist (20 mg Pondimin) for satiety. Average weight loss averaged 0.23 kg/week compared to placebo. Weight losses level off after 6 months; drugs help to maintain lower body weight.	Not all individuals respond to drug therapy: in some individuals when medication is discontinued, weight is regained. BMI of 30 or greater; patients who are medically at risk because of their comorbid conditions.
5. Gastric surgery (long-term commitment and follow-up; attention to diet, behavior modification, and activity/exercise)	Vertical handed gastroplasty Roux-en-Y gastric bypass Substantial weight losses occur within 12 months with some of the weight regained within 2–5 years. (Amount of weight loss is directly proportional to the degree of obesity- average of 50% of excess weight lost) Estimates of 10% morbidity (leakage, stomal obstruction, marginal ulceration, anemia, neurological complications) and < 1% mortality have been associated with gastric restrictive surgery.	Significant improvement in comorbid conditions. Risks include micronutrient deficiencies, "dumping syndrome," vomiting, and late postoperative depression. Patients who have failed with non-surgical measures, who are well informed and motivated. BMI > 40 (severe obesity) BMI 35 to 40 with high-risk comorbid conditions and/or physical problems.

*All approaches should include attention to diet, activity/exercise, and behavior modification for long-term life-style changes. Source: Adapted from *Weighing the Options: Criteria for Evaluating Weight-Management Programs* by the Committee to Develop Criteria for Evaluating the Outcomes of Approaches to Prevent and Treat Obesity, Food and Nutrition Board, Paul R Thomas, ed, Institute of Medicine, with permission of National Academy Press, © 1995.

to implement preventative public health measures that will decrease the overall prevalence of overweight and, thus, related morbidity and mortality from related diseases.

References

1. Brownell KD, Wadden TA. Etiology and treatment of obesity: understanding a serious, prevalent and refractory disorder. *J Consult Clin Psychol.* 1992;60:505–517.

2. Colditz GA. Economic costs of obesity. *Am J Clin Nutr.* 1992;55:503S–507S.

3. Public Health Service. *Healthy People 2000: National Health Promotion and Disease Prevention Objectives.* Washington, DC: Government Printing Office; 1991. U.S. Department of Health and Human Services Publication (PHS) 91-50212.

4. Kuczmarski RJ, Flegal KM, Campbell SM, Johnson CL. Increasing prevalence of overweight among US adults. *JAMA.* 1994;272:205–211.

5. Kumanyika SK. Special issues regarding obesity in minority populations. *Ann Intern Med.* 1993;119:650–654.

6. Melnyk MG, Weinstein E. Preventing obesity in black women by targeting adolescents: a literature review. *J Am Diet Assoc.* 1994;94:536–540.

7. Hubert HB, Feinleib M, McNamara PM, Castelli WP. Obesity as an independent risk factor for cardiovascular disease: a 26 year follow-up of participants in the Framingham Heart Study. *Circulation.* 1983;67:968–977.

8. Collins KS, Rowland D, Salganicoff A, Chait E. Assessing and Improving Women's Health. A Women's Health Report of the Women's Research and Education Institute. New York: Women's Research and Education Institute; 1994:1–53.

9. Pi-Sunyer FX. Medical hazards of obesity. *Ann Intern Med.* 1993;119(7 pt 2):655–660.

10. St. Jeor ST. The role of weight management in the health of women. *J Am Diet Assoc.* 1993;93:1007–1012.

11. Blackburn GL, Dwyer J, Flanders WH, et al. Report of the American Institute of Nutrition (AIN) Steering Committee on Healthy Weight. *J Nutr.* 1994;124:2240–2243.

12. Simopoulos AP, Van Itallie TB. Body weight, health and longevity. *Ann Intern Med.* 1984; 100:285–295.

13. Van Itallie TB. Health implications of overweight and obesity in the United States. *Ann Intern Med.* 1985;103:983–988.

14. Manson JE, Colditz GA, Stampfer MJ, et al. A prospective study of obesity and risk of coronary heart disease in women. *N Engl J Med.* 1990;322:882–889.

15. Bjorntorp P. "Portal" adipose tissue as a generator of risk factors for cardiovascular disease and diabetes. *Arteriosclerosis.* 1990;10:493–496.

16. Hartz AJ, Rupley DC Jr, Kalkhoff RD, Rimm AA. Relationship of obesity to diabetes: influence of obesity level and body fat distribution. *Prev Med.* 1983;12:351–357.

17. Garfinkel L. Overweight and cancer. *Ann Intern Med.* 1985;103:1034–1036.

18. Lubin F, Ruder AM, Wax Y, Modan B. Overweight and changes in weight throughout adult life in breast cancer etiology. A case-control study. *Am J Epidemiol.* 1985;122:579–588.

19. National Task Force on Prevention of Obesity. Weight cycling. *JAMA.* 1994;272:1196–1202.

20. Rodin J. Cultural and psychosocial determinants of weight concerns. *Ann Intern Med.* 1993;119:643–645.

21. Andersen AE. Gender differences in eating disorders. Scientific Symposium on Eating Disorders, National Institute of Mental Health, Chicago, Illinois; May 7–8, 1993. Abstract.

22. Serdula MK, Collins ME, Williamson DF, Anda RF, Pamuk E, Byers TE. Weight control practices of U.S. adolescents and adults. *Ann Intern Med.* 1993;119:667–671.

23. Horm J, Anderson K. Who in America is trying to lose weight? *Ann Intern Med.* 1993;119:672–676.

24. Forman MR, Trowbridge FL, Gentry EM, Marks JS, Hogelin GC. Overweight adults in the United States: the behavioral risk factor surveys. *Am J Clin Nutr.* 1986;44:410–416.

25. St Jeor ST, Brunner RL, Scott BJ, Harrington M. Dieting behaviors in women and men. Obesity update: assessment and treatment of the patient with medically significant obesity. North American Association for the Study of Obesity and University of California, Davis; October 18–28, 1991.

26. Brownell KD. Whether obesity should be treated. *Health Psychol.* 1993;12:339–441.

27. Jeffery RW, Adlis SA, Forster JL. Prevalence of dieting among working men and women: the Healthy Worker Project. *Health Psychol.* 1991;10:274–281.

28. Foreyt JP, Goodrick GK. Evidence for success of behavior modification in weight loss and control. *Ann Intern Med.* 1993;119:698–701.

29. Green M. A weighty issue: dangers and deceptions of the weight loss industry. An investigative report by the New York City Department of Consumer Affairs; June 1991.

30. Frank A. It's time to regulate the diet industry. *Med Econ.* 1993;70(5):23–30.

31. Wadden TA. The treatment of obesity. An overview. In: Stunkard AJ, Wadden TA, eds. *Obesity: Theory and Therapy. 2nd ed.* New York, NY: Raven Press; 1993:197–217.

32. National Task Force on the Prevention and Treatment of Obesity. Very low-calorie diets. *JAMA.* 1993;270:967–974.

33. Weintraub M. Long-term weight control study: conclusions. *Clin Pharmacol Ther.* 1992;51:642–646.

34. St. Jeor ST, Brownell KD, Atkinson RL, et al. Obesity. Workshop III. AHA Prevention Conference III. Behavior change and compliance: keys to improving cardiovascular health. *Circulation.* 1993;88:1391–1396.

35. Bray GA. Use and abuse of appetite-suppressant drugs in the treatment of obesity. *Ann Intern Med.* 1993;119:707–713.

36. Atkinson RL, Hubbard VS. Report on the NIH Workshop on Pharmacologic Treatment of Obesity. *Am J Clin Nutr.* 1994;60:153–156.

37. National Institutes of Health. Gastrointestinal surgery for severe obesity: National Institutes of Health Consensus Development Conference Statement. March 25–27, 1991. *Am J Clin Nutr.* 1992;55:615S–619S.

38. Kral JG. Overview of surgical techniques for treating obesity. *Am J Clin Nutr.* 1992;55:552S–555S.

39. Brolin RE. Critical analysis of results: weight loss and quality of data. *Am J Clin Nutr.* 1992;55:577S–581S.

40. National Task Force on Prevention and Treatment of Obesity. *Understanding Adult Obesity.* U.S. Department of Health and Human Services, Public Health Service, National Institutes of Health; 1993:1–6. NIH Publication no. 94-3680.

41. Willett WC, Stampfer M, Manson JA, VanItallie T. New weight guidelines for Americans: justified or injudicious? *Am J Clin Nutr.* 1991;53:1102–1103.

42. Weigley ES. Average? Ideal? Desirable? A brief overview of height-weight tables in the United States. *J Am Diet Assoc.* 1984;84:417–423.

43. Callaway W. Weight standards: their clinical significance. *Ann Intern Med.* 1984;100:296–298.

44. Himes JH, Bouchard C. Do the new Metropolitan Life Insurance weight-height tables correctly assess body frame and body fat relationships? *Am J Public Health.* 1985;75:1076–1079.

45. Colliver JA, Frank S, Frank A. Similarity of obesity indices in clinical studies of obese adults: a factor analytic study. *Am J Clin Nutr.* 1983;38:640–647.

46. Lee L, Kolonel LN, Hinds MW. Relative merits of the weight-corrected-for-height indices. *Am J Clin Nutr.* 1981;34:2521–2529.

47. Schulz LO. Obese, overweight, desirable, ideal: where to draw the line in 1986? *J Am Diet Assoc.* 1986;86:1702–1704.

48. Bray GA. Fat distribution and body weight. *Obes Res.* 1993;1:203–205.

49. U.S. Department of Health and Human Services. *The Surgeon General's Report on Nutrition and Health.* Washington, DC: Public Health Service, U.S. Department of Health and Human Services; 1988, DHHS (PHS) Publication. no. 88-50210.

50. Metropolitan Life Foundation. New weight standards for men and women. *Stat Bull Metropol Life Insur Co.* 1959;40:1–4.

51. Committee on Diet and Health, Food and Nutrition Board. Obesity and eating disorders. In: *Diet and Health. Implications for Reducing Chronic Disease.* Washington, DC: National Academy Press; 1989; 565.

52. van der Kooy K, Leenen R, Seidell JC, Deurenberg P, Droop AN, Bakker CJG. Waist-hip ratio is a poor predictor of changes in visceral fat. *Am J Clin Nutr.* 1993;57:327–333.

53. Scott BJ, Brunner RL, St. Jeor ST. A closer inspection of the predictive value of waist to hips ratio for cardiovascular risk. *Int J Obes.* 1991;15:57. Abstract.

54. Bjorntorp P. Classification of obese patients and complications related to the distribution of surplus fat. *Am J Clin Nutr.* 1987;45:1120–1125.

55. Folsom AR, Kaye SA, Sellers TA, et al. Body fat distribution and 5 year risk of death in older women. *JAMA.* 1993;269:483–487.

56. Bjorntorp P. Visceral obesity: a "civilization syndrome." *Obes Res.* 1993;1:206–222.

57. Rodin J. Determinants of body fat localization and its implications for health. *Ann Behav Med.* 1992;14:275–281.

58. Kirschner MA, Samojlik E, Drejka M, Szmal E, Schneider G, Ertel N. Androgen-estrogen metabolism in women with upper body vs lower body obesity. *J Clin Endocrinol Metab.* 1990;70:473–479.

59. Parnham ES. The context of weight changes: factors associated with weight changes in adult women. *J Am Diet Assoc.* 1988;88:1539–1544.

60. Adams N, Ferguson J, Stunkard AJ, Agras S. The eating behavior of obese and nonobese women. *Behav Res Ther.* 1978;16:225–232.

61. Jenkins DJA, Wolever TMS, Vuksan V, et al. Nibbling versus gorging: metabolic advantages of increased meal frequency. *N Engl J Med.* 1989;321:929–934.

62. Edelstein SL, Barrett-Connor EL, Wingard DL, Cohn BA. Increased meal frequency associated with decreased cholesterol concentrations; Rancho Bernardo, CA 1984–1987. *Am J Clin Nutr.* 1992;55:664–669.

63. Hill JO, Peters JC, Reed GW, Schlundt DG, Sharp T, Greene HL. Nutrient balance in humans: effects of diet composition. *Am J Clin Nutr.* 1991;54:10–17.

64. Sheppard L, Kristal AR, Kushi LH. Weight loss in women participating in a randomized trial of low-fat diets. *Am J Clin Nutr.* 1991;54:821–828.

65. Leibel RL, Hirsch J, Appel BE, Checani GC. Energy intake required to maintain body weight is not affected by wide variation in diet composition. *Am J Clin Nutr.* 1992;55:350–355.

66. Swinburn B, Ravussin E. Energy balance or fat balance. *Am J Clin Nutr.* 1993:57(suppl):766S–771S.

67. Hill JO, Drougas H, Peters JC. Obesity treatment: can diet composition play a role? *Ann Intern Med.* 1993;119:694–697.

68. Scott BJ, St. Jeor ST. Using food records to identify eating patterns of women and men. Proceedings of the 18th National Databank Conference, Baton Rouge, La; 1993.

69. Kinsella KG. Changes in life expectancy 1900–1990. *Am J Clin Nutr.* 1992;55:1196S–1202S.

70. Food and Nutrition Board, Committee on Nutrition of the Mother and Preschool Child. Summary of a workshop. Fetal and infant nutrition, and susceptibility to obesity. National Research Council, National Academy of Sciences; 1978:1–9.

71. Dietz WH. Critical periods in childhood for the development of obesity. *Am J Clin Nutr.* 1994;59:955–959.

72. Frisch RE, McArthur JW. Menstrual cycles: fatness as a determinant of minimum weight for height necessary for the maintenance or onset. *Science.* 1974;185:949–951.

73. Berg FM. Health risks of obesity. 1993 special report. North Dakota. *Obes Health.*1993;128.

74. Frisch RE, Wyshak G, Vincent L. Delayed menarche and amenorrhea in ballet dancers. *N Engl J Med.* 1980;303:17–19.

75. Frisch RE, Gotz-Welbergen AV, McArthur JW, et al. Delayed menarche and amenorrhea of college athletes in relation to age of onset of training. *JAMA.* 1981;246:1559–1563.

76. Frisch RE. The right weight: body fat, menarche and ovulation. *Baillieres-Clin-Obstet-Gynaecol.* 1990;4:419–439. Abstract.

77. Garn SM, LaVelle M, Rosenberg KR, Hawthorne VM. Maturational timing as a factor in female fatness and obesity. *Am J Clin Nutr.* 1986;43:879–883.

78. Guo SS, Roche AF, Chumlea WC, Gardner JD, Siervogel RM. The predictive value of childhood body mass index values for overweight at age 35 y. *Am J Clin Nutr.* 1994;59:810–819.

79. Gortmaker SL, Dietz WH, Sobol AM, Wehler CA. Increasing pediatric obesity in the United States. *Am J Dis Child.* 1987;141:535–540.

80. Must A, Jacques PF, Dallal GE, Bajema CJ, Dietz WH. Long-term morbidity and mortality of overweight adolescents. *N Engl J Med.* 1992;327:1350–1355.

81. Braddon FEM, Rodgers B, Wadsworth MEJ, Davies JMC. Onset of obesity in a 36 year birth cohort study. *BMJ.* 1986;293:299–303.

82. Epstein L. New developments in childhood obesity. In: Stunkard AJ, Wadden TA, eds. *Obesity Theory and Therapy.* 2nd ed. New York, NY: Raven Press; 1993;301–312.

83. Bouchard C. Current understanding of the etiology of obesity: genetic and nongenetic factors. *Am J Clin Nutr.* 1991;53:1561S–1565S.

84. Mellin L. To: President Clinton Re: Combating childhood obesity. *J Am Diet Assoc.* 1993;93:265–266.

85. Berg F. Young adults risk major weight gain. *Obes Health.*1990;83–85.

86. Williamson DF, Kahn HS, Remington PL, Anda RF. The 10-year incidence of overweight and major weight gain in U.S. adults. *Arch Intern Med.* 1990;150:665–672.

87. Williamson DF, Kahn HS, Byers T. The 10-y incidence of obesity and major weight gain in black and white US women aged 30–55 y. *Am J Clin Nutr.* 1991;53:1515S–1518S.

88. Brown JE, Kaye SA, Folsom AR. Parity-related weight change in women. *Int J Obes.*1992; 16:627–631.

89. Food and Nutrition Board. *Nutrition during Pregnancy.* Washington, DC: National Academy Press; 1990.

90. Keppel KG, Taffel SM. Pregnancy-related weight gain and retention: implication of the 1990 Institute of Medicine Guidelines. *Am J Public Health.*1983;83:1100–1103.

91. Grodner M. "Forever dieting": chronic dieting syndrome. *J Nutr Educ.* 1992;24:207–210.

92. VanItallie TB. The perils of obesity in middle-aged women. *N Engl J Med.* 1990;322:928–929.

93. Wing RR, Matthews KA, Kuller LH, Meilahn EN, Plantinga PL. Weight gain at the time of menopause. *Arch Intern Med.* 1991;151:97–102.

94. Tayback M, Kumanyika S, Chee E. Body weight as a risk factor in the elderly. *Arch Intern Med.* 1990;150:1065–1071.

95. Brownell KD, Wadden TA. The heterogeneity of obesity: fitting treatments to individuals. *Behav Ther.* 1991;22(2):153–177.

96. Weinsier RL, Wadden TA, Ritenbaugh C, Harrison GG, Johnson FS, Wilmore JH. Recommended therapeutic guidelines for professional weight control programs. *Am J Clin Nutr.* 1984;40:865–872.

97. Berg F. Recommendations for adult weight loss programs. Task force to establish weight loss guidelines for Michigan. *Obes Health.* 1994;27–29.

98. Drewnowski A (chair), Task Force to Establish Weight Loss Guidelines, Michigan Health Council. *Toward Safe Weight Loss. Recommendations for Adult Weight Loss Programs in Michigan.* Lansing: Michigan Department of Public Health; 1990.

99. Food and Nutrition Board. Institute of Medicine,. *Weighing the Options: Criteria for Evaluating Weight Management Programs.* Washington, DC: National Academy Press; 1995.

100. Foreyt JP, Brunner RL, Goodrick GK, Cutter G, Brownell KD, St. Jeor ST. Psychological correlates of weight fluctuation. *Int J Eating Disorders.* 1995; 17(3): 263–275.

13

&

Cardiovascular Disease

Debra A. Krummel

PREVALENCE

Despite improvements in mortality rates, cardiovascular diseases (CVD) remain the leading cause of death in women. Contrary to public belief, more women die from CVD than all other causes combined. Thus, CVD are prevalent in American women. Although no ethnic groups are immune from CVD, black women are most often affected. Overall, an estimated one in eight women older than 45 years of age has had a myocardial infarction or stroke.[1] Formation of atherosclerotic lesions in the intimal region of the artery starts to increase in men around the age of 25 to 30 years and in women at about 40 to 45 years.[2] At all ages, women have greater lesion involvement (surface area) in the aorta compared to the carotid or coronary arteries.[2]

Coronary heart disease (CHD) is the second most prevalent (behind hypertension) of all CVD. In women, the incidence of CHD begins to rise around menopause and then rapidly increases after age 65.[3] Compared with men, women are most often diagnosed with chronic rather than acute disease. When myocardial infarction or CHD is diagnosed, the prognosis is poorer in women than men. Women are more likely than men to have a recurrent attack and to die in the recovery period.[1] Thus, prevention of CVD is critical to promote the health and well-being of women.

RISK FACTORS FOR CORONARY HEART DISEASE

Many risk factors for CHD have been identified (Table 13-1). Although some confer risk in both sexes (e.g., low high-density lipoprotein-cholesterol [HDL-C]), others (menopausal status) are unique to women. The prevalence of the

Table 13-1 Major Risk Factors for CHD in Women

Risk Factor	Cut-Point Associated with Increased Risk
Modifiable	
Total cholesterol	>240 mg/dL
LDL-C	>160 mg/dL
Low HDL-C	<50 mg/dL
High triglyceride level	>400 mg/dL
Hypertension	
Systolic blood pressure	>140 mm Hg or on antihypertensive medications
Diastolic blood pressure	> 90mm Hg
Cigarette smoking	Use of cigarettes
Diabetes mellitus	Diagnosis
Overweight	BMI >27.3
Sedentary	Lack of at least 30 min of light-to-moderate activity 5 times per week
Waist-to-hip-ratio	>0.8
Nonmodifiable	
Age	>55 years
Family history	Clinical evidence in male/female first degree relative

major risk factors increases with age (Table 13-2). Hence, more postmenopausal women than premenopausal women have hypercholesterolemia and/or hypertension, obesity, or diabetes.

Age

Across all races, CVD mortality increases with age. Because of the importance of aging, age was considered to be a risk factor in the Second Adult Treatment Panel II (ATP II).[4] For women, being older than the age of 55 is considered a major risk factor. In younger, premenopausal women, CHD is less prevalent except in women with multiple risk factors (i.e., smokers and oral contraceptive users,[5] smokers with elevated apolipoprotein B[6]).

Family History

Family history for premature CVD is a strong risk factor for women. A positive family history is defined as clinical evidence of CHD, a myocardial infarction, or sudden death in male first-degree relatives younger than age 55 or female first-degree relatives younger than age 65.[7] A positive family history along with an elevated low-density lipoprotein-cholesterol (LDL-C) may indicate a heritable dyslipoproteinemia.

Table 13-2 Prevalence of Selected Major Risk Factors among Women, by Ethnicity and Age

	Non-Hispanic White		Non-Hispanic Black		Mexican American	
	Younger[a] (%)	Older[a] (%)	Younger[a] (%)	Older[a] (%)	Younger[a] (%)	Older[a] (%)
High blood cholesterol[b–d]	37	76	39	77	36	74
Overweight[e–g]	30	50	48	58	48	57
Smoking[h–j]	27	25	35	23	18[j]	NA
Diabetes[k,l]	2	15	4	25	NA	NA
High blood pressure[m,n]	26	59	46[o]	78	20[o]	NA

NA, data not available.
[a]See superscripts below for specific ages.
[b]Younger, <50 years; older, ≥50 years.
[c]Greater than 200 mg/dL.
[d]*Source:* Sempos C. NHANES III Phase 1 1988–91, NCHS.
[e]Younger, 30–39 years; older, 50–59 years.
[f]BMI ≥27.3 kg/m².
[g]*Source: JAMA.* 272:208, 1994.
[h]Younger, 35–44 years; older, 45–64 years.
[i]*Source:* Health United States, 1992.
[j]All Hispanic females (*Med Clin North Am.* 76:289, 1992).
[k]Younger, 20–44 years; older, 55–64 years.
[l]*Source: Diabetes.* 36:523, 1987.
[m]Younger, 35–44 years; older, 55–64 years.
[n]*Source:* Health United States,1992.
[o]NHANES III data (20–74 years old).
Source: Reprinted with permission from Krummel DA and Kris-Etherton PM, Nutrition and Prevention of Cardiovascular Disease in Women, *Nutrition and the MD* (1994;20:1–4), Copyright © 1994, PM Inc.

Premature Menopause

In the 1950s, bilateral oophorectomy was associated with accelerated atherosclerosis. Since then, it has been shown that the lack of endogenous estrogen is associated with risk of CHD. Women undergoing partial hysterectomy or surgical menopause have higher rates of CHD than their age-matched premenopausal counterparts.[8] The ATP II defines premature menopause without hormone replacement therapy as a risk factor. Menopause is associated with increased risk because of (1) estrogen deficiency, (2) aging, and (3) worsening or addition of other risk factors.

Hypercholesterolemia

Both elevated total cholesterol and LDL-C levels are risk factors for women. The lipid levels to differentiate risk are the same for men and women (see Table

13-1). Although LDL-C is used for screening and intervention goals, the association between LDL-C and CHD risk in epidemiologic studies of women is unclear (i.e., some population studies have not found a relationship between LDL-C and CHD). One explanation for this lack of an association in women is the heterogeneity in LDL particles. Small LDL particles are associated with increased risk,[9] and postmenopausal women are more likely to have these smaller particles.[10] Also, it may be that LDL-C is weakened as a predictor because estrogen prevents the oxidative modification of LDL-C necessary for atherogenesis.[11,12]

High total cholesterol and LDL-C are common in U.S. women and the prevalence increases with age across all races (Table 13-2). It is unknown if diet interventions can prevent the age-related rise in blood cholesterol levels. Based on LDL-C levels seen in the National Health and Nutrition Examination Survey 1988 to 1991 (NHANES III), 27% of all women and 50% of women aged 55 to 74 years would need diet intervention for hypercholesterolemia.[13]

Low High-Density Lipoprotein-Cholesterol

Throughout the life cycle, HDL-C levels in women average about 10 mg/dL higher than men. HDL-C is inversely related to CHD in both men and women. In population studies, it is a strong and independent predictor of CHD in women.[14] A 1-mg/dL increase in HDL-C is predictive of a 3.2% decrease in CHD risk in women.[15] The exact cut-point for HDL-C that is associated with the lowest risk in women is unknown. While the ATP II defines low HDL-C as less than 35 mg/dL, this value represents the 5th percentile for women.[16] In the Framingham study, women with CHD had an average HDL-C level of 53 mg/dL.[17] A more recent analysis of the Lipid Research Clinics (LRC) Follow-up Study showed that at all levels of LDL-C, an HDL-C less than 50 mg/dL was associated with three to four times the CVD mortality rate compared with women with higher HDL-C.[18] Furthermore, in these women aged 50 to 69 years, HDL-C was a stronger predictor of disease than total cholesterol levels. Thus, women with high total cholesterol (>240 mg/dL) and low HDL-C (<50 mg/dL) were at greatest risk. ATP II now subtracts one risk factor if HDL-C is more than 60 mg/dL (between the 50th and 75th percentile for white females). HDL-C levels are negatively correlated with body mass index (BMI) and waist-to-hip ratio in black and white women.[19] Cigarette smoking, no leisure-time physical activity, and education level were also negatively related to HDL-C in white women. Age was unrelated to HDL-C in either race.

Hypertriglyceridemia

High triglyceride levels are more predictive of CVD risk in women than in men.[20] In the Framingham and the LRC Follow-up Study, women with higher triglyceride levels (>400 mg/dL) concomitant with low HDL-C (<50 mg/dL) had higher rates of CVD.[18,21] Thus, the lipid profile most associated with risk was normal LDL-C, low HDL-C, and high triglyceride levels. Although these women would be at increased risk, they would not be picked up with the usual cholesterol screen. This common pattern is often seen in patients with android obesity, glucose intolerance, and hypertension. At triglyceride levels greater than 150 mg/dL, the triglyceride content of the intermediate-density lipoproteins (IDL) and LDL fractions increases.[21,22] These are the small, dense, more atherogenic β-very low-density lipoprotein (β-VLDL) and LDL particles that are predictive of CHD in women.[9,23] For screening purposes, a triglyceride level greater than 150 mg/dL with an HDL-C less than 40 mg/dL in the absence of vegetarianism suggests that the more atherogenic lipoproteins will be present.[21]

Hypertension

Stage 1 hypertension (140 to 159 mm Hg/90 to 99 mm Hg) is the most common form of hypertension seen in adults and thus most associated with risk of CHD or stroke.[24] Fifty percent of all women older than the age of 20 have hypertension.[25] The prevalence of hypertension is higher in older women (Table 13-2). This age-related increase in blood pressure is believed to be preventable.[26] Black women of any age are at greatest risk for developing hypertension.

Cigarette Smoking

One-fifth of CVD deaths can be linked to smoking and about 25% of U.S. women smoke cigarettes. The *Healthy People 2000* objective is to have no more than 15% of the population as smokers [27](Table 13-3). Over the past 20 years, there has been a fall in the numbers who smoke. However, the decline has been greater for men than women. The benefits of smoking cessation far outweigh the risks of a small weight gain (average, 2 to 3 kg).[28] In a large prospective study, the risk of stroke in smokers disappeared within 4 years after smoking cessation.[29] Thus, former smokers had the same risk of having a stroke as nonsmokers. This benefit was not dependent on the number of cigarettes smoked per day or the number of years as a smoker.

Overall, older women are less likely to smoke than younger women (see Table 13-2). Also, the prevalence of smoking is higher in women with less education and lower socioeconomic status (SES).[30] As with other risk factors, being a smoker in conjunction with other risk factors multiplies the risk of CVD development. In particular, the combination of smoking and oral contraceptive use mark-

Table 13-3 Status of Women Meeting Healthy People 2000 Objectives

	Baseline	1991	Target 2000
Overweight prevalence (20–74 yr) (%)			
All females	27	35	20
Low-income females	37	—	25
Black females	44	48	30
Hispanic females	27	—	25
Mexican-American	39	47	25
Cuban	34	—	25
Puerto Rican	37	—	25
Hypertension (%)			
All females (20–74 yr)	50	—	41
Dietary fat intake			
Females (>20 yr)	36	34	30
Total fat (% energy)	13	12	10
Saturated fat (% energy)			
Fruit and vegetable intake (servings)			
20–39 yr	3.4	—	5
40–59 yr	4.0	—	5
>60 yr	3.9	—	5
19–50 yr	2.5	—	5
Grain intake (servings)			
19–50 yr	3.0	—	6
Salt and sodium (%)			
No added salt food preparation	54	43	65
Avoid salt at table	68	—	80
Purchase lower-sodium foods	20	—	40
Smoking (>20 yr) (%)	27	24	15
Females reproductive ages 18–44 yr	29	27	12

Source: Reprinted with permission from Lewis CJ, Crane NT, Moore BJ, and Hubbard VS, Healthy People 2000. Report on the 1994 Nutrition Progress Review, *Nutrition Today* (1992;29[6]:6–14), Copyright © 1992, Williams & Wilkins.

edly increases risk (39-fold) in women younger than 50 years[31,32]; 26% of American women use both oral contraceptive agents (OCA) and cigarettes.[33]

Diabetes Mellitus

The prevalence of diabetes is highest in American Indians, Puerto Ricans, and Mexican-Americans. Blacks have higher rates than whites. In all races, more older women have diabetes than younger women.

Irrespective of other risk factors, diabetes is a strong predictor of CVD mortality in premenopausal[34] and postmenopausal women.[35,36] Diabetic women develop CHD and have mortality rates similar to men.[37] Women with diabetes in combination with other risk factors (smoking, hypertension, and obesity) are at highest risk for developing CVD.[38] Thus, having diabetes removes any protective effect of sex hormones or other factors in women.

The typical lipoprotein profile in women with diabetes is (1) an elevated triglycerides (but usually <250 mg/dL); (2) normal LDL-C; and (3) reduced HDL-C.[39] Ten to fifteen percent of women with non–insulin-dependent diabetes mellitus (NIDDM) in NHANES II had HDL-C less than 35 mg/dL; the average HDL-C for white diabetic women was 50 mg/dL.[40]

Obesity and Central Adiposity

All levels of overweight are associated with an increased risk of CHD in women, with the superobese (BMI>29) at highest risk.[41–43] Often, carrying excess weight is concurrent with having other risk factors such as hypertension, hypercholesterolemia, and diabetes (Table 13-4). In black and white women, 35% and 21% of CHD incidence, respectively, is attributable to being obese.[44]

The *Healthy People 2000* goal is to reduce overweight in women to no more than 20% of the population.[27] At last evaluation, instead of decreasing prevalence, an increase of 8% occurred between NHANES II (1976 to 1980) and NHANES III (1988 to 1991) (see Table 13-3). Thus, more than half of white women (>50 years) and about 60% of black and Mexican women are overweight (BMI >27.3).[45]

The incidence of overweight (i.e., the number of women gaining weight each year) is highest in younger women. Thirty-seven percent of U.S. women (25 to 44 years old) gained 5 to 15% of their body weight over a 10-year period.[46] Major weight gains of about 30 lb occurred in 8% of women aged 25 to 34 years old[47] (Table 13-5). Black women are 60% more likely to become obese than white women.[44] Other factors predictive of weight gain are low education level (less

Table 13-4 Prevalence of Selected Multiple Risk Factors in All Women

Risk Factors	Percentage of Women
Overweight and hypertension	52
Overweight and hypercholesterolemia	38
Overweight and diabetes	35
Smoking and oral contraceptive use	26

Source: Reprinted with permission from Krummel DA and Kris-Etherton PM, Nutrition and Prevention of Cardiovascular Disease in Women, *Nutrition and the MD* (1994;20:1–4), Copyright © 1994, PM Inc.

Table 13-5 Incidence of a Large Weight Gain[a] in Women over a 10-Year Period[b]

Age (yr)	%
25–34	8.4
35–44	7.2
45–54	3.8
55–64	1.7
65–74	0.9

[a]Major weight gain is defined as an increase in BMI of 5 kg/m^2 or more/m^2 or $\geq$ 30-lb increase for average adult.
[b]1971–1975 to 1982–1984.
Source: Interagency Board for Nutrition Monitoring and Related Research. Ervin B, Reed D, eds. Nutrition Monitoring in the United States. Chartbook I: Selected Findings from the National Nutrition Monitoring and Related Research Program. Hyattsville, Md: Public Health Service; 1993.

than college), lower SES, and sedentary life style.[48,49] For primary prevention of overweight, intervention efforts need to be targeted to adolescent and young women. Adverse effects of weight loss efforts do not outweigh the benefits of moderate weight loss in obese individuals.[50,51]

In addition to total body fat, how that fat is distributed is also predictive of CHD risk. Abdominal or android obesity, commonly seen in postmenopausal women, is associated with a worsening of the lipoprotein profile and glucose metabolism.[52] Other factors that cause this type of fat distribution are smoking, physical inactivity, and alcohol consumption.[53] Combined estrogen/progesterone (hormone replacement therapy [HRT]) prevents android obesity in postmenopausal women.[54]

Physical Inactivity

A sedentary life style, the most prevalent of all risk factors, is positively associated with CVD risk.[55] Sixty percent of U.S. women report either no or irregular physical activity.[56] The prevalence of an inactive life style increases with age and is inversely related to income.[57] Given the rising prevalence of overweight, the numbers of sedentary women are of great concern. Clearly, much needs to be done to reach the *Healthy People 2000* objective of less than 15% of the population being sedentary.

Low Education Level

Less than 12 years of education is strongly associated with CHD risk in women.[58,59] Low education levels are confounded by low SES and likelihood of smoking and being overweight.

FACTORS IN FEMALES THAT AFFECT THE LIPOPROTEIN PROFILE

Many factors affect blood lipids in women. What is unique to women is the many changes in sex hormones during a lifetime. Both endogenous and exogenous sex hormones affect blood lipids and must be considered in nutrition assessment.

Endogenous Hormones

Adolescence

After sexual maturation, gender-specific HDL-C levels appear for the first time. In boys, HDL-C falls to an average of 45 mg/dL; in girls, it stays around 52 mg/dL.[16] In the Bogalusa Heart Study, correlations between endogenous hormones and blood lipids were reported.[60] Testosterone was negatively correlated with HDL-C in pubertal boys whereas estradiol was positively correlated with HDL-C. Estrogen stimulates VLDL catabolism by transferring surface components to HDL-C, thereby increasing HDL-C levels.[61] Total cholesterol and LDL-C increase with age in both genders. Usually women have lower LDL-C, possibly because estradiol stimulates lipoprotein lipase and enhances hepatic uptake of LDL-C for a net effect of lower LDL-C.

Normal Menstrual Cycle

The four phases of the menstrual cycle are the (1) menstrual (day when menstruation begins), (2) follicular (from menstruation through ovulation), (3) ovulation (around day 14; when egg is released), and (4) luteal (from ovulation until menstruation) phases. To briefly summarize cyclical hormonal changes, estrogen peaks before ovulation, falls, and then increases slightly during the luteal phase (see Figure 5-1). Progesterone concentrations are low before ovulation and then rise rapidly, peak in the luteal phase, then drop as menstruation approaches. Thus, menstrual changes in blood lipids could be a function of either changes in estrogen, progesterone, or both.

In a cross-sectional study of premenopausal women, progesterone concentrations were negatively correlated with total cholesterol and LDL-C in the luteal phase.[62] Thus, when progesterone concentrations were highest (luteal phase), total cholesterol and LDL-C were lowest.[62,63] Six of nine prospective studies also reported a fall in total cholesterol or LDL-C (both were not measured in all studies) during the luteal phase[64-69] (Table 13-6). Blood cholesterol levels fall during the luteal phase when women consume either a high-fat or low-fat diet.[66] On average, total cholesterol levels were 6 to 11% lower during the luteal phase as compared with the follicular phase. The fall in total cholesterol reflects the

Table 13-6 Total Cholesterol Levels at Different Stages of the Menstrual Cycle

Study	Sample Size	Total Cholesterol Level (mg%) Follicular	Luteal	Difference (%)
Kim and Kalkhoff (1979)[64]	14	205	183	11[a]
Demacker et al (1982)[71]	10	205	202	NS
Woods et al (1987)[70]	15	169[c]	170[c]	NS
		190[b]	178[b]	6
Jones et al (1988)[66]	31	192[c]	174[c]	9
		171[d]	159[d]	7
Lebech et al (1990)[72]	37	179	168[e]	NS
Lussier-Cacan et al (1991)[67]	18	184	170[f]	8
Tangney et al (1991)[68]	9	176	163	9
Schijf et al (1993)[69]	54	212	199	6

[a] $p < .01$.
[b] Baseline diet.
[c] High-fat diet (40% of energy from fat).
[d] Low-fat diet (20% of energy from fat).
[e] Early luteal phase.
[f] Menstrual phase.
NS = not significant.

increased uptake for sex hormone synthesis. The lowest cholesterol levels are during the onset of menstruation; within 3 days after blood cholesterol levels begin rising.[68] Possible reasons for lack of significant findings in the three studies include (1) methods to characterize samples and different times within a phase for sampling, (2) small sample sizes with lack of power, and (3) only measuring blood lipids during one cycle even though intraindividual variability in women is high. Overall, the magnitude of lipid variation is great enough that the menstrual phase should be controlled when determining serum lipids in premenopausal women during interventions.[69] If not controlled, a woman may be inappropriately classified or appear noncompliant.

Other lipids vary less consistently during the menstrual cycle. Two studies[64,70] found that triglyceride levels were highest at ovulation, and three groups[63,64,66] found that they were lower during the luteal phase. Others[67,69,71–73] found no effect of menstrual phase on triglyceride levels. Similarly, most of these studies did not find any fluctuations in HDL-C related to the menstrual cycle. The two that reported differences in HDL-C were in conflict (i.e., one found it elevated in the follicular phase[65] and the other during the luteal phase[66]).

Pregnancy

In pregnancy, normolipemic women become hyperlipemic. All lipids and lipo-proteins increase—total cholesterol (by 25%), LDL-C (1.6-fold), HDL-C (1.5-fold, then declines to 1.1-fold), and triglycerides (2.5-fold)—above prepregnant values.[61] This hyperlipemic response is considered a normal physiologic response to supply placental steroidogenesis. Because of these alterations, cholesterol screening in pregnant women is inappropriate. After pregnancy, most values return to baseline levels, although triglyceride levels take longer than 6 weeks postpartum to normalize.[74] Similarly, HDL-C was found to be lower than prepregnant levels at 1-year postpartum.[75]

Lower HDL-C has also been associated with parity in epidemiologic studies. In the Rancho Bernardo study, postmenopausal women who had at least five pregnancies had HDL-C levels that were on average 5 mg/dL lower than women with four or fewer pregnancies.[76] The effects of parity were seen after controlling for other factors known to affect HDL-C levels (i.e., age, obesity, diabetes, alcohol and cigarette use, exercise, and estrogen use). No other lipid levels were related to parity in these women.

Multiparity has been associated with a small increase in CHD and CVD risk in two large prospective studies.[77] Women who had more than six pregnancies had 1.5 to 1.6 times the risk of a woman who was never pregnant. The increased risk was not diminished after adjustment for other risk factors. It is unknown whether multiparity itself is a risk factor or a marker for some other risk factor. This area needs further investigation.

Perimenopausal Period

The time around menopause has been associated with negative changes in serum lipids[78–81] (Table 13-7). A large cohort of women, premenopausal at base-line, were followed for 2.5 years; 69 women became menopausal.[78] The women going through menopause had a fall in HDL-C (mean, 3.5 mg/dL) and a rise in LDL-C (mean, 12 mg/dL). In the 8-year perimenopausal period (2 years before and 6 years after), women experienced a 19% increase in total cholesterol levels.[81] Interestingly, women who increased their intake of polyunsaturated fatty acids (from 6 to 8% of energy) during this 8-year period had a significantly lower increase in total cholesterol, 19 mg/dL versus 25 mg/dL, respectively. Whether diet or other interventions can impact these adverse postmenopausal changes in lipids is unknown.

Table 13-7 Changes in Total Cholesterol Levels in the Perimenopausal/Postmenopausal Period

Study	Sample Size	Total Cholesterol Level[a] (mg%)		Difference (%)
		Peri/Pre[a]	Post	
Matthews et al (1989)[78]	541	193	203	5
Demirovic et al (1992)[79]				
Blacks	344	188	194	7
Whites	474	189	204	15
Stevenson et al (1993)[80]	542	192	218	14
van Beresteijn et al (1993)[81]	167	225	268	19

[a]Peri, perimenopausal period; pre, premenopausal period; post, postmenopausal period.
[b]$p <.05$.
[c]$p <.0003$.
[d]$p <.001$.
[e]$p <.01$.
Numbers without superscripts were not significant.

Menopause

Around menopause, the postmenopausal woman will experience a 5 to 19% increase in total cholesterol levels (Table 13-7). Concomitantly, LDL-C concentrations rise and for the first time in the life cycle surpass levels in men.[82] Total triglycerides also increase and HDL-C and HDL$_2$-C decrease.[80] These adverse changes in the lipid profile are associated with a 25% increase in CVD risk, independent of other risk factors.[83]

Exogenous Hormones

The effects of exogenous hormones on serum lipids depend on the source, formulation, mode of administration, dose, androgenicity of the progesterone, and age of the users. Usually, oral estrogen has several positive effects on lipoprotein metabolism.[84] First, it increases LDL receptor activity, resulting in a lower LDL-C level. Second, it stimulates production of HDL particles and delays catabolism, thereby increasing HDL-C levels. On the negative side, estrogen increases plasma triglyceride levels by increasing synthesis of VLDL. However, the VLDL are the large buoyant type, which are not associated with increased CVD risk. By contrast, progestin causes no change or slight increase in total cholesterol, an increase in LDL-C, a decrease in HDL-C, and a decrease in total triglycerides.

Oral Contraceptives

In epidemiologic studies, oral contraceptive use was associated with increased total cholesterol, triglycerides, HDL-C, and apolipoprotein AI.[85] The formulation of the oral contraceptive agent (OCA) determines specific changes in blood lipids. Estrogen-dominant formulations decrease LDL-C and apolipoprotein B and increase apolipoprotein AI, and progestin-dominant formulas decrease or have no effect on HDL-C and apolipoprotein AI.[85,86] Lipids begin falling after discontinuation of OCA therapy; however, at 1 month post-therapy, they have not returned to baseline.[67]

OCAs have been associated with increased thrombosis. Low-dose OCA users have one-third the risk of having a cerebral thromboembolic attack as high-dose users.[87] Thus, low-dose users are not risk-free as once believed. However, most population studies show that OCAs do not increase CVD risk in the absence of other risk factors. In studies in which a relationship was observed, the women were on high-dose preparations and had multiple risk factors, especially increased age, hypertension, glucose intolerance, and hyperlipidemia.[88] An algorithm for the appropriateness of OCA use based on LDL-C and other risk factor status has been developed (Table 13-8). Essentially, women older than 35 years old who smoke (more than ten cigarettes per day) or have elevated LDL-C with zero or one other risk factor should use alternative methods of birth control. Other women should use the lowest dose possible.

Hormone Replacement Therapy

Unopposed estrogen as HRT increases HDL-C and triglycerides and decreases LDL-C and total cholesterol in users.[89] In dyslipidemic postmenopausal women, large changes occur—increases in HDL-C by 24%, triglyceride by 30%, VLDL-C by 12%, apolipoprotein AI by 56%; and decreases in total cholesterol by 13%,

Table 13-8 Suggested Algorithm for Oral Contraceptive Use Based on the Number of Risk Factors

	Risk Factors			
	<35 years		≥35 years	
LDL-C(mg/dL)	0 or 1	2 or more	0 or 1	2 or more
<130	Yes	Yes	Yes[a]	Yes[a]
130–160	Yes	Yes with diet	Yes with diet[a]	No
160–190	Yes with diet	No	No	No
>190	No	No	No	No

[a]Not recommended for women over 35 years of age who smoke.
Source: Reprinted with permission from Knopp RH, LaRosa JC, and Burkman RT, Contraception and Dyslipidemia, *American Journal of Obstetrics and Gynecology* (1993;168:1994-2005), Copyright © 1993, Mosby-Year Book.

LDL-C by 27%, and apolipoprotein B by 13%.[90] These changes were produced while the women were following a Step Two diet. Therefore, these positive effects on the lipid profile were a function of both diet and exogenous hormones. Lipid changes at these levels would decrease CVD risk by 50%. Other epidemiologic studies have confirmed that low-dose (0.625 mg/day) noncontraceptive estrogen use is associated with a reduction in the incidence of myocardial infarction,[91] stroke,[92] and CHD and CVD mortality in women.[93–95] Less is known about the effects of combination therapy on lipid levels or CVD risk.[96] However, as with OCAs, the progestin with the least negative effects is recommended. In the United States, this is medroxyprogesterone acetate.[83] HRT may be clinically indicated for women with hypercholesterolemia, low HDL-C without hypertriglyceridemia, risk for CVD, or established CVD.[84]

Diet

Many dietary components affect blood lipids and lipoprotein metabolism.[97] Epidemiologic studies have shown that dietary factors are predictive of blood lipids in women. Saturated fatty acids are significant negative predictors of total cholesterol, LDL-C, and HDL-C in premenopausal women.[98,99] Similarly, changes in saturated fatty acid intakes over a 10-year period were correlated with changes in total cholesterol and triglyceride levels in elderly women.[100] In the Framingham study, dietary cholesterol was the only significant predictor of total cholesterol levels in premenopausal women. By contrast, protein (animal) intake was the only variable significantly related to serum cholesterol in postmenopausal women.[101]

In intervention studies, low- to moderate-fat diets that are low in saturated fatty acids and high in carbohydrate produce positive changes in premenopausal women's blood lipids (Table 13-9). LDL-C is decreased by 9 to 32%, HDL-C is decreased by 1 to 10% or increased by 6%, and triglycerides are increased by 8 to 30% or decreased by 2 to 11%.[102–109] The greatest response is seen in those with moderate-to-severe hypercholesterolemia.[109] This hyperresponsiveness is above what is due to regression to the mean.[110] Individuals with mean cholesterol levels of 280 mg/dL had an 18% reduction in serum cholesterol on a low-saturated fatty acid (SFA) diet compared with an 11% reduction seen in those with a mean cholesterol level of 155 mg/dL. Also, a higher response was shown when phase of the menstrual cycle was controlled for blood measurement.[103]

Dietary responsiveness is similar in premenopausal and postmenopausal women[102,107] and in men and women.[109] Interestingly, on a low-fat diet, total cholesterol levels are lowest during the luteal phase.[104] A high-fat diet shifts the whole curve upward, but the effects of menstrual cycle remain (Figure 13-1).

Table 13-9 Lipoprotein Response to a Low- to Moderate-Fat Diet in Women

Study/Reference	No.	Diet	LDL-C PreM	LDL-C Post-M[a]	HDL-C PreM	HDL-C PostM	Triglycerides PreM	Triglycerides PostM
			(% Change)					
Hallfrisch et al (1985)[102]	19 PreM 14 PostM	Fat 35 en%, CHO 50 en%, PRO 15 en%, 300 mg cholesterol	-14^b	-5^b	-10^b	-8	$+8$	<1
Kohlmeier et al (1985)[103]	12^e	Fat 31 en%, CHO 56 en%, PRO 13 en%, 13 mg cholesterol, P:S ratio 3.2, fiber 43.5 g	-32	NA	-16	NA	$+29$	NA
Jones et al (1987)[104]	31PreM	Fat 19 en%, CHO 64 en%, PRO 17 en%, 230 mg cholesterol, P:S ratio 0.3	NA	NA	-6^b	NA	$+18^c$	NA
Jones et al (1987)[104]	31 PreM	Fat 19 en%, CHO 64 en%, PRO 17 en%, 200 mg cholesterol, P:S ratio 1.0	NA	NA	<1	NA	$+9$	NA
Wahrburg et al (1992)[105]	18 PreM	Fat 33 en%, SFA 10 en%, MUFA 16 en%, PUFA 4 en%, CHO 51 en%, PRO 15 en%, 30 mg cholesterol, 41 g dietary fiber	-15^c	NA	-7^b	NA	-2	NA
Wahrburg et al (1992)[105]	18 PreM	Fat 33 en%, SFA 10 en%, MUFA 10 en%, PUFA 10 en%, CHO 51 en%, PRO 15 en%, 30 mg cholesterol, 41 g dietary fiber	-13^c	NA	-10^d	NA	-7	NA
Cole et al (1992)[106]	19 PreM^f	Fat 21 en%, SFA 5 en%, MUFA 6 en%, PUFA 8 en%, CHO 60 en%, PRO 19 en%, 100 mg cholesterol, 21 g fiber	10^b	NA	-5–10	NA	$+20$–30	NA
Mata et al (1992)[107]	13 PreM 8 PostM	Fat 35 en%, SFA 10 en%, MUFA 21 en%, PUFA 3 en%, CHO 48 en%, PRO 16 en%, 410 mg cholesterol, 23 g fiber	-20^e	16	$+6^e$	$+4$	$+12^e$	$+9$
Mata et al (1992)[107]	13 PreM 8 PostM	Fat 35 en%, SFA 10 en%, MUFA 12 en%, PUFA 12 en%, CHO 49 en%, PRO 16 en%, 415 mg cholesterol, 23 g fiber	-15^e	14	-5^e	-7	-3^e	$+4$
Kasim et al (1993)[108]	34 PreM	Fat 18 en%, P:S ratio 0.75, 146 mg cholesterol	-13^b	NA	-8^b	NA	$+17$	NA
Geil et al (1995)[109]	76^g	Fat 30 en%, CHO 50–60 en%, PRO 10–20 en%, <300 mg cholesterol	-9^b	NA	-4^b	NA	-11^b	NA

CHO, Carbohydrate; SFA, Saturated fatty acid; Pro, protein; P:S ratio; MUFA, monounsaturated fatty acid; PUFA, polyunsaturated fatty acid; en%= % of total energy from fat; P:S ratio = polyunsaturated to saturated fatty acid ratio.
[a]PreM, premenopausal women; PostM, postmenopausal women.
[b]$p < .05$.
[c]$p < .01$.
[d]$p < .001$.
[e]Menstrual phase was controlled, but exact phase not reported.
[f]Menopausal status not controlled (women were 22–47 years of age); assumed premenopausal.
[g]Not separated by menstrual phase or menopausal status.

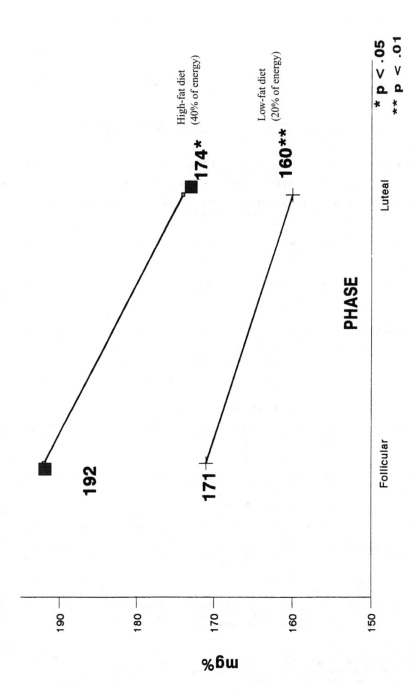

Figure 13-1 Total Cholesterol during the Menstrual Cycle Controlling for Diet. *Source:* Reprinted with permission from Jones DY, Judd JT, Taylor PR et al, Menstrual Cycle Effect on Plasma Lipids, *Metabolism: Clinical and Experimental* (1988;37:1–2), Copyright © 1988, WB Saunders.

Body Weight

Carrying excess body weight adversely affects the lipoprotein profile in women. Premenopausal women with a high BMI (27 to 30) have higher blood cholesterol (18 mg/dL) and LDL-C (17 mg/dL) levels than women with a normal BMI (21 to 23).[111] Although a similar pattern was observed in postmenopausal women, the differences were much lower. An even more striking relationship was observed for BMI and triglyceride levels (35 to 48 mg/dL increase with higher BMI). In all women, higher BMI was associated with higher triglyceride levels (+35 to 48 mg/dL) and lower HDL-C levels (-5 to 9 mg/dL). Along with the deleterious effects of body weight on serum lipids, there are some data to suggest that obese subjects (BMI >30) may have a lessened response to a low-fat diet than leaner subjects.[106] This area needs further research.

Exercise

The effects of exercise on plasma lipids in women are inconsistent. In cross-sectional studies, more active women have higher HDL-C levels than inactive counterparts.[112] However, only about half of the intervention studies in women produced a rise in HDL-C (average around 18%). Reasons for the discrepancies in the literature include (1) not controlling for menstrual phase when measuring blood lipids, (2) inadequate type, duration, and intensity of exercise intervention, and (3) not controlling for baseline HDL-C. Duncan et al[113] demonstrated the importance of controlling for menstrual phase. They conducted a randomized trial of mild-to-moderate walking in premenopausal women and were the first group to show that intensity was not related to increases in HDL-C levels. Lipid responsiveness to exercise interventions in premenopausal and postmenopausal women is an emerging area of investigation. Irrespective of lipid response, activity is critical for women for normalization of other risk factors (i.e., body weight, blood glucose, and blood pressure).

INTERVENTION STRATEGIES IN WOMEN

Because CVD morbidity is high in women, especially older women, intervention strategies for primary prevention of CVD need to be developed. Diet plays a major role in the primary and secondary prevention of CVD in both men and women.[114] Primary prevention of myocardial infarction (MI) in women can be substantially reduced by life-style changes.[32]

Knowledge and Attitudes

Knowledge about diet, risk factors, and CVD relationships has improved over time in the American population.[115,116] Women have slightly higher[115,117] or equivalent knowledge scores when compared with men.[118–120] White men and women scored highest on cardiovascular knowledge in the National Health Interview Survey (NHIS).[117] However, the strongest predictor of knowledge was education level.[115,117–119] Lower education levels were associated with poorer scores on knowledge items. Women with other risk factors such as diabetes had more knowledge than lower-risk women. With all the factors studied, only a small part of the variance in knowledge score was explained (8%).[117] Therefore, other variables affect the acquisition or retention of CVD knowledge. With respect to food composition, more subjects were knowledgeable about fat (43%) than fiber (11%) content of selected foods.[119] Interestingly, women have more misconceptions about diet and CVD relationships than men.[120] For example, more women believe changing to oil from other fats would decrease total fat intake.

Over the past 12 years, there has been an increased awareness about blood cholesterol levels, risk factors, and dietary variables related to CVD risk.[116] This increased knowledge, however, has not resulted in behavior modification. Individuals were not more likely to self-initiate dietary changes in later surveys compared with an earlier survey.[116] This is not surprising because gaining knowledge is only one component of behavior change. Skills and motivation are two other integral parts to facilitate change. Individuals need to know the benefits of change as well as the mechanisms for getting there. In a survey of cancer prevention knowledge and attitudes, the two knowledge and attitude barriers to making change were that people enjoyed eating and did not want to sacrifice the pleasurable side of food and that the number of recommendations was overwhelming to differentiate the relative importance.[121]

College women's knowledge, attitudes, and behavior were assessed in the context of the two behavior change models (Health Belief Model and Social Cognitive Theory).[122] Although young, these women had a high knowledge about the relationship between diet, risk factors, and CHD. They also had desirable attitudes about susceptibility to CVD with different life styles. On the negative side, these women had little knowledge about food composition and perceived poor control over environmental constraints on food consumption (i.e., influence of friends and foods served in the dormitory). Thus, self-efficacy and motivation to change were low. As seen by others, positive attitudes and knowledge did not correlate with positive behaviors such as reading the food label.

Behaviors

Although progress has been made, women are still consuming diets that are too high in total fat and SFA (see Table 13-3). Two food groups that may be related to fat consumption are fruits and vegetables and grains. Average intakes for all of these groups were below recommended levels. Most adults consume less than one daily serving of fruit.[25] Less than about 20% of women consume 55% of energy from carbohydrate or less than 30% of energy from fat (Table 13-10). Even fewer (less than 5%) consume the recommended level of fiber.

Several studies using very different methodologies indicate women can make "heart-healthy" diet changes. In the Rancho Bernardo study, women of all ages were more likely to self-report increasing exercise, changing diet, and reading self-help materials for the previous 15 years than men.[123] However, by design, one cannot discern if the women actually made more positive changes or they were just more likely to say they did. Husbands' premature MI produced positive changes in their spouse's diets but only in the short term. As length of time post-MI increased, recidivism occurred in the women but not in the men.[124] Women in the Women's Health Trial, a dietary intervention to reduce breast cancer incidence, received intensive instruction for fat reduction from 39% of energy to 20%.[125] The intervention focused on the major sources of fat in the diet that would also decrease CVD risk (added fats and oil, red meat, and dairy products). At 3 months, subjects had lowered their fat intake from 39% of energy to 22%; this low-fat diet was maintained at 24 months. Both short- and long-term changes in fat consumption were positively related to meals missed per week and negatively related to responsibility for food. However, only 12% of variance was explained; hence other variables affect dietary behavior change. Providing skills for planning is important for behavior maintenance. Also, inclusion of the meal preparer is critical to the success of the intervention.

The stages of change model categorizes individuals into stages that describe their readiness to make behavior changes. Stages are precontemplation, contemplation, preparation, action, maintenance, and relapse. Interventions to facilitate behavior change may be more successful if the participant's stage is assessed and the intervention modified accordingly. For each stage, strategies have been identified that should increase efficacy (Table 13-11).[126] Greene et al[127] developed a methodology for defining stage of change for decreasing fat intake to less than

Table 13-10 Percentage of Women Meeting Recommended Consumption Levels

	Age (yr)				
Recommendation	*30–39*	*40–49*	*50–59*	*60–69*	*≥ 70*
≤30% kcal from fat	15	15	18	20	19
≤10% of kcal from SFA	14	16	23	21	20
<300 mg cholesterol/day	72	75	70	74	81
>55% of kcal from CHO	16	18	13	17	23
≈25 g fiber/day	2	<1	5	1	2

SFA, Saturated fatty acids; CHO, carbohydrates.
Source: Reprinted with permission from Kris-Etherton PM and Krummel D, Role of Nutrition in the Prevention and Treatment of Coronary Heart Disease in Women, *Journal of the American Dietetic Association* (1993;93:987–993), Copyright © 1993, American Dietetic Association.

30% of energy. Five food markers emerged to indicate which people were in the action stage (i.e., with a commitment to change). These markers were use of low-fat cheese; eat bread, rolls, and muffins without butter or margarine; take skin off chicken; use low-calorie dressings on salads; and eat vegetables for snacks.

Maintenance

In the Women's Health Trial, women most successful at lowering fat intake made changes within 6 months of initiation and were able to maintain these

Table 13-11 Application of the Stage of Change Model to Level and Form of Nutrition Intervention

Stage	Goal	Strategies
Precontemplation	Personalize risk	1. Create supporting climate for change 2. Discuss personal aspects of poor-eating behavior 3. Assess nutrition knowledge and beliefs in myths 4. Build on prior nutrition knowledge
Contemplation	Increase self-efficacy	1. Identify problematic behaviors 2. Prioritize behaviors to change 3. Discuss coping strategies 4. Discuss motivations 5. Identify barriers to change and possible solutions 6. Elicit support from family and friends
Preparation	Initiate change	1. Encourage initial small steps to change 2. Discuss earlier attempts to change and ways to succeed
Action	Commitment to change	1. Reinforce decision 2. Encourage self-rewarding behavior 3. Discuss relapse and coping strategies 4. Reinforce self-confidence
Maintenance/ habituation	Continued commitment	1. Plan follow-up to support changes 2. Reinforce self-rewarding behaviors 3. Increase coping skills 4. Discuss relapse and techniques
Relapse	Reinforce commitment	1. Reassess motivation and barriers 2. Discuss importance of maintaining change 3. Explore new coping strategies

Source: Reprinted from Sandoval WM, Heller KE, Wiese WH, and Childs DA. Stages of Change: A Model for Nutrition Counseling, *Topics in Clinical Nutrition* (1994;9[3]:67), Copyright © 1994, Aspen Publishers, Inc.

behaviors at 24 months.[128] The behavior changes that women were most successful at modifying were decreasing fats and oils, red meat, and whole-fat dairy groups. All women had a difficult time increasing fruits, vegetables, and grains. Many factors affect adherence to dietary changes. What subjects believed to be barriers to dietary change were what was reported in an intervention to reduce dietary fat.[129] The barriers encountered were poorer taste of low-fat foods and the diet in general, decrease in convenience, lack of support system, and inability to estimate total fat intake. Thus, both cognitive and social issues needed to be addressed. McMurray et al[130] composed a problem-solving model to facilitate heart-healthy eating patterns (Figure 13-2). Women need to learn coping skills and move toward self-efficacy to achieve dietary recommendations to reduce CVD risk. Nutrition counselors need to empower women to make changes.

RECOMMENDATIONS FOR WOMEN

The Step One diet is recommended for all women for primary prevention and for hypercholesterolemic women as the first line of therapy (Table 13-12). The Step Two diet is for those who do not meet lipid goals after 6 months of a compliant Step One diet. Food choices for the diets are shown in Table 13-13 and sample menus for women in Exhibit 13-1. The Step One and Step Two diets can help women to lose or maintain body weight. With appropriate planning, most women can meet the Recommended Dietary Allowance for nutrients on the Step One diet (see Chapter 19 for calculations). Postmenopausal women consuming lower caloric intakes may have difficulty ensuring adequate calcium intakes. Supplements may be appropriate if needs cannot be met by dietary intake.

Table 13-12 Diet for the Prevention and Treatment of High Blood Cholesterol

Nutrient[a]	Step I Diet	Recommended Intake	Step II Diet
Total fat		≤30% of total calories	
Saturated fatty acids	8–10% of total calories		<7% of total calories
Polyunsaturated fatty acids		≤10% of total calories	
Monounsaturated fatty acids		≤15% of total calories	
Carbohydrates		≥55% of total calories	
Protein		~15% of total calories	
Cholesterol	<300 mg/day		<200 mg/day
Total calories		To achieve and maintain desirable weight	

[a]Calories from alcohol not included.
Source: Reprinted from National Cholesterol Education Program, Second Report of the Expert Panel on Detection, Evaluation, and Treatment of High Blood Cholesterol in Adults, National Heart Lung and Blood Institute, NIH Pub No 93-3095, 1993.

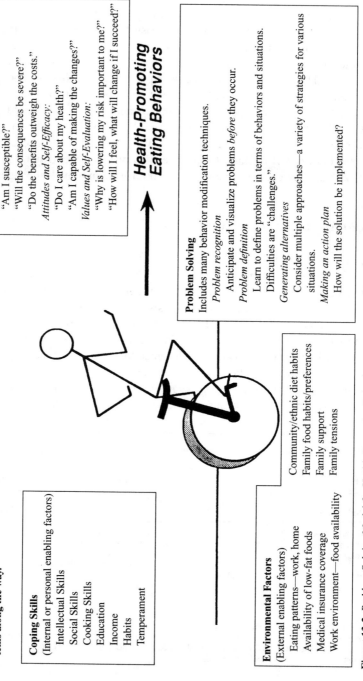

The key to increasing healthy eating behavior is not so much knowing what to do, but being able to avoid the obstacles and solve the problems along the way.

Coping Skills
(Internal or personal enabling factors)
Intellectual Skills
Social Skills
Cooking Skills
Education
Income
Habits
Temperament

Environmental Factors
(External enabling factors)
Eating patterns—work, home
Availability of low-fat foods
Medical insurance coverage
Work environment—food availability
Community/ethnic diet habits
Family food habits/preferences
Family support
Family tensions

Motivational Factors
(Predisposing factors and reinforcing factors)
Beliefs and Outcome Expectancy:
"Am I susceptible?"
"Will the consequences be severe?"
"Do the benefits outweigh the costs."
Attitudes and Self-Efficacy:
"Do I care about my health?"
"Am I capable of making the changes?"
Values and Self-Evaluation:
"Why is lowering my risk important to me?"
"How will I feel, what will change if I succeed?"

Health-Promoting Eating Behaviors

Problem Solving
Includes many behavior modification techniques.
Problem recognition
Anticipate and visualize problems *before* they occur.
Problem definition
Learn to define problems in terms of behaviors and situations.
Difficulties are "challenges."
Generating alternatives
Consider multiple approaches—a variety of strategies for various situations.
Making an action plan
How will the solution be implemented?

Figure 13-2 Problem-Solving Model for Health-Promoting Behaviors. *Source:* Reprinted with permission from McMurray MP, Hopkins PN, Gould R et al, Family-oriented Nutrition Intervention for a Lipid Clinic Population, *Journal of the American Dietetic Association* (1991;91:57–65), Copyright © 1991, American Dietetic Association.

Table 13-13 Daily Food Choices for the Step One and Step Two Diets

Food Group	No. of Servings	Serving Size	Some Suggested Foods
Vegetables	3–5	1 cup leafy/raw 1/2 cup other	Leafy greens, lettuce Corn, peas, green beans, broccoli, carrots, cabbage, celery, tomato, spinach, squash, bok choy, mushrooms, eggplant, collard and mustard greens
		3/4 cup juice	Tomato juice, vegetable juice
Fruits	2–4	1 piece fruit 1/2 cup diced fruit	Orange, apple, applesauce, pear, banana, grapes, grapefruit, tangerine, plum, peach, strawberries and other berries, melons, kiwi, papaya, mango, lychee
		3/4 cup fruit juice	Orange juice, apple juice, grapefruit juice, grape juice, prune juice
Breads, cereals, pasta, grains, dry beans, peas, potatoes, and rice	6–11	1 slice	Wheat, rye or enriched breads/rolls, corn and flour tortillas
		1/2 bun, bagel, muffin	English muffin, bagel, muffin, cornbread
		1 oz dry cereal	Wheat, corn, oat, rice, bran cereal, or mixed grain cereal
		1/2 cup cooked cereal	Oatmeal, cream of wheat, grits
		1/2 cup dry beans or peas	Kidney beans, lentils, split peas, black-eyed peas
		1/2 cup potatoes	Potato, sweet potato
		1/2 cup rice, noodles, barley, or other grains	Pasta, rice, macaroni, barley, tabbouli
		1/2 cup bean curd	Tofu
Skim/low-fat dairy products	2–3	1 cup skim, 1% milk	Low/nonfat yogurt, skim milk, 1% milk, buttermilk
		1.0 oz low-fat, fat-free cheese	Low-fat cheeses
Lean meat, poultry, and fish		≤6 oz day—Step I Diet ≤5 oz day—Step II Diet	Lean and extra lean cuts of meat, fish, and skinless poultry, such as sirloin, round steak, skinless chicken, haddock, cod
Fats and oils	≤6–8[a]	1 teaspoon soft margarine 1 tablespoon salad dressing	Soft or liquid margarine, vegetable oils
		1 oz nuts	Walnuts, peanuts, almonds, pecans
Eggs		≤4 yolks/week—Step I ≤2 yolks/week—Step II	Used in preparation of baked products
Sweets and snack foods		In moderation	Cookies, fortune cookies, pudding, bread pudding, rice pudding, angel food cake, frozen yogurt, candy, punch, carbonated beverages Low-fat crackers and popcorn, pretzels, fat-free chips, rice cakes

[a]Includes fats and oils used in food preparation, also salad dressings and nuts.
Source: Reprinted from National Cholesterol Education Program, Second Report of the Expert Panel on Detection, Evaluation, and Treatment of High Blood Cholesterol in Adults, National Heart Lung and Blood Institute, NIH Pub No 93-3095, 1993.

Exhibit 13-1 Ethnic Step One and Step Two Diets for Women

Step I Sample Menu for Asian-American Cuisine for Women Aged 25–49 Years

Breakfast
   Banana **(1 medium)**
   Whole wheat bread (2 slices)
    Margarine (2 tsp)
   Orange juice (3/4 cup)
   Milk, **1%** (1 cup)

Lunch
   Beef noodle soup, canned, low-sodium (1/2 cup)
   Chinese noodle and beef salad
    Lean roast beef (3 oz)
    Peanut oil **(1 1/2 tsp)**
    Soy sauce, low-sodium (1 tsp)
    Carrots (1/2 cup)
    Squash (1/2 cup)
    Onion (1/4 cup)
    Chinese noodles, soft-type (1/4 cup)
   Steamed white rice (1/2 cup)
   Apple (1 medium)
   Tea, unsweetened (1 cup)

Dinner
   Pork stirfry with vegetables
    Pork cutlet **(3 oz)**
    Peanut oil **(1 1/2 tsp)**
    Soy sauce, low-sodium (1 tsp)
    Broccoli (1/2 cup)
    Carrots (1/2 cup)
    Mushrooms (1/4 cup)
   Steamed white rice (1/2 cup)
   Milk, **1%** (3/4 cup)
   Tea, unsweetened (1 cup)

Snack
   Wonton soup, prepared with low-sodium broth (1/2 cup)
   Tea, unsweetened (1 cup)

Calories:	1853	Total Carb, % kcals:	51
Total Fat, % kcals:	30	Simple Carb, % Carb:	34
Saturated Fatty Acid, % kcals:	9	Complex Carb, % Carb:	66
Cholesterol, mg:	207	* Sodium, mg:	1323
Protein, % kcals:	19		

continues

Exhibit 13-1 Ethnic Step One and Step Two Diets for Women (continued)

Step I Sample Menu for Mexican-American Cuisine for Women Aged 25–49 Years

Breakfast
  Cantaloupe (1/2 cup)
  Farina, prepared with **1%** milk (3/4 cup)
  White bread (1 slice)
    Margarine (1 tsp)
    Jelly (1 tsp)
  Orange juice (3/4 cup)
  Hot cocoa, prepared with **1%** milk (3/4 cup)

Lunch
  Beef enchilada
    Tortilla, corn (2 tortillas)
    Lean roast beef **(3 oz)**
    Vegetable oil (2/3 tsp)
    Cheddar cheese, low-fat and low-sodium (1/2 oz)
    Onion (1/8 cup)
    Tomato (1/8 cup)
    Lettuce (1/4 cup)
    Chili peppers (2 tsp)
  Refried beans **(1/2 cup)**, prepared with vegetable oil
  Carrots (4 sticks), celery (4 sticks)
  Milk, **1%** (1/2 cup)

Dinner
  Chicken taco
    Tortilla, corn (1 tortilla)
    Chicken breast, without skin (3 oz)
    Vegetable oil (2/3 tsp)
    Cheddar cheese, low-fat and low-sodium (1/2 oz)
    Guacamole (1 T)
    Salsa (1 T)
  Corn (1/2 cup), seasoned with margarine (1/2 tsp)
  Spanish rice (1/2 cup), prepared with margarine
  Banana **(1/2 medium)**
  Coffee (1 cup)
    Milk, **1%** (1/2 cup)

Snack
  Ice Milk (1/2 cup)

Calories:	1852	Total Carb, % kcals:	51
Total Fat, % kcals:	29	Simple Carb, % Carb:	41
Saturated Fatty Acid, % kcals:	8.5	Complex Carb, % Carb:	59
Cholesterol, mg:	169	* Sodium, mg:	1429
Protein, % kcals:	20		

Exhibit 13-1 Ethnic Step One and Step Two Diets for Women (continued)

Step II Sample Menu for Asian-American Cuisine for Women Aged 25–49 Years

Breakfast
  Banana **(1/2 medium)**
  Whole wheat bread (2 slices)
    Margarine (2 tsp)
  Orange juice (3/4 cup)
  Milk, **skim** (1 cup)

Lunch
  Beef noodle soup, canned, low-sodium (1/2 cup)
  Chinese noodle and beef salad
    Sirloin steak (3 oz)
    Peanut oil **(1 T)**
    Soy sauce, low-sodium (1 tsp)
    Carrots (1/2 cup)
    Squash (1/2 cup)
    Onion (1/4 cup)
    Chinese noodles, soft-type (1/4 cup)
  Steamed white rice (1/2 cup)
  Apple (1 medium)
  Tea, unsweetened (1 cup)

Dinner
  Pork stirfry with vegetables
    Pork cutlet **(2 oz)**
    Peanut oil **(1 T)**
    Soy sauce, low-sodium (1 tsp)
    Broccoli (1/2 cup)
    Carrots (1/2 cup)
    Mushrooms (1/4 cup)
  Steamed white rice (1/2 cup)
  Milk, **skim** (3/4 cup)
  Tea, unsweetened (1 cup)

Snack
  Wonton soup, prepared with low-sodium broth (1/2 cup)
  Tea, unsweetened (1 cup)

Calories:	1815	Total Carb, % kcals:	52
Total Fat, % kcals:	29	Simple Carb, % Carb:	33
Saturated Fatty Acid, % kcals:	6.8	Complex Carb, % Carb:	67
Cholesterol, mg:	176	* Sodium, mg:	1300
Protein, % kcals:	19		

continues

Exhibit 13-1 Ethnic Step One and Step Two Diets for Women (continued)

Step II Sample Menu for Mexican-American Cuisine for Women Aged 25–49 Years

Breakfast
  Cantaloupe (1/2 cup)
  Farina, prepared with **skim** milk (3/4 cup)
  White bread (1 slice)
      Margarine (1 tsp)
      Jelly (1 tsp)
  Orange juice (3/4 cup)
  Hot cocoa, prepared with **skim** milk (3/4 cup)

Lunch
  Beef enchilada
      Tortilla, corn (2 tortillas)
  Lean roast beef **(2 oz)**
      Vegetable oil (2/3 tsp)
      Cheddar cheese, low-fat and low-sodium(1/2 oz)
      Onion (1/8 cup)
      Tomato (1/8 cup)
      Lettuce (1/4 cup)
      Chili peppers (2 tsp)
  Refried beans **(2/3 cup)**, prepared with vegetable oil
  Carrots (4 sticks), celery (4 sticks)
  Milk, **skim** (1/2 cup)

Dinner
  Chicken taco
      Tortilla, corn (1 tortilla)
  Chicken breast, without skin (3 oz)
      Vegetable oil (2/3 tsp)
      Cheddar cheese, low-fat and low-sodium (1/2 oz)
      Guacamole (1 T)
      Salsa (1 T)
  Corn (1/2 cup), seasoned with margarine (1/2 tsp)
  Spanish rice (1/2 cup), prepared with margarine
  Banana **(1 medium)**
  Coffee (1 cup)
      Milk, **skim** (1/2 cup)

Snack
  Popcorn (1 cup)
      Margarine (1 tsp)

Calories:	1860	Total Carb, % kcals:	53
Total Fat, % kcals:	28	Simple Carb, % Carb:	36
Saturated Fatty Acid, % kcals:	6.2	Complex Carb, % Carb:	64
Cholesterol, mg:	127	* Sodium, mg:	1450
Protein, % kcals:	19		

100% RDA met for all nutrients except zinc 90%.
Boldface food items represent differences between the Step I and Step II Diets. See companion menu.
*No salt is added in recipe preparation or as seasoning. All margarine is low-sodium.
Source: Reprinted from National Cholesterol Education Program, Second Report of the Expert Panel on Detection, Evaluation, and Treatment of High Blood Cholesterol in Adults, National Heart Lung and Blood Institute, NIH Pub No 93-3095, 1993.

For overweight women, the goals for successful weight management are (1) long-term weight loss defined as loss of at least 5% of body weight or a reduction in BMI of 1 unit or more for a 1-year period, (2) improvement in obesity-related comorbidities (i.e., hypertension, dyslipidemia, NIDDM), and (3) improvement in health practices such as meeting recommendations of Food Guide Pyramid on 4 of 7 days or walking 30 minutes or more four or more times per week.[51] For many obese clients, reaching desirable body weight may be unattainable. Thus, one approach to weight management is to lose weight in increments of Δ5 BMI or Δ11.6 kg.[43] Losing this amount of weight will often normalize other risk factors. For further discussion on weight management, see Chapter 12. For normal-weight women, the American Institute of Nutrition recommends that women be monitored so that (1) not more than 10 to 15 lb be gained after the age of 21 years, and (2) waist measure does not increase by more than 2 to 3 in. after age 21.[131] Maintaining a healthy body weight for prevention of obesity, hypertension, and glucose intolerance will reduce risk of MI by 35 to 55%.[32]

SUMMARY

Women are at risk for CVD and experience greater morbidity than men. Thus, primary prevention is critical for maintenance of quality of life, especially in the golden years. CVD risk and blood lipids in women are affected by endogenous and exogenous sex hormones. Both must be considered when designing intervention studies in women. Many risk factors in women can be prevented by nutrition intervention. Strategies to promote and maintain behavior change need to be developed. Only then will CVD in women be decreased.

References

1. American Heart Association. *Heart and Stroke Facts: 1995 Statistical Supplement.* Dallas, Tex.: 1994.

2. Blankenhorn DH, Hodis HH. Arterial imagery and atherosclerosis reversal. *Arterioscler Thromb.* 1994;14:177–192.

3. Massachusetts Medical Society. Coronary heart disease incidence, by sex—United States, 1971–1987. *MMWR.* 1992;41:526.

4. National Cholesterol Education Program. Summary of the second report of the National Cholesterol Education Program (NCEP) Expert Panel on Detection, Evaluation, and Treatment of High Blood Cholesterol in Adults (Adult Treatment Panel II). *JAMA.* 1993;269:3015–3023.

5. Jick H, Dinan B, Herman R, Rothman K. Myocardial infarction and other vascular diseases in young women. *JAMA.* 1978;240:2548–2552.

6. Kwiterovich PO, Coresh J, Smith HH, Bachorik PS, Derby CA, Pearson TA. Comparison of the plasma levels of apolipoproteins B and A-1, and other risk factors in men and women with premature coronary artery disease. *Am J Cardiol.* 1992;69:1015–1021.

7. National Cholesterol Education Program. *Second Report of the Expert Panel on Detection, Evaluation, and Treatment of High Blood Cholesterol in Adults.* Bethesda, Md.: National Institutes of Health. National Heart, Lung, and Blood Institute; 1993.NIH Publication no. 93-3095.

8. Stampfer MJ, Colditz GA, Willett WC. Menopause and heart disease. *Ann NY Acad Sci.* 1990;599:193–203.

9. Austin MA, Breslow JL, Hennekens CH, Buring JE, Willet WC, Krauss RM. Low-density lipoprotein subclass patterns and risk of myocardial infarction. *JAMA.* 1988;260:1917–1921.

10. Campos H, McNamara JR, Wilson PW, Ordovas J, Schaefer EJ. Differences in low density lipoprotein subfractions and apolipoproteins in premenopausal and postmenopausal women. *J Clin Endocrinol Metab.* 1988;67:30–35.

11. Rifici VA, Khachadurian AK. The inhibition of low-density lipoprotein oxidation by 17-B estradiol. *Metabolism.* 1992;41:1110–1114.

12. Maziere C, Auclair M, Ronveaux M-F, Salmon S, Santus R, Maziere J-C. Estrogens inhibit copper and cell-mediated modification of low density lipoprotein. *Atherosclerosis.* 1991;89:175–182.

13. Sempos CT, Cleeman JI, Carroll MD, et al. Prevalence of high blood cholesterol among US adults. *JAMA.* 1993;269:3009–3014.

14. Bush TL, Fried LP, Barrett-Connor E. Cholesterol, lipoproteins, and coronary heart disease in women. *Clin Chem.* 1988;34:B60–B70.

15. Gordon DJ, Probstfield JL, Garrison RJ, et al. High-density lipoprotein cholesterol and cardiovascular disease. Four prospective American studies. *Circulation.* 1989;79:8–15.

16. Lipid Research Clinics. *Population Studies Data Book, 1. The Prevalence Study.* U.S. Department of Health and Human Services, Public Health Service, Bethesda, Md: National Institutes of Health; 1980. NIH Publication no. 80-1527.

17. Kannel WB, Wilson PW. Efficacy of lipid profiles in prediction of coronary disease. *Am Heart J.* 1992;124:768–774.

18. Bass KM, Newschaffer CJ, Klag MJ, Bush TL. Plasma lipoprotein levels as predictors of cardiovascular death in women. *Arch Intern Med.* 1993;153:2209–2216.

19. Heath GW, Macera CA, Croft JB, et al. Correlates of high-density lipoprotein cholesterol in black and white women. *Am J Public Health.* 1994;84:98–101.

20. Austin MA, Hokanson JE. Epidemiology of triglycerides, small dense low-density lipoprotein, and lipoprotein (a) as risk factors for coronary heart disease. *Med Clin North Am.* 1994;78:99–115.

21. Castelli WP. Epidemiology of triglycerides: a view from Framingham. *Am J Cardiol.* 1992;70:3H–9H.

22. Knopp RH, LaRosa JC, Burkman RT. Contraception and dyslipidemia. *Am J Obstet Gynecol.* 1993;168:1994–2005.

23. Reardon MF, Nestel PJ, Craig IH, et al. Lipoprotein predictors of the severity of coronary artery disease in men and women. *Circulation.* 1985;71:881–888.

24. Joint National Committee on the Detection, Evaluation, and Treatment of Blood Pressure. Fifth report (JNC V). *Arch Intern Med.* 1993;153:154–183.

25. Lewis CJ, Crane NT, Moore BJ, Hubbard VS. Healthy People 2000. Report on the 1994 nutrition progress review. *Nutr Today.* 1994;29(6):6–14.

26. Stamler J, Stamler R, Caton J. Blood pressure, systolic, diastolic, and cardiovascular risks. *Arch Intern Med.* 1993;153:598.

27. Healthy People 2000. *National Health Promotion and Disease Prevention Objectives.* Hyattsville, Md.: Department of Health and Human Services; 1990. DHHS Publication no. (PHS) 91-50213.

28. Williamson DV, Madans J, Anda RF, et al. Smoking cessation and severity of weight gain in a national cohort. *N Engl J Med.* 1991;324:739–745.

29. Kawachi I, Colditz GA, Stampfer MJ, et al. Smoking cessation and decreased risk of stroke in women. *JAMA.* 1993;269:232–236.

30. Fiore MC. Trends in cigarette smoking in the United States. *Med Clin North Am.* 1992;76:289–303.

31. Rosenberg L, Kaufman D, Helmrich S, et al. Myocardial infarction and cigarette smoking in women younger than 50 years of age. *JAMA.* 1985;253:2965–2969.

32. Manson JE, Tosteson H, Ridker PM, et al. The primary prevention of myocardial infarction. *N Engl J Med.* 1992;326:1406–1416.

33. National Center for Health Statistics. Healthy People 2000 Review. Hyattsville, Md.: Public Health Service; 1994.

34. Perlman JA, Wolf PH, Ray R, Lieberknecht A. Cardiovascular risk factors, premature heart disease, and all-cause mortality in a cohort of northern California women. *Am J Obstet Gynecol.* 1988;158:1568–1574.

35. Barrett-Connor EL, Cohn BA, Wingard DL, Edelstein SL. Why is diabetes mellitus a stronger risk factor for fatal ischemic heart disease in women than in men? *JAMA.* 1991;265:627–631.

36. Donahue RP, Goldberg RJ, Chen Z, et al. The influence of sex and diabetes mellitus on survival following acute myocardial infarction: a community-wide perspective. *J Clin Epidemiol.* 1993;46:245–252.

37. Liao Y, Cooper RS, Ghali JK, Lansky D, Cao G, Lee J. Sex differences in the impact of coexistent diabetes on survival in patients with coronary heart disease. *Diabetes Care.* 1993;16:708–713.

38. Manson JE, Colditz GA, Stampfer MJ, et al. A prospective study of maturity-onset diabetes mellitus and risk of coronary heart disease and stroke in women. *Arch Intern Med.* 1991;151:1141–1147.

39. Brown WV. Lipoprotein disorders in diabetes mellitus. *Med Clin North Am.* 1994;78:143–161.

40. Cowie CC, Howard BV, Harris MI. Serum lipoproteins in African Americans and whites with non–insulin-dependent diabetes in the US population. *Circulation.* 1994;90:1185–1193.

41. Hubert HB, Feinleib M, McNamara PM, Castelli WP. Obesity as an independent risk factor for cardiovascular disease: a 26-year follow-up of participants in the Framingham Heart Study. *Circulation.* 1983;67:968–977.

42. Manson JE, Colditz GA, Stampfer MF, et al. A prospective study of obesity and risk of coronary heart disease in women. *N Engl J Med.* 1990;322:882–889.

43. Blackburn GL, Kanders BS. Medical evaluation and treatment of obese patients with cardiovascular disease. *Am J Cardiol.* 1987;60:55G–58G.

44. Williamson DF, Kahn HS, Byers T. The 10-y incidence of obesity and major weight gain in black and white US women aged 30–55 y. *Am J Clin Nutr.* 1991;53:1515S–1518S.

45. Kuczmarski RJ, Flegal KM, Campbell SM, Johnson CL. Increasing prevalence of overweight among US adults. *JAMA.* 1994;272:205–211.

46. Williamson DF. Descriptive epidemiology of body weight and weight change in U.S. adults. *Ann Intern Med.* 1993;119:646–649.

47. Ervin B, Reed D, eds. *Nutrition Monitoring in the United States. Chartbook I: Selected findings from the National Nutrition Monitoring and Related Research Program.* Hyattsville, Md.: Interagency Board for Nutrition Monitoring and Related Research, Public Health Service; 1993.

48. Kahn HS, Williamson DF, Stevens JA. Race and weight change in US women: the roles of socioeconomic and marital status. *Am J Public Health.* 1991;81:319–323.

49. Williamson DF, Madans J, Anda RF, Kleinman JC, Kahn HS, Byers T. Recreational physical activity and ten-year weight change in a US national cohort. *Int J Obesity.* 1993b;17:279–286.

50. National Task Force on the Prevention and Treatment of Obesity. Weight cycling. *JAMA.* 1994;272:1196–1202.

51. Committee to Develop Criteria for Evaluating Outcomes of Approaches to Prevent and Treat Obesity, Food and Nutrition Board, Institute of Medicine, National Academy of Science. Summary: Weighing the options—criteria for evaluating weight-management programs. *J Am Diet Assoc.* 1995;95:96–105.

52. Soler JT, Folsom AR, Kushi LH, Prineas RJ, Seal US. Association of body fat distribution with plasma lipids, lipoproteins, apolipoproteins AI and B in postmenopausal women. *J Clin Epidemiol.* 1988;41:1075–1081.

53. Emery EM, Schmid TL, Kahn HS, Filozof PP. A review of the association between abdominal fat distribution, health outcome measures, and modifiable risk factors. *Am J Health Promot.* 1993;7:342–353.

54. Haarbo J, Marslew U, Gotfredsen A, Christiansen C. Postmenopausal hormone replacement therapy prevents central distribution of body fat after menopause. *Metabolism.* 1991;40:1323–1326.

55. Powell KE, Thompson PD, Caspersen CJ, Kendrick JS. Physical activity and the incidence of coronary heart disease. *Annu Rev Public Health.* 1987;8:352–387.

56. Public health focus: physical activity and the prevention of coronary heart disease. *JAMA.* 1993;270:1529–1530.

57. Prevalence of sedentary lifestyle—behavioral risk factors surveillance system, United States, 1991. *MMWR.* 1993;42:576–579.

58. Matthews KA, Kelsey SF, Meilahn EN, Kuller LH, Wing RR. Educational attainment and behavioral and biologic risk factors for coronary heart disease in middle-aged women. *Am J Epidemiol.* 1989;129:1132–1144.

59. Winkleby MA, Jatulis DE, Frank E, Fortmann SP. Socioeconomic status and health: how education, income, and occupation contribute to risk factors for cardiovascular disease. *Am J Public Health.* 1992;82:816–820.

60. Srinavasan SR, Sundaram GS, Williamson GD, Webber LS, Berenson GS. Serum lipoproteins and endogenous sex hormones in early life: observations in children with different lipoprotein profiles. *Metabolism.* 1985;34:861–867.

61. Knopp RH. Cardiovascular effects of endogenous and exogenous sex hormones over a woman's lifetime. *Am J Obstet Gynecol.* 1988;158:1630–1643.

62. Krummel DA, Mashaly MA, Kris-Etherton PM. Prediction of plasma lipids in a cross-sectional sample of young women. *J Am Diet Assoc.* 1992;92:942–948.

63. Hemer AH, Valles de Bourges V, Ayala JJ, Brito G, Diaz-Sanchez V, Garza-Flores J. Variations in serum lipids and lipoproteins throughout the menstrual cycle. *Fertil Steril.* 1985;44:80–84.

64. Kim H-K, Kalkhoff RK. Changes in lipoprotein composition during the menstrual cycle. *Metabolism.* 1979;23:663–668.

65. Tikkanen MJ, Kuusi T, Nikkila EA, Stenman U-H. Variation of postheparin plasma hepatic lipase by menstrual cycle. *Metabolism.* 1986;35:99–104.

66. Jones DY, Judd JT, Taylor PR, et al. Menstrual cycle effect on plasma lipids. *Metabolism.* 1988;37:1–2.

67. Lussier-Cacan S, Xhignesse M, Desmarais J-L, et al. Cyclic fluctuations in human serum lipid and apolipoprotein levels during the normal menstrual cycle: comparison with changes occurring during oral contraceptive therapy. *Metabolism.* 1991;40:849–854.

68. Tangney C, Brownie C, Wu S-M. Impact of menstrual periodicity on serum lipid levels and estimates of dietary intakes. *J Am Coll Nutr.* 1991;10:107–113.

69. Schijf CP, van der Mooren MJ, Doesburg WH, et al. Differences in serum lipids lipoproteins, sex hormone binding globulin and testosterone between the follicular and the luteal phase of the menstrual cycle. *Acta Endocrinol.* 1993;129:130–133.

70. Woods M, Schaefer EJ, Morrell A, et al. Effect of menstrual cycle phase on plasma lipids. *J Clin Endocrinol Metab.* 1987;65:321–323.

71. Demacker PN, Schade RW, Stalenhoef AF, Stuyt PM, Laar AV. Influence of contraceptive pill and menstrual cycle on serum lipids and high-density lipoprotein cholesterol concentrations. *BMJ.* 1982;284:1213–1215.

72. Lebech AM, Kjaer A, Lebech PE. Metabolic changes during the menstrual cycle: a longitudinal study. *Am J Obstet Gynecol.* 1990;163:414–416.

73. Brideau MA, Forest J-C, Lemay A, Dodin S. Correlation between ovarian steroids and lipid fractions in relation to age in premenopausal women. *Clin Endocrinol.* 1992;37:437–444.

74. Knopp RH, Bergelin RO, Wahl PW, Walden CE. Effects of pregnancy, postpartum lactation, and oral contraceptive use on the lipoprotein cholesterol/triglyceride ratio. *Metabolism.* 1985;34:893–899.

75. van Stiphout WA, Hofman A, de Bruijn AM. Serum lipids in young women before, during, and after pregnancy. *Am J Epidemiol.* 1987;126:922–928.

76. Kritz-Silverstein D, Barrett-Connor E, Wingard DL. The relationship between multiparity and lipoprotein levels in older women. *J Clin Epidemiol.* 1992;45:761–767.

77. Ness RB, Harris T, Cobb J, et al. Number of pregnancies and the subsequent risk of cardiovascular disease. *N Engl J Med.* 1993;328:1528–1533.

78. Matthews KA, Meilahn E, Kuller LH, et al. Menopause and risk factors for coronary heart disease. *N Engl J Med.* 1989;321:641–646.

79. Demirovic J, Sprafka JM, Folsom AR, et al. Menopause and serum cholesterol: differences between blacks and whites. *Am J Epidemiol.* 1992;136:155–164.

80. Stevenson JC, Crook D, Godsland IF. Influence of age and menopause on serum lipids and lipoproteins in healthy women. *Atherosclerosis.* 1993;98:83–90.

81. van Beresteijn ECH, Korevaar JC, Huijbregts PCW, et al. Perimenopausal increase in serum cholesterol: a 10-year longitudinal study. *Am J Epidemiol.* 1993;137:383–392.

82. Matthews KA, Wing RR, Kuller LH, et al. Influence of the perimenopause on cardiovascular risk factors and symptoms of middle-aged women. *Arch Intern Med.* 1994;154:2349–2355.

83. Miller VT. Lipids, lipoproteins, women and cardiovascular disease. *Atherosclerosis.* 1994;108:S73–S82.

84. Knopp RH, Zhu X, Bonet B. Effects of estrogens on lipoprotein metabolism and cardiovascular disease in women. *Atherosclerosis.* 1994;110:S83–S91.

85. Vaziri SM, Evans JC, Larson MG, Wilson PW. The impact of female hormone usage on the lipid profile. *Arch Intern Med.* 1993;153:2205–2206.

86. Godsland IF, Crook D, Simpson R, et al. The effects of different formulations of oral contraceptive agents on lipid and carbohydrate metabolism. *N Engl J Med.* 1990;323:1375–1381.

87. Lidegarrd O. Oral contraception and risk of cerebral thromboembolic attack: results of a case-control study. *BMJ.* 1993;306:956–963.

88. Sullivan JM, Lobo RA. Considerations for contraception in women with cardiovascular disorders. *Am J Obstet Gynecol.* 1993;168:2006–2011.

89. Lobo R. Effects of hormonal replacement on lipids and lipoproteins in postmenopausal women. *J Clin Endocrinol Metab.* 1991;73:925–930.

90. Granfone A, Campos H, McNamara JR, et al. Effects of estrogen replacement on plasma lipoproteins and apolipoproteins in postmenopausal, dyslipidemic women. *Metabolism.* 1992;41:1193–1198.

91. Psaty BM, Heckbert SR, Atkins D, et al. The risk of myocardial infarction associated with the combined use of estrogens and progestins in postmenopausal women. *Arch Intern Med.* 1994;154:1333–1339.

92. Finucane FF, Madans JH, Bush TL, et al. Decreased risk of stroke among postmenopausal hormone users. *Arch Intern Med.* 1993;153:73–79.

93. Bush TL, Barrett-Connor E, Cowan LD, et al. Cardiovascular mortality and noncontraceptive use of estrogen in women: results from the Lipid Research Clinics program follow-up study. *Circulation.* 1987;75:1102–1109.

94. McFarland KF, Boniface ME, Hornung CA, et al. Risk factors and noncontraceptive estrogen use in women with and without coronary disease. *Am Heart J.* 1989;117:1209–1213.

95. Stampfer MJ, Colditz GA, Willett WC, et al. Postmenopausal estrogen therapy and cardiovascular disease. *N Engl J Med.* 1991;325:756–762.

96. Psaty BM, Heckbert SR, Atkins D, et al. A review of the association of estrogens and progestins with cardiovascular disease in postmenopausal women. *Arch Intern Med.* 1993;153:1421–1427.

97. Kris-Etherton PM, Krummel DA, Russell ME, et al. The effect of diet on plasma lipids, lipoproteins, and coronary heart disease. *J Am Diet Assoc.* 1988;88:1373–1400.

98. Van Horn L, Ballew C, Liu K, et al. Diet, body size, and plasma lipids/lipoproteins in young adults: differences by race and sex. *Am J Epidemiol.* 1991;133:9–23.

99. Krummel DA, Mashaly MM, Kris-Etherton PM. Prediction of plasma lipids in a cross-sectional sample of young women. *J Am Diet Assoc.* 1992;92:942–948.

100. Garry PJ, Hunt WC, Koehler KM, et al. Longitudinal study of dietary intakes and plasma lipids in healthy elderly men and women. *Am J Clin Nutr.* 1992;55:682–688.

101. Posner BM, Cupples LA, Miller DR, et al. Diet, menopause, and serum cholesterol levels in women: the Framingham Study. *Am Heart J.* 1993;125:483–489.

102. Hallfrisch J, West S, Fisher C, et al. Modification of the United States' diet to affect changes in blood lipids and lipoprotein distribution. *Atherosclerosis.* 1985;57:179–188.

103. Kohlmeier M, Stricker G, Schlierf G. Influences of "normal" and "prudent" diets on biliary and serum lipids in healthy women. *Am J Clin Nutr.* 1985;42:1201–1205.

104. Jones DY, Judd JT, Taylor PR, et al. Influence of caloric contribution and saturation of dietary fat on plasma lipids in premenopausal women. *Am J Clin Nutr.* 1987;45:1451–1456.

105. Wahrburg U, Martin H, Sandkamp M, et al. Comparative effects of a recommended lipid-lowering diet vs. a diet rich in monounsaturated fatty acids on serum lipid profiles in healthy young adults. *Am J Clin Nutr.* 1992;56:678–683.

106. Cole TG, Bowen PE, Schmeisser D, et al. Differential reduction of plasma cholesterol by the American Heart Association phase 3 diet in moderately hypercholesterolemic, premenopausal women with different body mass indexes. *Am J Clin Nutr.* 1992;55:385–394.

107. Mata P, Garrido JA, Ordovas JM, et al. Effect of dietary monounsaturated fatty acids on plasma lipoproteins and apolipoproteins in women. *Am J Clin Nutr.* 1992;56:77–83.

108. Kasim SE, Martino S, Paik-Nyon K, et al. Dietary and anthropometric determinants of plasma lipoproteins during a long-term low-fat diet in healthy women. *Am J Clin Nutr.* 1993;57:146–153.

109. Geil PB, Anderson JW, Gustafson NJ. Women and men with hypercholesterolemia respond similarly to an American Heart Association step 1 diet. *J Am Diet Assoc.* 1995;95:436–441.

110. Denke MA, Frantz ID. Response to a cholesterol-lowering diet: Subjects even after adjustment for regression to the mean. *Am J Med.* 1993;94:626–631.

111. Denke MA, Sempos CT, Grundy SM. Excess body weight. An under-recognized contributor to dyslipidemia in white American women. *Arch Intern Med.* 1994;154:401–410.

112. Krummel DA, Etherton TD, Peterson S, Kris-Etherton PM. Effects of exercise on plasma lipids and lipoproteins of women. *PSEBM.* 1993;204:123–137.

113. Duncan JJ, Gordon NF, Scott CB. Women walking for health and fitness. How much is enough? *JAMA.* 1991;266:3295–3299.

114. Kris-Etherton PM, Krummel DA. Role of nutrition in the prevention and treatment of coronary heart disease in women. *J Am Diet Assoc.* 1993;93:987–993.

115. Frank E, Winkleby MA, Fortmann SP, et al. Improved cholesterol-related knowledge and behavior and plasma cholesterol levels in adults during the 1980s. *JAMA.* 1992;268:1566–1572.

116. Schucker B, Wittes JT, Santanello NC, et al. Change in cholesterol awareness and action. *Arch Intern Med.* 1991;151:888–973.

117. Ford ES, Jones DH. Cardiovascular health knowledge in the United States: findings from the National Health Interview Survey, 1985. *Prev Med.* 1991;20:725–736.

118. Hyman DJ, Simons-Morton DG, Ho K, et al. Cholesterol-related knowledge, attitudes, and behaviors in a low-income, urban patient population. *Am J Prev Med.* 1993;9:282–289.

119. Cremer SA, Kessler LG. The fat and fiber content of foods: what Americans know. *J Nutr Ed* 1992;24:149–152.

120. Auld GW, Achterberg C, Durrwachter J, Novak J. Gender differences in adults' knowledge about fat and cholesterol. *J Am Diet Assoc.* 1991;91:1391–1397.

121. Cotugna N, Subar AF, Heimemdinger J, Kahle L. Nutrition and cancer prevention knowledge, beliefs, attitudes, and practices: the 1987 National Health Interview Survey. *J Am Diet Assoc.* 1992;92:963–968.

122. Blake AJ, Melton RA. Dimensions of knowledge, attitudes, and behavior of diet and cardiovascular disease based on principles of diet and disease behavior change model criteria. *Nutr Res.* 1992;12:1295–1313.

123. Ferrini RL, Edelstein SL, Barrett-Connor E. Factors associated with health behavior change among residents 50 to 96 years of age in Rancho Bernardo, California. *Am J Prev Med.* 1994;10:26–30.

124. Russell BS, Harris BV, Huster GA, Sprecher DL. Effect of premature myocardial infarction in men on the eating habits of spouses and offspring. *J Am Diet Assoc.* 1994;94:859–864.

125. Bowen DJ, Henry H, Burrows E, et al. Influences of eating patterns on change to a low-fat diet. *J Am Diet Assoc.* 1993;93:1309–1311.

126. Sandoval WM, Heller KE, Wiese WH, Childs DA. Stages of change: a model for nutrition counseling. *Top Clin Nutr.* 1994;9:64–69.

127. Greene GW, Ross SR, Reed GR, et al. Stages of change for reducing dietary fat to 30% of energy or less. *J Am Diet Assoc.* 1994;94:1105–1110.

128. Burrows ER, Henry HJ, Bowen DJ, Henderson MM. Nutritional applications of a clinical low fat dietary intervention to public health change. *J Nurs Ed.*1993;25:167–175.

129. Lloyd HM, Paisley CM, Mela DJ. Barriers to the adoption of reduced-fat diets in a UK population. *J Am Diet Assoc.* 1995;95:416–422.

130. McMurray MP, Hopkins PN, Gould R, et al. Family-oriented nutrition intervention for a lipid clinic population. *J Am Diet Assoc.* 1991;91:57–65.

131. Report of the American Institute of Nutrition (AIN) Steering Committee on Healthy Weight. *J Nutr.* 1994;124:2240–2243.

14

ða

Osteoporosis

Robert P. Heaney

DEFINITION

Osteoporosis is technically defined as a condition in which the bone is excessively fragile. The fragility is the result of decreased bone mass and of accumulated microarchitectural damage to the bone tissue. Most of the resulting fractures occur among the elderly.

Fractures of the vertebral bodies, wrist, and hip are usually spoken of as typical osteoporotic fractures, but that approach overlooks the fact that virtually every bone in the body becomes fragile in patients with osteoporosis, and fractures of every bony site increase. Ribs, humerus, pelvis, tibia, hands, and feet are also common sites for fractures in patients with osteoporosis. Fractures of osteoporosis are typically of the low-trauma variety, such as those incurred in a fall from standing height. Although true as far as it goes, that approach also overlooks the full impact of the bony fragility. Fractures from all kinds of trauma increase. Simply put, a fragile skeleton is more likely to break than a strong skeleton.

Often termed a *silent epidemic,* osteoporosis typically produces no symptoms until a fragility fracture occurs. Exact prevalence of even symptomatic osteoporosis is uncertain. Osteoporosis is commonly considered to affect 20 to 25 million Americans, 80% of them women. Although it is more common in underweight women and in white women of northern European ancestry, it occurs in all racial and ethnic groups. After menopause a woman faces a 32% chance of sustaining a vertebral fracture before she dies, a 16% chance of a hip fracture, and a 15% chance of a wrist fracture.[1] In aggregate, her chances of developing some sort of osteoporosis are close to 50%—a risk, incidentally, that is substantially greater than her chances of developing breast cancer.

Financial costs of osteoporosis are currently estimated to be approximately $10 billion per year in the United States, most of this for hip fracture. Estimates of the degree of morbidity and disability produced by osteoporosis vary widely. For example, about 40% of vertebral fractures detectable on x-ray are effectively

418

silent. But at the other extreme, women can lose many inches of height and be severely disabled by multiple vertebral fractures. Hip fracture is the best studied manifestation of osteoporosis in this regard. It carries a 16% excess mortality and a huge cost in terms of loss of independence: about half of all hip fracture survivors lose the ability to live independently.

PATHOGENESIS OF FRACTURES

Osteoporosis is multifactorial in origin. Whether a bone fractures or not depends not only on intrinsic bony fragility but on the number of falls an older person sustains, how much soft tissue padding she/he has over the point of impact, and how well her protective reflexes keep her from striking particularly vulnerable parts of the skeleton.

The bony fragility itself is also multifactorial (as the definition implies) and arises not only from decreased bone mass but also from microarchitectural damage, specifically loss of critical connections between trabecular elements, as well as an accumulation of the fatigue damage that occurs in any structural unit as a result of use over the years (and which, for one reason or another, is not adequately repaired). Low bone mass itself has several causes, including decreased physical activity, gonadal hormone loss, poor nutrition (chiefly inadequate calcium intake and vitamin D status), and various life-style and medical causes as well. Although nutrition comes into the picture mainly by influencing bone mass, it also influences the tendency to fall,[2] and it plays an obvious role in maintaining enough soft tissue mass to protect bony parts when they are struck in a fall.

Genetic factors are also important and have been estimated to account for 20 to 80% of the variation in bone mass in the population. They influence not only the tendency to be "heavy-boned" (i.e., how much bone a person is able to accumulate) but, perhaps as important, determine the shape of various bones. Asians, for example, have only about half the hip fracture rate of whites, even though their bone mass is at least as low as that of whites in Europe and North America, and they lose bone at essentially the same rate with age. This has recently been shown to be explained by the fact that they have a substantially shorter relative distance between the lateral surface of the hip and the head of the femur (hip axis length).[3] Recall that the upper end of the femur is sharply angled, and the longer that angled segment, the weaker the structure. Thus, whites, with a greater hip axis length, require a greater bone density than Asians if their femora are to be of equal strength.

Recently, allelic differences on the chromosome where the vitamin D receptor gene is located have been found.[4] Individuals with one allele have been found by some investigators to have higher average bone mass than those with the other allele. The mechanisms are unknown, but the connection with the vitamin D receptor is interesting, particularly in a nutritional context.

Although we cannot alter our genetics, we can control our nutrition. Basically, our personal and professional objectives should be to make certain that diet provides sufficient nutrients during growth for bone building, both to achieve the full genetic program for bone mass and to offset daily losses. At maturity, the role of nutrition is primarily to preserve the bone mass one has achieved and secondarily to help the skeleton recover from the inevitable periods of disability, injury, or illness that an adult experiences periodically throughout life. Finally, nutrition plays an important role in susceptibility to fragility fractures in the elderly (particularly hip fractures) and in recovery from fracture. Table 14-1 briefly summarizes the most important of these influences.

Although good nutrition will not offset the negative skeletal effects of non-nutritional problems, it does help ensure that the impact of these other factors is not made worse by a superimposed calcium deficiency (for example). So, regardless of what a woman's baseline risk might be for genetic and other reasons, good nutrition helps to reduce the risk of fracture, and poor nutrition increases it.

How much of an effect does nutrition have? The available evidence suggests that ensuring sufficiency of both calcium and vitamin D throughout life could reduce the fracture burden due to osteoporosis by as much as 50%, perhaps even more. But even if the eventual benefit turns out to be as small as 10 to 20%, the associated reduction in cost and disability would be substantial. Hence, ensuring adequate nutrition must be an important women's health goal.

Table 14-1 Influences Affecting Acquisition, Maintenance, and Loss of Bone

Acquisition/Maintenance	Loss
Normal gonadal hormone levels	Gonadal hormone deficiency
Adequate calcium intake	Menopause
Exercise	Athletic amenorrhea
Growth hormone	Anorexia nervosa
Fluoride (in therapeutic doses)	Castration (males)
Parathyroid hormone	Corticosteroids
	Immobility
	Paralysis
	Illness
	Sedentariness
	Space flight
	Excess thyroid hormone
	Alcoholism
	Smoking
	Thinness
	Calcium deficiency

Many nutritional factors are required to build and maintain a healthy skeleton. These include calcium, phosphorus, protein, vitamins C, D, and K, and the trace minerals manganese, zinc, and copper, among others. But the nutrients most likely to be in short supply in the diets of North American and European women are calcium during growth, and calcium and vitamin D during maturity and the declining years of life. Thus, it is these nutrients that will be discussed in this chapter.

It is important to note that bone health is much like a three-legged stool. The three legs of this stool are nutrition (mainly calcium), hormones (mainly estrogen), and lifestyle (mainly exercise). Each is essential: one cannot substitute for another or make up for a deficiency of another. It takes three legs to support the stool. In practical terms, this means that a high-calcium diet will not prevent the bone loss of menopause or immobilization, just as estrogen or exercise will not allow us to make or sustain bone without adequate dietary calcium.

CLINICAL MEASUREMENT OF BONE MASS AND DENSITY

Because so much of the osteoporosis literature describes results of measurement of bone mass and density, it is essential to understand what these terms mean, and how they are used—and misused—in papers describing studies of nutrition and bone status. With most of the current techniques, a high-energy beam of ionizing radiation is passed through the body. The instruments measure and record how much of that beam is absorbed. This tells us about the bone because bone mineral absorbs more of the radiation than does soft tissue (just as it does with an ordinary x-ray film). However, instead of an image on a photographic emulsion, the bone absorptiometric methods yield a number—the quantity of bone mineral in the path of the beam. The principal methods used for this work today are dual energy x-ray absorptiometry (DEXA), single photon absorptiometry (SPA), and quantitative computed tomography (QCT). Each technique effectively scans back and forth across a body region and measures bone mass at many thousands of points.

There are two ways of summarizing these thousands of values. One is as bone mineral content (BMC), or simply bone mass (i.e., how much bony tissue there is in the region scanned). The other is bone mineral density (BMD). To complicate matters further, there are actually two density measures in common use: (1) areal density, or BMC divided by the area of the shadow cast by the bone as the beam scans across it, and (2) true density, or BMC divided by the volume of the scanned region. DEXA and SPA are capable of yielding only areal density, whereas QCT gives true density. Bearing in mind that bones are typically hollow or honey-combed, one can summarize these approaches by noting that mass is a measure of how much bone tissue is present, and density, a measure of how tightly it is packed. For reasons related to their use in diagnosis of bone disease, the available methods have tended to emphasize density over mass (or BMD over BMC), although both outputs are nearly always provided by the various instruments if the user chooses to take advantage of them.

The choice of density is a poor one for nutritional purposes, especially during growth, when what we are acquiring is skeletal *mass*. During growth, our bones, of course, expand in three dimensions. An areal density eliminates two of those, and QCT, all three. Hence, any density measure eliminates most or all of the actual bone tissue gain occurring during growth. The preferred measure in all growth studies must, therefore, be BMC. Unfortunately, much of the published literature is confused on this point.

Even after growth has ceased, BMC will often be the superior measure, in part because bone size is an important determinant of bone strength (and BMD normalizes all measurements effectively to the same size) and in part, also, because skeletal dimensions change slowly with age and can cause us to draw wrong conclusions if we use only BMD values. An example is the common observation that true vertebral density (by QCT) declines steadily after about age 20. However, it would be a mistake to conclude from this observation that bone strength is reduced accordingly. Vertebral bodies actually expand slowly with age during this period, and the available bony tissue is simply redistributed over a larger volume. That is why density declines. But content or mass does not decline (and may even increase somewhat). Because of the shape change, the bone actually gets stronger (not weaker, as BMD would have led us to conclude).

NATURAL INTAKE OF CALCIUM AND VITAMIN D

Vitamin D is produced normally in the skin by a photochemical reaction in which ultraviolet light from the sun changes 7-dehydrocholesterol into provitamin D. As the human species evolved in equatorial East Africa, with ample sunlight year-round, two mechanisms were developed to prevent building up an excess of vitamin D. One was skin pigmentation, which blocked the ultraviolet rays before they could act on 7-dehydrocholesterol, and the second was the fact that, as provitamin D built up in the skin, it shunted the photochemical reaction in the direction of inert products. As a result, after a few minutes of sun exposure, vitamin D synthesis simply stops. As races have moved farther and farther away from the equator and needed all the ultraviolet light they could get, their skin pigmentation became lighter and lighter. Even so, in latitudes such as that of Boston and farther north, the sun is so low in the sky in winter that effectively none of the responsible ultraviolet rays gets through the atmosphere, even on a sunny day.[5]

Vitamin D tends to be a scarce nutrient in northern latitudes, and without careful attention to maintaining adequacy, varying degrees of vitamin D insufficiency will be common. More than 80% of the children dying in northern Europe in the late 19th century showed evidences of rickets at autopsy—often severe. This matter is made even worse by air pollution, which further blocks the critical ultraviolet wavelengths.

One might argue that vitamin D ought not be considered a nutrient at all, because it is not a constituent of most foods and is naturally synthesized in our skin, given adequate solar exposure; but it was grouped accidentally with the other vitamins (nutrients in the strict sense) in the early days of development of nutritional science, and that is how we think about it today. That is not just an historical curiosity. Nutritionists in the past have often held that one can get all the nutrients one needs from a balanced, varied diet and have been slow to embrace the notions of engineered foods and food fortification. That clearly is a misguided approach to an accidental nutrient such as vitamin D. As the human species moved out of equatorial regions, we did not hesitate to develop warm clothing and shelter to protect us from the cold environment. For vitamin D, at least, we need to take the same approach, now that we understand the biochemistry involved. We have done that for infants and children for the past 60+ years, and rickets is rare today in the industrialized nations, but vitamin D insufficiency is still common among adults—particularly among the elderly.

Calcium, too, was present in abundance in the environment in which the human species evolved. The natural foods eaten by hunter-gatherers provided a calcium intake that, adjusted for differences in body size, would be in the range of 2000 to 3000 mg/day for us.[6,7] (Contrast that figure with the median value for women 20 and older in the United States in the NHANES II study: in the range of 500 mg/day.)[8] These sources included a very large number of greens, tubers, roots, nuts, and berries, many of them with very high-calcium nutrient densities.[7] Cultivated plants, by contrast, have augmented levels of carbohydrate and/or fat without a proportionate increase in trace nutrients and thus almost always have lower calcium densities than do the wild varieties.

In fact, primitive diets were so calcium-rich that, to protect against too much calcium, the body developed an intestinal absorptive barrier. At the same time, our physiologies failed to develop mechanisms to conserve calcium once absorbed (because there was no need to conserve in the face of environmental surfeit). We typically absorb only about 25 to 35% of the calcium in our diets, and we are very inefficient at retaining it once absorbed. Thus, net retention of a dietary calcium increment is in the range of only 5 to 10%. Furthermore, we have completely unregulated dermal losses of calcium and do a poor job of conserving calcium at the kidney as well. These are precisely the physiologic patterns one would expect with an environmentally abundant nutrient.

It is instructive to compare the body's handling of calcium with that of sodium, which was an environmentally scarce nutrient during human evolution. In contrast to calcium, 100% of dietary sodium is absorbed, and dermal and renal sodium losses can be reduced to near zero. The problem is that, as we developed industrialized societies, we adopted a diet high in sodium and low in calcium, and our physiologies are not adapted to these conditions. These are the reasons why, despite a high standard of living and the potential to nourish ourselves at a level never previously achieved in history, our present diets tend to be deficient in precisely these two critical nutrients, calcium and vitamin D.

CALCIUM

Calcium and Growth

What happens if we do not get enough calcium during growth? And why do we continue to need calcium after growth has been completed?

The answer to the first question is fairly straightforward. Calcium is the principal cation of bone; it is an element, and therefore we cannot manufacture it; if we do not get sufficient calcium in our diets, we cannot build an adequate skeletal mass. Does that mean that growth will be stunted? Usually not. What occurs is that the body takes the limited amount of calcium that is available and spreads it over the growing skeleton. The result is that all the bones tend to be somewhat flimsy, with thin, porous cortices and sparse trabeculae, even though, externally, they are usually of normal size and shape.

This redistribution of bony mineral is accomplished by adjusting the balance of the processes of bone resorption and bone formation, which tear down and rebuild bone, respectively. Together, these processes are termed modeling (during growth) and remodeling (after growth has been completed). The two are coupled in different ways during growth and maturity, which is why they are given different names, but for our purposes, they amount to the same thing. Both processes are extremely active while we are young, and in the face of inadequate dietary calcium to support the demands of growth, comparatively minor adjustments suffice to tear down some of the bony tissue recently deposited on the insides of growing bones and to redistribute its raw materials to accommodate growth in length and in external diameter.

There is general agreement among osteoporosis experts that one of the most important protections against fragility fractures in old age is building the largest peak bone mass possible within the limits of the genetic program. Charles Dent,[9] many years ago, commented that osteoporosis was a pediatric disease that did not manifest itself until old age.

There has been some uncertainty about the age when peak bone mass is achieved, but it now appears that the answer is at different times for different bones.[10] The skull continues to increase in density throughout life and never really does "peak." Density at the hip, by contrast, probably peaks in the late adolescent years and declines slowly thereafter. The cortex of long bones such as the radius peaks in the mid- to late 20s. Vertebral bodies probably peak in the mid- to late 20s also, and their mass remains constant (or may increase slightly) until menopause.

Recker et al[11] found continuing gain in bone mass in the spine, forearm, and total body in nearly 200 healthy women in their 20s, and Matkovic and Heaney,[12] in a meta-analysis of published balances, were able to show that healthy women from ages 18 to 30 were able to store significant quantities of calcium (i.e., they were able to build bone) if the calcium intake was high enough. In the study of Recker et al, the rate of gain was inversely proportional to age; no further gain could be found after about age 29 to 31. Thus, it appears that the window of opportunity for achieving peak bone mass remains at least partially open to about age 30.

The importance of calcium intake during growth was highlighted in the study of Recker et al,[11] who found that the principal determinant of the amount of bone gained in third-decade women was the calcium:protein ratio of the diet (that is, the calcium content of the diet adjusted for its protein content—see below). The quantity of calcium required to reach the genetic potential, given typical American diets, was analyzed by Matkovic and Heaney in their meta-analysis of more than 500 published balances.[12] They used a threshold model illustrated in Figure 14-1, which recognizes that more calcium will produce more bone only up to a point where the genetic potential is fully saturated and that intakes above that level produce no further benefit. (Exactly the same phenomenon pertains to iron and hemoglobin.) Thus, in a curve relating bone gain (or calcium balance) to intake, the optimal intake is one just at or above the point where the ascending portion of the curve joins the horizontal segment. For children aged 2 to 8, that optimal intake was found to be about 1100 mg/day, for adolescents up through age 18, 1600 mg/day, and for young adults to age 30, 1100 mg/day. The first two figures are substantially above the Recommended Dietary Allowance (RDA)[13] for the ages concerned in the United States.

That a high-calcium diet could augment bone mass accumulation during growth is suggested by two randomized controlled trials in which growing children were given extra calcium.[14,15] In both trials, the calcium-supplemented children gained more bone than the placebo-treated controls. More to the point, the control intake in both studies was close to, or even above, the relevant RDA, so in a sense, these investigations amounted to a test of the current RDA.

Calcium and Bone Health in the Mature Adult

During the adult years, there is a continuing calcium need not only for the obvious demands of a woman's reproductive life (pregnancy and lactation) but for the simple reason that we are losing calcium every day. Shed skin, hair, nails, and